T0309651

Computational Models of Conditioning

Since first described, multiple properties of classical conditioning have been discovered, establishing the need for mathematical models to help explain the defining features. The mathematical complexity of the models puts our understanding of their workings beyond the ability of our intuitive thinking and makes computer simulations irreplaceable. The complexity of the models frequently results in function redundancy, a natural property of biologically evolved systems that is much desired in technologically designed products. Featuring contributions from experts in the field, this book discusses the latest advancements and presents detailed descriptions of how the models simulate conditioned behavior and its physiological bases. It offers advanced students and researchers examples of how the models are used to analyze existing experimental results and design future experiments. This volume is of great interest to psychologists and neuroscientists, as well as computer scientists and engineers searching for ideas applicable to the design of robots that mimic animal behavior.

NESTOR SCHMAJUK is Professor of Psychology and Neuroscience at Duke University. He has developed and tested several neural network models of classical conditioning, operant conditioning, animal communication, creativity, spatial learning, cognitive mapping, and prepulse inhibition. His previous books include *Animal Learning and Cognition: A Neural Network Approach* (Cambridge University Press, 1997), *Latent Inhibition and its Neural Substrates* (Kluwer Academic, 2002), and *Mechanisms in Classical Conditioning: A Computational Approach* (Cambridge University Press, 2010).

Computational Models of Conditioning

Edited by

NESTOR SCHMAJUK
Duke University

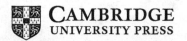

CAMBRIDGE
UNIVERSITY PRESS

University Printing House, Cambridge CB2 8BS, United Kingdom

One Liberty Plaza, 20th Floor, New York, NY 10006, USA

477 Williamstown Road, Port Melbourne, VIC 3207, Australia

314-321, 3rd Floor, Plot 3, Splendor Forum, Jasola District Centre, New Delhi - 110025, India

79 Anson Road, #06-04/06, Singapore 079906

Cambridge University Press is part of the University of Cambridge.

It furthers the University's mission by disseminating knowledge in the pursuit of education, learning and research at the highest international levels of excellence.

www.cambridge.org
Information on this title: www.cambridge.org/9780521113649

© Cambridge University Press 2010

This publication is in copyright. Subject to statutory exception and to the provisions of relevant collective licensing agreements, no reproduction of any part may take place without the written permission of Cambridge University Press.

First published 2010

A catalogue record for this publication is available from the British Library

Library of Congress Cataloging in Publication data
Computational models of conditioning / [edited by] Nestor Schmajuk.
    p. cm.
  Includes bibliographical references and index.
  ISBN 978-0-521-11364-9
  1. Paired-association learning–Congresses. 2. Cognition–Congresses. 3. Eyelid conditioning–Congresses. I. Schmajuk, Nestor A. II. Title.
  BF319.5.P34C66 2010
  153.1–dc22
  2010022337

ISBN 978-0-521-11364-9 Hardback

Cambridge University Press has no responsibility for the persistence or accuracy of URLs for external or third-party internet websites referred to in this publication, and does not guarantee that any content on such websites is, or will remain, accurate or appropriate.

Contents

v

Contributors

José E. Burgos
University of Guadalajara, Mexico

Joseph Dunsmoor
Department of Psychology and Neuroscience, Duke University, USA

Justin A. Harris
School of Psychology, University of Sydney, Australia

Richard A. Hullinger
Indiana University, Bloomington, USA

John K. Kruschke
Indiana University, Bloomington, USA

Munir G. Kutlu
Department of Psychology and Neuroscience, Duke University, USA

José A. Larrauri
Department of Psychology and Neuroscience, Duke University, USA

Michael E. Le Pelley
School of Psychology, Cardiff University, Cardiff, UK

Michael D. Mauk
Center for Learning and Memory and Section of Neurobiology, University of Texas, Austin, USA

Ralph R. Miller
Department of Psychology, State University of New York, Binghamton, USA

Nestor A. Schmajuk
Department of Psychology and Neuroscience, Duke University, USA

Edgar H. Vogel
Universidad de Talca, Talca, Chile

Allan R. Wagner
Yale University, New Haven, Connecticut, USA

James E. Witnauer
Department of Psychology, State University of New York,
Binghamton, USA

Introduction

This book contains the presentations given during the Duke Symposium on Computational Models of Conditioning, which took place between May 15th and May 17th of 2009 at the Duke Campus in Durham, N.C. The meeting was sponsored by the Duke Department of Psychology and Neuroscience, the Duke Office of the Vice Provost for International Affairs, and the Duke Arts and Sciences Research Council. All the participants and I are indebted for their generous support.

The meeting was organized with the assistance of my friend and former Ph.D. advisor Professor John Moore (University of Massachusetts at Amherst). I am particularly thankful to John for helping me in finding a group of participants who contributed both well-established and novel theories of classical conditioning. I am also grateful to Munir Gunes Kutlu for his help in running many aspects of the meeting.

The models

John Kruschke and Rick Hullinger (Indiana University, USA) prepared the chapter on "The evolution of learned attention." In this chapter, the authors use simulated evolution, with adaptive fitness measured as overall accuracy during a lifetime of learning, and show that evolution converges to architectures that incorporate attentional learning. They also describe the specific training environments that encourage this evolutionary trajectory, and how we assess attentional learning in the evolved learners. Interestingly, the resulting attentional mechanism is similar to that proposed by Mackintosh (1975).

A question regarding the evolution of complex systems is whether a simple, basic associative system first evolves, and then attentional (and also configural)

1

mechanisms would appear in later stages of the simulated evolution. The plausi-
bility of such a process is partly supported by the observation that most ver-
tebrates share a basic brain structure that is supplemented by more complex
processing brain areas (like the neocortex) in certain species (Romer, 1970).

Justin A. Harris (University of Sydney, Australia) contributed the chapter
on "The arguments of associations." In this chapter, Harris demonstrates that,
although it is commonly assumed that the solution to patterning and biconditional discriminations requires "configural" elements, these discriminations
can be solved by assuming that some elements of each stimulus are inhibited
when two stimuli are presented in compound.

Harris's approach is similar, in some respects, to that introduced by Grossberg
(1975) and further developed by Schmajuk and Di Carlo (1989), although neither of these authors applied this "normalization" mechanism to discrimination problems. It also interesting that when a configural model is used (e.g.,
Schmajuk & Di Carlo, 1992), the configurations produced by the model in its
"hidden layer" look very much like those suggested by Harris. In addition, this
normalization mechanism might have an important role as a "front end" for
a competitive network (e.g., Rescorla & Wagner, 1972) when a large number
of stimuli are used which might overwhelm the network, thereby destabil-
izing the algorithm. Despite all its positive properties, the fact that Harris's
(2006) model cannot describe some occasion-setting paradigms (e.g., like those
in which the feature is weaker than the target, such as positive-feature, simultaneous discriminations with a weak feature, motivational learning or contextual learning) suggests that configural mechanisms cannot be completely
discarded.

Michael Le Pelley (Cardiff University, United Kingdom) wrote the chapter
on "The hybrid modeling approach to conditioning." In this chapter, Le Pelley
describes his "hybrid" model of associative learning which incorporates two
associabilities; α defined as in Mackintosh's (1975) theory, and σ defined as in
the Pearce–Hall model, with the overall learning rate for a stimulus being determined by $\alpha \times \sigma$. The chapter discusses evidence from recent studies of animal
conditioning and discrimination learning that provides support for the hybrid
modeling approach. Common to both Le Pelley's (2004) hybrid model and the
Schmajuk, Lam and Gray (1996) SLG model, is that blocking is the result of two
mechanisms simultaneously at work (Schmajuk & Larrauri, 2006).

Ralph Miller and James Witnauer (Binghamton University, USA) provided
the chapter on "The role of within-compound associations in cue interactions:
models and data." In this chapter, the authors use computational modeling
to review and simulate experiments related to the role of within-compound
associations in negative mediation, positive mediation, and counteraction.

A mathematical model that attributes all cue interactions to within-compound associations was shown to provide a better fit to some negative mediation phenomena than a model that attributes negative mediation effects to variations in outcome processing. Overall, the results of this analysis suggest that within-compound associations are important for cue competition, conditioned inhibition, counteraction effects, retrospective revaluation, and second-order conditioning.

Some similarities between the role of CX–CS and CS–CX associations in Miller's comparator model (Miller & Schachtman, 1985), Wagner's (1981) Sometimes Opponent Process (SOP), and Schmajuk et al.'s (1996) SLG model should be noted. For instance, in all three models these associations decrease responding. In the comparator model, the CS–CX association activates the CX–US association, which subtracts from the CS–US association, thereby decreasing the output of the comparator. In the SOP and SLG models the CR is attenuated by decreasing the activation of the CS–US association when the CS is predicted by the CX.

Allan R. Wagner (Yale University, USA) and Edgar Vogel (Universidad de Talca, Chile) contributed the chapter on "Associative modulation of US processing: implications for understanding of habituation." In this chapter, the authors analyze, in the light of data from their and other laboratories, Wagner's (1976, 1979) suggestion that long-term habituation might be the result of an associative process by which stimuli come to be "expected" in the context in which they have been exposed. The authors indicate that one complication is that extended contexts (as well as discrete cues) can control response-potentiating, conditioned-emotional tendencies, in addition to the presumed decremental effects. They describe experiments that separate these effects and illustrate how the approach offered by SOP and AESOP (Wagner, 1981; Wagner & Brandon, 1989) describes those results.

The Wagner and Vogel chapter has some commonalities with Stout and Miller's (2007) modeling of the extended comparator hypothesis. In their chapter, Miller and Witnauer indicate that the comparator sometimes subtracts and at other times adds the CS–US associations, in order to explain why sensory preconditioning training results in responding to the non-reinforced CS with a few CS1–CS2 and CS1–US alternated trials (a potentiating effect), but results in the CS being inhibitory with an increasing number of trials (a decremental effect).

Together with Munir Gunes Kutlu, Joey Dunsmoor, and Jose Larrauri (Duke University, USA), we wrote the chapter on "Attention, associations, and configurations in conditioning." This chapter describes a number of computational mechanisms (associations, attention, configuration, and timing) that first seemed necessary to explain a small number of conditioning results, and then proved able to account for a large part of the extensive body of conditioning data. The chapter first presents Schmajuk *et al.*'s (1996) SLG model, a neural-network theory that includes attentional and associative mechanisms, and applies it to the description of compound conditioning with different initial associative values, extinction of the conditioned excitor decreasing the retardation of conditioning of its conditioned inhibitor (conditioned inhibition as a slave process), facilitation of conditioning by context preexposure, recovery and absence of recovery from blocking, latent inhibition–overshadowing synergism and antagonism, summation tests in the context of extinction, and spontaneous recovery. Although other models can increase processing when the predictor of a CS disappears and the CS is presented by itself (change of CX in latent inhibition), only the SLG model can increase attention to a CS upon presentation of another, novel stimulus (e.g., presenting a novel stimulus preceding an extinguished CS to produce disinhibition). Also, the SLG model is unique in yielding mediated attentional changes, whenever a CS_A predicted by a CS_B is absent when the CS_B is presented by itself, thereby increasing Novelty and attention to the predicted, absent CS_A.

The chapter also introduces the Schmajuk, Lamoureux and Holland (1998) SLH model, a neural network that incorporates configural mechanisms, and applies it to the description of response form in occasion setting. Finally, it is shown how the combination of configural and timing mechanisms describes timing of occasion setting, and how the combination of attentional, associative, and configural mechanisms describes causal learning. Because these computational mechanisms were implemented by artificial neural networks, which can be mapped onto different brain structures, the approach permits the establishment of brain–behavior relationships, like the Burgos and Mauk models described in the next two chapters.

Michael Mauk (University of Texas, USA) contributed the chapter on "Computer simulation analysis of cerebellar mechanisms of eyelid conditioning." This chapter first outlines work that identifies the essential principles of cerebellar learning and lays down the foundation for simulating cerebellar function. Then it describes a number of new computational findings that offer a relatively accurate description of the essential computational unit of the cerebellum and how it works in a noisy input background.

José E. Burgos (Universidad de Guadalajara, Mejico) wrote the chapter "The operant/respondent distinction: a computational neural-network analysis." This chapter outlines a neural-network interpretation of the distinctions between types of stimulus–response relations (operant versus classical), reinforcement contingencies (response-dependent versus stimulus-dependent), and their effects. The operant–classical distinction is interpreted in terms of the difference between two types of input–output relations that involve different types of input units, as well as different types of output units. The distinction between different types of contingencies is interpreted in terms of the difference between two types of training protocols (S-dependent versus R-dependent). The distinction between the effects of the contingencies is interpreted in terms of the difference between changes in the different types of output units in the presence of S activations. Finally, the chapter suggests possible roles of hippocampal and dopaminergic systems in conditioning.

Using the same nomenclature used in the rest of the book, the Burgos model can be re-described as follows. In classical conditioning, presentation of the unconditioned stimulus (US, S*) activates the unconditioned response UR (R*) which strengthens its connection with the conditioned stimulus (CS, S). Subsequent presentations of the CS (S) will activate the CR (R*). In operant conditioning, generation of an arbitrary response R will result in the delivery of the US (S*), which will strengthen the connection with the S present at the time. Subsequent presentations of the CS (S) will activate the operant R. In this way, the network clarifies the differences and similarities between classical and operant mechanisms and how they interact.

Beyond parsimony: redundancy and reliability

Most chapters in this book seem to reinforce the notion that more than one mechanism is needed to account for the reported results on classical conditioning. Conditioning can be described by a rather complex combination of different mechanisms. At the Duke Meeting, Mike LePelley's talk title pointed out that "parsimony is overrated."

Overall, they suggest that simple notions like Mackintosh's (1975) attentional theory, Rescorla–Wagner's (1972) delta rule, Pearce and Hall's (1980) attentional model, Miller and Schachtman's (1985) first comparator hypothesis, or Grossberg's (1975) attentional competition model failed to explain important aspects of conditioning. Instead, the field has moved to increasingly complex models that have incorporated those ideas. Even these models have limitations and might require the incorporation of additional mechanisms to provide a complete account of associative learning. It is apparent that the complexity of these models puts them beyond the ability of our intuitive thinking and makes computer simulations irreplaceable.

The content of this book suggests that the different mechanisms required for a full description of the data can be analyzed separately and then combined into an integrated model. As indicated before (Schmajuk, 2010), the method is reminiscent of the Wright brothers' approach to airplane design, which consisted of the independent development and testing of the individual components of the plane before assembling them together into a flying machine

(Padfield & Lawrence, 2003). Interestingly, that approach was based on a study of bird flight by George Cayley (1773–1857), who realized that the lift function and the thrust function of bird wings were separate and distinct, and could be imitated by separate systems on a fixed-wing craft. Imitation of each separate, relatively simple function permits the explanation of how each function is achieved.

If more than one mechanism is required for a full description of classical conditioning, therefore making parsimony unrealistic, it is possible that some of the properties provided by these mechanisms might overlap. As mentioned above, both Le Pelley's (2004) hybrid model and the SLG model describe blocking as the result of two mechanisms. That is, multiple, complex mechanisms might provide redundancy and increased reliability, which is a much-desired property of both technologically designed products and biologically evolved systems. In sum, computational models might be becoming less parsimonious, but the added redundancy increases reliability. A clear demonstration of such increased reliability is that some functions (like blocking) can survive the effect of hippocampal lesions (Holland & Fox, 2003).

Evaluation of the models

In order to quantify the quality of a model's simulated results, some chapters (e.g., Miller and Witnauer's) have used correlations. Alternative methods have been used in the past, for instance, Schmajuk *et al.* (2001) used χ^2, and Schmajuk and Larrauri (2006) applied analysis of variance using the actual variance of the experimental subjects. Of these alternative methods we prefer to use correlations because, although they disregard the importance of the variance in the data, they indicate when to reject the null hypothesis (that simulated values and experimental data are not correlated). Instead, χ^2 indicates when to accept the null hypothesis (that simulated values and experimental data are equivalent). Finally, the analysis of variance used in Schmajuk and Larrauri (2006) requires knowledge of the values of the variance of the data, which is not always reported in the experimental studies.

Evaluation of the data

In addition to the question of the evaluation of the models, the issue of the robustness of the data was an important concern during our discussions. For example, the Schmajuk *et al.* chapter refers to the contradictory results regarding the combined effect of preexposure, which usually yields latent inhibition, and compound training, which usually results in overshadowing. As indicated in that chapter, it has been reported that preexposure and compound training can add and cancel each other. Because the SLG model (Schmajuk *et al.*, 1996) explains away these contradictions in terms of differences in experimental parameters used in the different reports, parametric studies are needed to test those explanations. Most important, in addition to testing the model, these parametric studies would serve to determine the range in which some reported results are valid and can be replicated.

Future challenges

A general problem of the models presented in this book is that most of them, with the exception of Mauk's, neither take into account any specific preparation (e.g., rabbit's eyeblink conditioning, rat's conditional emotional response, taste aversion, human ratings), nor the different experimental values (e.g., duration of the CS, salience of the CS, the duration and strength of the US, context salience, intertrial interval, trials to criterion) used in the experiments run with those preparations. Therefore, most models are "generic" models of classical conditioning. We expect that future models will (1) adopt parameters appropriate for specific preparations, and (2) use simulation values (e.g., stimulus duration and salience, trials to criterion) that are scaled to those used in the corresponding experiments. The resulting models will provide more accurate descriptions of the data.

Society for Computational Modeling of Associative Learning

One important achievement of the Duke meeting was the creation by all the participants of the Society for Computational Modeling of Associative Learning. The purpose of the Society is to (1) foster communication about computational models of associative learning among those who do computational modeling, between those who create models and those who might be instructed by them, and between those who do experiments on associative learning and those whose models might be instructed; and (2) to promote the use of computational models for addressing conceptual issues in associative learning. After the meeting, a number of researchers were invited to become members and at the time of this writing the society has more than 30 members.

References

Grossberg, S. (1975). A neural model of attention, reinforcement, and discrimination learning. *International Review of Neurobiology*, **18**, 263–327.

Harris, J. A. (2006). Elemental representations of stimuli in associative learning. *Psychological Review*, **113**, 584–605.

Holland, P. C. & Fox, G. D. (2003). Effects of hippocampal lesions in overshadowing and blocking procedures. *Behavioral Neuroscience*, **117**(3), 650–656.

Le Pelley, M. E. (2004). The role of associative history in models of associative learning: a selective review and a hybrid model. *The Quarterly Journal of Experimental Psychology*, **57B**, 193–243.

Mackintosh, N. J. (1975). A theory of attention: variations in the associability of stimuli with reinforcement. *Psychological Review*, **82**, 276–298.

Miller, R. R. & Schachtman, T. (1985). Conditioning context as an associative baseline: implications for response generation and the nature of conditioned inhibition. In R. R. Miller and N. E. Spear, eds., *Information Processing in Animals: Conditioned Inhibition*. Hillsdale, NJ: Erlbaum, pp. 51–88.

Padfield, G. D. & Lawrence, B. (2003). The birth of flight control: an engineering analysis of the Wright brothers' 1902 glider. *The Aeronautical Journal*, December, 697–718.

Pearce, J. M. & Hall, G. (1980). A model for Pavlovian conditioning: variations in the effectiveness of conditioned but not unconditioned stimuli. *Psychological Review*, **87**, 332–352.

Rescorla, R. A. & Wagner, A. (1972). A theory of Pavlovian conditioning: variations in the effectiveness of reinforcement and non-reinforcement. In A. H. Black and W. F. Prokasy, eds., *Classical Conditioning II: Current Research and Theory*. New York: Appleton–Century–Crofts, pp. 64–99.

Romer, A. S. (1970). *The Vertebrate Body*. Philadelphia: W. B. Saunders.

Schmajuk, N. A. (2010). *Mechanisms in Classical Conditioning: A Computational Approach*. Cambridge: Cambridge University Press.

Schmajuk, N. A. & Di Carlo, J. J. (1989). A neural network approach to hippocampal function in classical conditioning. *Behavioral Neuroscience*, **105**, 82–110.

Schmajuk, N. A. & Di Carlo, J. J. (1992). Stimulus configuration, classical conditioning, and the hippocampus. *Psychological Review*, **99**, 268–305.

Schmajuk, N. A. & Larrauri, J. A. (2006). Experimental challenges to theories of classical conditioning: application of an attentional model of storage and retrieval. *Journal of Experimental Psychology: Animal Behavior Processes*, **32**, 1–20.

Schmajuk, N. A., Cox, L. & Gray, J. A. (2001). Nucleus accumbens, entorhinal cortex and latent inhibition: a neural network approach. *Behavioral Brain Research*, **118**, 123–141.

Schmajuk, N. A., Lam, Y. & Gray, J. A. (1996). Latent inhibition: a neural network approach. *Journal of Experimental Psychology: Animal Behavior Processes*, **22**, 321–349.

Schmajuk, N. A., Lamoureux, J. A. & Holland, P. C. (1998). Occasion setting: a neural network approach. *Psychological Review*, **105**, 3–32.

Stout, S. C. & Miller, R. R. (2007). Sometimes-competing retrieval (SOCR): a formalization of the comparator hypothesis. *Psychological Review*, **114**, 759–783.

Wagner, A. R. (1976). Priming in STM: an information-processing mechanism for self-generated or retrieval-generated depression in performance. In T. J. Tighe and R. N. Leaton, eds., *Habituation: Perspectives from Child Development, Animal Behavior, and Neurophysiology*. Hillsdale, NJ: Erlbaum, pp. 95–128.

Wagner, A. R. (1979). Habituation and memory. In A. Dickinson and R. A. Boakes, eds., *Mechanisms of Learning and Motivation*. Hillsdale, NJ: Lawrence Erlbaum.

Wagner, A. R. (1981). SOP: A model of automatic memory processing in animal behavior. In N. E. Spear and R. R. Miller, eds., *Information Processing in Animals: Memory Mechanisms*. Hillsdale, NJ: Erlbaum, pp. 5–47.

Wagner, A. R. & Brandon, S. E. (1989). Evolution of a structured connectionist model of Pavlovian conditioning (AESOP). In S. B. Klein and R. R. Mowrer, eds., *Contemporary Learning Theories: Pavlovian Conditioning and the Status of Traditional Learning Theory*. Hillsdale, NJ: Erlbaum, pp. 149–189.

1

Evolution of attention in learning

JOHN K. KRUSCHKE AND RICHARD A. HULLINGER

Abstract

A variety of phenomena in associative learning suggest that people and some animals are able to learn how to allocate attention across cues. Models of attentional learning are motivated by the need to account for these phenomena. We start with a different, more general motivation for learners, namely, the need to learn quickly. Using simulated evolution, with adaptive fitness measured as overall accuracy during a lifetime of learning, we show that evolution converges to architectures that incorporate attentional learning. We describe the specific training environments that encourage this evolutionary trajectory and we describe how we assess attentional learning in the evolved learners.

Birds do it, bees do it; maybe ordinary fleas do it. They all learn from experience. But why is learning so ubiquitous? Why not just be born already knowing how to behave? That would save a lot of time and a lot of error. Presumably, we are born ignorant either because evolution is unfinished or because what we need to know is too complex to be fully coded in the genome. Either way, it seems that evolution has cleverly found a mechanism for dealing with the birth of ignorance; a mechanism that we call learning.

Of course, it may be that learning is merely something that organisms do for fun in their spare time. Perhaps there is not much adaptive value in learning, and little cost, and therefore no selective pressure on the mechanisms of learning. To the contrary, there is good evidence that learning is metabolically costly (Mery & Kawecki, 2003) and, therefore, it is probably achieving something of reproductive value (Johnston, 1982).

Importantly, what matters is not merely the ability to learn slowly and eventually. What matters is learning quickly. As just one recent example of this fact, Raine and Chittka (2008) showed that different hives of honeybees learned about sources of food at different rates, and those hives that learned faster got significantly more food.

Fast learning favors selective attention

Given that faster learning is better learning, how should learning be speeded up? What sorts of learning mechanisms may have evolved which make learning faster? In this chapter we argue that "selective attention in learning" is a natural consequence of evolutionary pressure to learn quickly in certain environments. We show through simulations that merely by giving a reproductive advantage to organisms that learn faster, an attentional mechanism evolves. Attentional processes yield faster learning in particular environments, and much of our chapter is devoted to describing a range of environments that encourage the evolution of attention in learning.

This perspective, that selective attention is adaptive and beneficial for learning, contrasts with the intuitive view that selective attention is merely an unfortunate side effect of limited-capacity processing. If attention were merely the consequence of capacity limitations then selective attention should go away when capacity increases. We show the opposite: even when there is no metabolic penalty for high learning rates, speed of learning favors selective attention.

The second main purpose of the chapter is to remind readers that some apparent infelicities in learning are, in fact, a natural consequence of having evolved to learn fast. In particular, the "highlighting effect," which will be described in detail later in the chapter, seems irrational from a normative statistical perspective, but is a natural consequence of a mechanism for learning quickly, namely attention shifting and learning (for a review see Kruschke, 2009). The highlighting effect should not be construed as an error in an otherwise rational learner. Instead, highlighting should be understood as a signature of a learner who is well adapted to learning quickly in particular environments. The benefits of fast learning outweigh the costs of "irrational" generalization, which might never actually be tested in the real world.

The highlighting effect has been explained by a theory of attentional shifting and learning (Kruschke, 1996a, 2001, 2003, 2009). The idea is that when a cue–outcome event occurs that contradicts previously learned expectations, attention shifts away from cues that cause error, toward other cues. The reallocation of attention becomes a learned response to those cues. Various data converge on that explanation, including eye tracking data (Kruschke, Kappenman, & Hetrick, 2005). No other theory has yet been able to account for the highlighting effect in as much detail. Therefore, we use the highlighting effect as a strong signature of attentional shifting during learning. One of the main findings of this chapter is that learners who have evolved to learn fast (in certain environments) also exhibit highlighting as a side effect.

The chapter is organized as follows. First, we describe the particular type of training environment in which the simulated learners will evolve. Essentially, the environment implements context-dependent cue relevances, with contexts changing through time. Then we describe a class of learning agents that will be explored. We use variants of backpropagation networks (Rumelhart, Hinton, & Williams, 1986) as a representative class of associative learning models. We then show results from "intelligent design," by which we humorously refer to the process whereby we establish intuitively reasonable architectures (instead of randomly searching for architectures) and use hill-climbing optimization to find optimal learning rates. In all cases, the learning rates that learn the training environments fastest also show robust highlighting. Next, we report results from genetic algorithms that searched the space of architectures and learning rates simultaneously. Again, the best learners show highlighting. We conclude with a discussion of other training environments conducive to learned attention.

Fast learning *of what* favors selective attention *to what?*

We have made the skeletal claim in the introduction that fast learning favors selective attention. To flesh out the claim, we need to define what environmental situations are being learned and what aspects are attended to.

Attention to what? The representation

If the need for speed is paramount in learning, then why not just evolve a high-capacity memorizer? This would be analogous to a high-speed, high-resolution video camera that has yottabytes[1] of memory, recording every moment instantly. It seems that this might be the optimal learner, subject only to costs of hardware. To the contrary, such a system is far from optimal, even if the hardware is free. The problem comes in using the stored information. To use the memory for anticipating outcomes in new situations, either the new situation must retrieve an *exact match* in the vast memory to determine the exact outcome that occurred before, or the new situation must retrieve many *similar* memories and the system must somehow integrate across those

---

[1] A yottabyte is 10^{24} bytes, i.e., one trillion terabytes.

memories to anticipate a likely outcome. In the real world there is never an *exact* repetition of a situation. For example, recognizing a person from day to day demands imperfect matching to memory of the person from previous days, because the person's appearance and behavior are never exactly the same from day to day. Therefore, memory retrieval that is based on exact matching would be useless in practice, even if the hardware were available in principle.

Instead of exact matches to memory, retrieval must be based on some form of similarity between stimulus and memories. Similarity can be defined many different ways, and only in the context of specific representational formats. In any case, the point is that the mind has some representational format that is not a mere copy of the sensory surface. The representation is a transformation of the sensory information into a format that has various useful components.

It is the components of the representation that can be selectively attended. By this we mean that the representational components can be selectively enhanced or suppressed. We will not be modeling the entire process of transforming a sensory surface into internal representations of perception, cognition, and action. Instead, our model starts with an input representation that already assumes considerable transformation from sensory input to percept. Specifically, we will assume that the learner's world consists of the presence or absence of various features, such as tones, lights, colors, etc. This sort of input representation is assumed by many venerable models of associative learning.

What makes this sort of feature-based representation so intuitive and effortless is that the features can be easily selectively attended by us. For example, we can talk about the presence/absence of a tone, or the presence/absence of a light, because they can be selectively attended. Aspects of the world that are difficult to selectively attend, such as brightness versus saturation of colors, are used less often in associative learning experiments. The selectively attendable features need not be conceptually simplistic, such as pure tones or lights. Instead, the features could be complex entities, such as the presence/absence of the word "radio," or the presence/absence of a picture of a fish. We assume that the learner has already acquired some internal representation of certain features, however simple or complex. Our models, to be described below, allow forms of selective attention to those features.

Learning of what? The environment

What is it that must be learned that we claim can be speeded by selective attention? We believe that a fundamental challenge faced by an organism is "context-dependent relevances of cues." The challenges posed by contextual dependencies have been recognized by machine learning researchers for decades (for a review see, e.g., Edmonds & Norling, 2007). Individual learners, such as humans, may be born into environments with cue relevances that change depending on the context. The context-specific relevances must be learned, and learned quickly for reproductive advantage.

Definition of context

The term "context" is used by different authors in different ways. In general, contextual cues may differ from non-contextual cues in their spatial or temporal arrangement, or in their contingent relationship with the outcomes. Contextual cues are sometimes thought of as spatially ambient rather than focal. For example, context may be the color of the background of a visual display (e.g., Dibbets, Maes, Boermans, & Vossen, 2001), or context may be the spatial constellation of items in an array (e.g., Chun, 2000). Contextual cues are sometimes supposed to be relatively static through time compared with focal cues. For example, the context may be the restaurant in which a sequence of different foods (the focal cues) is observed (e.g., Rosas & Callejas-Aguilera, 2006). Contextual cues are also often intended to be uncorrelated with the outcome, such that contextual information by itself is uninformative regarding what specific outcome to anticipate (e.g., Little & Lewandowsky, 2009; Yang & Lewandowsky, 2003). For our purposes, we define context as a cue that is not correlated with the outcome and that changes in time less frequently than other cues. In other words, we emphasize the temporal and contingency aspects of context, not its spatial aspect.

An environment with context-dependent relevance

Table 1.1 shows the standard training environment that we will use to instantiate context-dependent relevance. Cues arbitrarily denoted by labels "I" and "J" act as context cues. These context cues have zero correlation with the outcomes, but they do indicate which other cues are good predictors of the outcomes. When context cue I is present, focal cues A and B are perfect predictors of the outcomes, but focal cues C and D are uncorrelated with the outcomes. On the other hand, when context cue J is present, the roles of the focal cues are reversed, with cues C and D now being the perfect predictors of the outcomes, and cues A and B being uncorrelated with the outcomes.

During training, we will usually group together several consecutive trials that share the same context cue. Thus, several trials with context cue I will occur, followed by several trials with context cue J, and so forth. In this way, the context cues change less frequently than the other cues. The exact number of trials in one context or another will be manipulated in different simulations.

Neither the context nor focal cues have any spatial coding in the model. There is no distinction between context and focal cues other than their contingencies with other cues and the outcomes. The columns of Table 1.1 are labeled

Table 1.1 *A training environment that has context-dependent relevancies*

Context Cues		Focal Cues				Outcomes	
I	J	A	B	C	D	X	Y
1	0	1	0	1	0	1	0
1	0	1	0	0	1	1	0
1	0	0	1	1	0	0	1
1	0	0	1	0	1	0	1
0	1	1	0	1	0	1	0
0	1	1	0	0	1	0	1
0	1	0	1	1	0	1	0
0	1	0	1	0	1	0	1

Note: Presence of a cue or outcome is denoted by a 1, and absence is denoted by a 0. Each row denotes a different training trial.

separately (as context and focal cues) merely for the benefit of the reader; the simulations had no such benefit.

There is redundancy built into the structure of Table 1.1, with cue B being redundant with cue A, and cue D being redundant with cue C, and outcome Y being redundant with cue X. These redundancies are unnecessary for the basic demonstrations we report below, but the redundancies do provide symmetry that makes interpretation of the simulations easier.

The structure of Table 1.1 is also isomorphic to the structure denoted "Type III" in the monograph by Shepard, Hovland, and Jenkins (1961), which reported benchmark results regarding the relative difficulties of six different category structures. Unlike their work, our demonstrations do not assume that cues I-J, A-B, and C-D are alternative values of three distinct dimensions. Despite the fact that the cues in Table 1.1 are not dimensionalized, it may benefit understanding to display them as if they were, as shown in Figure 1.1. The items for which context cue I is present are shown on the left side of the figure, and the items for which context cue J is present are shown on the right side of the figure. The correct outcome is denoted by X and Y, along with grey shading in order to enhance the visual distinctiveness of outcome X. It can be seen that in context I, cues A and B are relevant to the outcome, but in context J, cues C and D are relevant to the outcome.

Designing fast learners

Our goal is to create fast learners of contextually dependent relevancies. We will use the structure of Table 1.1 as the test bed. The simulated

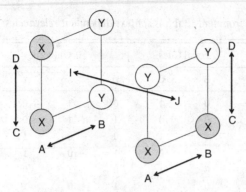

Figure 1.1 Spatial representation of the training structure in Table 1.1. Each circle represents a combination of cues A, B, C, D, I, and J. The letter in the circle, either X or Y, represents the correct outcome for that cue combination. The rhombus on the left has a letter I in its center to indicate that cue I is present, while the rhombus on the right has a letter J in its center to indicate that cue J is present. The upper circles have cue D present, while the lower circles have cue C present. The remaining dimension marks whether cue A or cue B is present. Although this diagram represents A–B, C–D, and I–J as if on dimensions, the basic structure does *not* encode or assume any dimensional relationship among the cues.

learners will be trained on several repeated blocks of the structure and the total accuracy during training will be used as a measure of reproductive fitness. We will explore various model architectures and temporal groupings of context trials. For each design, we will find learning rates that minimize the total error (i.e., maximize the total accuracy) during the lifetime of the learner.

Assessing selective attention: exhibiting highlighting

Having thereby designed optimal fast learners, we will then assess whether the learner has selective attention. There are many criteria one might establish for declaring that a learner possesses selective attention. The criterion we will use is that the learner exhibits "highlighting."

In the highlighting procedure (Kruschke, 2009), training begins with the presentation of two cues, denoted I and PE, leading to the outcome E. (Cue I here bears no relation to context I in the other structure; the shared label is accidental coincidence.) We denote such trials as I.PE→E. After this early training, occasional trials introduce a new case: I.PL→L. In later training, those cases predominate, so that the overall number of I.PE→E trials equals the overall number of I.PL→L trials. The outcomes are denoted E and L because they are "early trained" and "late trained," respectively. The cue PE is so labeled because it is a "perfect" predictor of the "early" outcome, and the cue PL is so labeled because it is a "perfect" predictor of the "late" outcome. The cue I is an "imperfect" predictor of the two outcomes.

Notice that the two outcomes have symmetric structure. Each outcome has one perfect predictor, and the outcomes share an imperfect predictor. Moreover, there are an equal number of trials of the two cases, overall. If people learn this simple symmetry, then the imperfect predictor should be equally (un-) associated with the two outcomes, and the two perfect predictors should be equally associated with their respective outcomes. This symmetry is easy to assess, as follows. After training, we test people with cue I by itself, asking people to respond with the outcome they think is most likely based on what they have learned. It turns out that people do not give 50/50 responding, but instead clearly prefer the early learned outcome E (roughly 70/30). This preference is not a mere primacy bias for any ambiguous test, however. When tested with the pair of cues PE.PL, people clearly prefer the later learned outcome L (roughly 65/35).

The "torsion" in preferences, wherein one ambiguous cue leads to a preference for E but another ambiguous cue leads to a preference for L, is called the highlighting effect. The highlighting effect has been found for many different stimuli, relative frequencies, cover stories, and so on. For a review, with data from a "canonical" experiment that has equal base rates for the various cases, see Kruschke (2009).

The highlighting effect is challenging to explain. Because of the simple symmetry in the structure, many formal models of learning predict symmetric response preferences. The Rescorla–Wagner (1972) model, for example, predicts symmetric associations (with sufficient training).

The most successful account of highlighting so far is an attentional account, suggested informally by Medin and Edelson (1988) and formalized by Kruschke (1996a, 2001). When people are learning the early cases I.PE→E, attention is allocated to both cues, because there is no reason not to do so. Consequently, moderate-strength associations are learned from both cues to outcome E. The associative strengths are only moderate because the two cues mutually support each other in generating the anticipation of the outcome. When subsequently learning cases of I.PL→L, however, attention rapidly shifts away from cue I, because it has already been learned to indicate something other than the correct outcome L. Attention therefore falls on the distinctive cue PL, and a strong association is learned from PL to outcome L. Thus, in learning I.PL→L, people have learned two things: first, they have learned to re-allocate attention away from I to PL. Second, they have learned to associate PL with L.

Because the attentional account of highlighting has been rather successful in quantitatively accounting for many variations of the highlighting design and other cue–outcome mappings (again, for a review, see Kruschke, 2009), we will treat the highlighting effect as a *behavioral* signature of attentional learning.

Other signatures of attentional learning?

There are other learning phenomena that have been explained in terms of attention, but we do not explore them in the present chapter for two different reasons. First, some of these other phenomena can be explained without appeal to attentional mechanisms. Second, some of these other phenomena require the ability to learn complex, non-linear relationships between cues and outcomes that the simple models we explore in this chapter cannot learn.

Consider the phenomenon known as "blocking," wherein an initial training stage involves trials of A→X, and a subsequent training stage involves trials with a redundant relevant cue, A.B→X (Kamin, 1969). In subsequent tests, the association from B to X appears to be weaker than it would have been if the initial phase with A alone had not been experienced. This relative weakness of B has been explained in attentional terms, such that there has been learned suppression of cue B (e.g., Kruschke, 2001; Kruschke & Blair, 2000; Kruschke *et al.*, 2005; Mackintosh, 1975). But the basic blocking effect can also be explained without appeal to attentional learning (e.g., Miller & Matzel, 1988; Rescorla & Wagner, 1972). Therefore, we have chosen not to use blocking, per se, as a signature of attentional learning.

Another phenomenon that has been explained in terms of attention is "latent inhibition" (Lubow, 1989; Schmajuk, 2002). In the basic procedure for latent inhibition, a cue is first presented with no notable outcome, in a set of trials called the preexposure phase. Subsequently, the cue is paired with a novel outcome. Latent inhibition occurs when learning of the novel cue–outcome association is retarded because of the preexposure phase. One explanation is that the preexposure phase produced learned attentional suppression of the cue, which lingered into the subsequent phase in which the cue was paired with an outcome (e.g., Kruschke, 2001; Schmajuk, Lam, & Gray, 1996). The phenomenon can be difficult to obtain in humans, however (but see Nelson & Sanjuan, 2006, for a recent example), and there are a variety of findings suggestive of different underlying mechanisms in latent inhibition. Therefore we have chosen not to use latent inhibition as a signature of attentional learning.

Another classic phenomenon that has been attributed to attentional learning is the advantage of "intradimensional shifts" relative to "extradimensional shifts" (e.g., Hall & Channell, 1985; Kruschke, 1996b; Slamecka, 1968). In these relevance-shift procedures, a learner is first trained on two-dimensional stimuli for which one dimension is perfectly predictive of the outcome and the other dimension is irrelevant to the outcome. For example, it could be that red circles or squares are mapped to outcome X, while green circles or squares are mapped to outcome Y. In this case, color is relevant while shape is irrelevant. In the shift phase, novel values of the dimensions are used: e.g., blue or yellow stars or triangles. When the same dimension is relevant in the shift phase, the shift is called an intradimensional shift. When the other dimension is relevant in the shift phase, the shift is called an extradimensional shift. Many experiments have demonstrated that for adult humans, intradimensional shift is easier to learn than extradimensional shift. This advantage for intradimensional shifts is naturally explained by attentional learning: in the initial phase, people have learned to attend to the relevant dimension and to ignore the irrelevant dimension. This attentional allocation persists into the shift phase. Whereas this is a strong indicator of attentional learning, a model of it requires representation of dimensions and values within dimensions: e.g., representation of red and green along with the dimension of color. In our modeling efforts, we opted to use a simpler representation that avoided assumptions about dimensions, and therefore this phenomenon of intradimensional shift advantage is beyond the scope of our present explorations (but see Kruschke, 1996b, for a related model).

Finally, in theories of category learning, attentional learning is used to explain the differential difficulties of various category structures. In particular, the relative ease of two structures introduced by Shepard et al. (1961) is naturally interpreted in terms of attentional learning. These structures involve three binary-valued dimensions, with the resulting eight instances mapped into two categories. One structure involves a non-linearly separable exclusive-OR on two dimensions, with the third dimension being irrelevant (called "Type II" by Shepard et al., 1961). The other structure is linearly separable, defined by two diametrically opposed prototypes whereby all three dimensions are relevant to distinguish the categories (called "Type IV" by Shepard et al., 1961). Despite the fact that the latter structure is linearly separable and the former structure is not, the latter category is harder to learn. Some theories assert that the latter structure is harder because it demands attention to all three dimensions, whereas the former category only demands attention to two dimensions (e.g., Kruschke, 1992; Nosofsky, Gluck, Palmeri, McKinley, & Glauthier, 1994; Shepard et al., 1961). Other theories use more rule-like representations to account for the relative difficulties (e.g., Goodman, Tenenbaum, Feldman, & Griffiths, 2008; Nosofsky, Palmeri, & McKinley, 1994), which might be re-construed in attention-like terms. Even among explicitly attentional approaches, modeling these structures appropriately requires representation of dimensions, and, as mentioned above, we have opted to use simpler representations in the current explorations.

Thus, of the many phenomena that may be considered as indicators of attentional learning, it is the highlighting phenomenon that is both structurally simple and uniquely explained (so far) by attentional learning. Therefore, we use highlighting as the behavioral signature of attentional learning.

Design space and functional desiderata

Given a design space consisting of backpropagation networks, we want to explore variations that may implement functional desiderata. One desideratum is that previous learning should be protected, as appropriate, when learning new associations. For example, there should not be catastrophic forgetting of the fact that 2 x 2 → 4 when subsequently learning the fact that 3 x 3 → 9 (McCloskey & Cohen, 1989). One way to help protect previous learning, when a new combination of cues is encountered, is by shifting the internal representation of the cues away from the conflicting, previously associated cues. In other words, if previous learning has associated a particular cue with a particular outcome, and new outcomes also include that previous cue among the presented cues, then the previous association from that cue can be protected by shifting attention away from it when learning the new outcome. Such a shift in internal representation can have an undesirable side effect, however, because the shift might generate arbitrary patterns of activation that correspond to nothing present in the cues. Loosely speaking, if you close your eyes to deflect your attention away from a previously learned cue, then you might imagine anything; an unconstrained shift of representation might cause "hallucinations." Therefore, a second functional desideratum is for the shift of representation to be constrained by the actually present cues.

These functional desiderata can be implemented in many ways. We considered the following possibilities. One way to keep the hidden-layer representation faithful to the actually presented cues is to establish hidden nodes that have fixed 1-to-1 connections from corresponding input cues. These 1-to-1 connections cause the corresponding hidden-node activations to start the training as approximate copies of the input-cue activations. This initial state can be eventually overruled by learned connections from other input cues, but at least there is an initial bias toward faithfulness to present cues. A second way to keep the hidden layer from hallucinating is to allow learning only for hidden nodes for which the corresponding input cue is activated. This method can be easily implemented by multiplying the hidden-node activation by the corresponding cue-node activation. The multiplicative product is large only if both the cue-node activation and the hidden-node activation are large.

The second desideratum, that is, protection of previous learning by a shift of hidden representation, can be achieved in different ways. One way is to do gradient descent on error with respect to the hidden weights first, before changing the output weights. In this way, the previously learned output weights are protected, if possible. After the hidden weights are shifted, then input is re-propagated to the hidden nodes and the output weights are learned. A second way to implement a shift is to have two sets of weights: one set is the regular type, the other set is "first and fast": first-updating but with fast decay to zero before the next trial begins (a related scheme for fast-decaying weights was proposed by Hinton & Plaut, 1987). Again, the first-fast weights protect the output weights from catastrophic forgetting, but in this case the slow hidden weights do not need to change radically to implement the protection.

Figure 1.2 illustrates all these design possibilities in a single network architecture. Not all of the options need to be implemented simultaneously. The diagram indicates that the hidden nodes and outcome nodes are standard backpropagation nodes that first sum their weighted inputs and then squash the sum with a sigmoid function. Formally, denote the activation of the ith input node as a_i^{in}, the activation of the jth output node as a_j^{out}, and the weight connecting node i to node j by w_{ji}. Then the sigmoidal activation function is given by

$$a_j^{out} = 1 \Big/ \left[1 + \exp\left(-\left[\sum_i w_{ji} a_i^{in} - \theta_j \right] \right) \right]$$

(1.1)

where θ_j is the "threshold" of the jth node. A graph of the sigmoidal output, as a function of the summed inputs, is a tipped "S" shape, as shown schematically inside the nodes of Figure 1.2. The sigmoid activation asymptotes at 1.0 as the summed input exceeds the threshold by a large positive amount, and the sigmoid activation asymptotes at 0.0 as the summed input is far below the threshold. When the summed input equals the threshold then the sigmoid activation is 0.5.

The dashed arrows in Figure 1.2 indicate learnable weights, all of which are initialized at zero. The solid arrows impinging upon the hidden nodes are fixed, non-learnable 1-to-1 connections that implement the idea that each hidden node starts as an approximate copy of the corresponding input cue. For purposes of demonstration in the simulations, the 1-to-1 connection weights were arbitrarily fixed at 10.0, with thresholds in the sigmoid function also set at 10.0. Consequently, in the naive network with all zero weights except the 1-to-1 connections, when an input cue is active, the corresponding hidden node has activation of 0.5, and when the input cue is not active, the corresponding hidden node has activation of nearly zero.

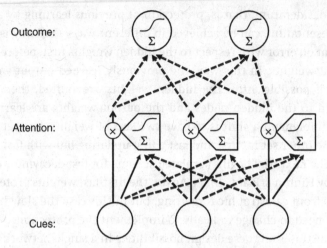

Outcome:

Attention:

Cues:

Figure 1.2 An architecture for exploring learning rates that minimize error.

Figure 1.2 also shows solid arrows from the input cues passing *beside* the hidden linear-sigmoid node, via a circle marked with a multiplication sign. These arrows indicate optional multiplication of the hidden-node activation by the corresponding input-cue activation.

Finally, the dashed arrows in Figure 1.2, which indicate learnable connections, each represent two different learnable connections. Both connections learn via the standard backpropagation algorithm but they can have different learning rates. Crucially, one connection is the traditional "slow" learner, whereas the other connection is a "first-fast" learner. The first-fast connection adjusts its weights before the slow connection, i.e., it learns *first*, and then activation is repropagated and error is recomputed before the slow connection is adjusted. Moreover, the first-fast weight decays to zero before the next trial starts, i.e., it is *fast* decaying, whereas the slow weight does not decay.

In summary, there are four learning rates in the architecture of Figure 1.2: the hidden, aka attention, nodes have incoming weights that have a slow learning rate and a first-fast learning rate. The outcome nodes also have slow and first-fast learning rates that can be different from the attention-node learning rates. If any of the learning rates is zero it is tantamount to that sort of learning being unavailable to the network. There is also an optional multiplicative "gating" of the input activation by the corresponding hidden activation.

Results: optimal learners exhibit highlighting

For each architectural option we used hill-climbing optimization to discover the learning rates that minimized the total error during training on the context-dependent-relevance structure in Table 1.1. It might seem that higher learning rates would always produce faster learning and smaller total error, but this is not the case. The reason is that learning rates that are too high cause the weights to overshoot the best values, thereby producing larger error on subsequent training trials. Thus, even though we allow the learning rates to be arbitrarily large as needed, the best learning rates turn out to be moderate in magnitude.

The main question is whether a network that has optimal learning rates also embodies selective attention. Selective attention is assayed behaviorally by exhibition of highlighting. For each architectural option, we found the optimal learning rates, then trained a naive network on the highlighting structure and tested whether the network exhibited highlighting.

In detail, the simulations proceeded as follows. In training the context-dependent-relevance structure, blocks of four consecutive trials used the same contextual cue (I or J). At the beginning of each block of four trials, there was a 50/50 chance of being trained in context I or context J. Each simulated network was trained on 20 random blocks, constituting 80 trials. For each simulated network, the total error across training was recorded. Fifty different random training sequences were averaged to compute the error for a given learning rate. Formally, denote the correct, "teacher," value at outcome node k on trial t in sequence s as T_{stk}, with $T_{stk} = 1$ if k is the correct outcome for the present cues, and $T_{stk} = 0$ otherwise. Then the overall error was measured as

$$\text{RMSD} = \left[\frac{1}{50 \times 80 \times 2} \sum_{\text{seq } s}^{50} \sum_{\text{trial } t}^{80} \sum_{\text{out } k}^{2} \left(T_{stk} - a_{stk}^{\text{out}} \right)^2 \right]^{1/2} \tag{1.2}$$

where the summations are over sequences, trials, and outcome nodes, respectively, and where a_{stk}^{out} is computed by the sigmoid activation function in Equation 1.1. The overall error in Equation 1.2 is also called the root-mean-squared deviation (RMSD) between the taught and generated values. As a reference for the magnitude of the RMSD, consider its value if the network learned nothing, so that the network's outcome activations were always exactly 0.5 (which is what the sigmoid activation function generates when all the weights are zero). In this case, because T is always zero or one, $T_{stk} - a_{stk}^{\text{out}}$ is always ±0.5. Hence the RMSD is 0.5 when there is no learning at all. The RMSD gets smaller than 0.5 when there is successful learning.

A hill-climbing optimization routine was used to find learning rates that produced the smallest possible error. The optimizer started with reasonable learning rates specified by the programmer and then incremented or decremented the various learning rates until adjustments no longer yielded any significant reduction in RMSD. (The arbitrary starting point for the learning rates was manually set at several different values for different runs, to gain confidence that a global minimum was achieved.) The hill-climbing optimizer found learning rates that minimized the RMSD.

Having converged to the optimal learning rates, the network was then reset to all-zero weights and tested on the highlighting structure. It began with 8 trials of I.PE→E, then a random mix of 12 trials of I.PE→E with 4 trials of I.PL→L, followed by a random mix of 8 trials of I.PE→E with 24 trials of I.PL→L. Notice that there were an equal number of I.PE→E and I.PL→L trials overall. After the training the network was tested with I.PE, I.PL, I alone, and PE.PL.

Different architectural options were used, with optimal learning rates determined for each. Figures 1.3 and 1.4 show the results when only slow-weight learning was permitted, with no multiplicative gating. In other words, the first-fast learning rates were fixed at zero, while the slow learning rates on both layers of nodes were allowed to be whatever values minimized the RMSD. Figure 1.3 shows the learned weights at the end of training for one representative network. The weights are displayed in matrix format, with the weight values indicated numerically and by the shading in the cells. The left matrix shows the weights to the hidden (attention) nodes from the cue nodes. Notice that the diagonal cells of the left matrix are all 10, reflecting the fact that the 1-to-1 connections are set permanently to 10 in these simulations. Of special interest is the lowest row of this matrix, which represents the weights from context cue I. The connections from context cue I to the hidden nodes corresponding to cues A and B have become *positive*, but the connections from context cue I to the hidden nodes corresponding to cues C and D have become *negative*. The weights from context cue J, in the next row up, show the opposite pattern. These weights suggest that the network has learned to allocate attention to A and B when context I is present, but to allocate attention to C and D when context J is present.

Figure 1.4 shows the result of subsequent testing of the network with the highlighting procedure. The same learning rates were used, but starting with a naive network. The figure shows the weights at the end of training on a typical run. It can be seen that the weight from PL to hidden-I is strongly negative, but the weight from PE to hidden-I is fairly positive. In other words, the network has learned to suppress attention to I when PL is present, but to attend to I when PE is present. The learned weights result in a strong highlighting effect: when presented with cue I by itself, the network produces a strong outcome preference for E, but when presented with cues PE.PL, the network produces a clear outcome preference for L. In summary, when the slow-weight learning rates are optimized so that the context-dependent-relevance structure is learned with least error, then the network exhibits robust highlighting.

We also found optimal learning rates when the architecture included first-fast learning on the input-to-hidden connections, and multiplication by the input

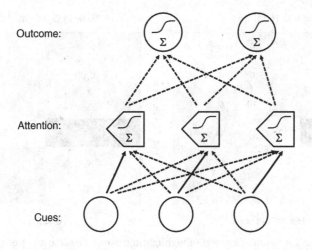

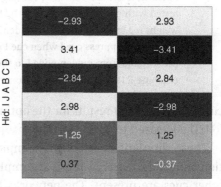

	Slow to Hid from In							**Slow to Out from Hid**	

In: I J A B C D

-1.29	1.19	-0.15	0.2	-0.01	10
-0.66	-2.22	0.26	0.09	10	-0.1
-1.7	-0.38	-0.01	10	-0.9	2.39
-0.26	-0.66	10	0	0.66	-1.72
0	10	-2.75	-2.16	3.49	3.75
10	0	2.86	2.44	-3.74	-3.08

Hid: I J A B C D

-2.93	2.93
3.41	-3.41
-2.84	2.84
2.98	-2.98
-1.25	1.25
0.37	-0.37

Out: X Y

Figure 1.3 Simulation results when there is only slow-weight learning on hidden and outcome layers, with no first-fast learning and no attentional multiplication, as suggested by the network diagram in the upper part of the figure. The network diagram shows only three cues, whereas the simulations involved six. The lower panel shows the weights at the end of training in a typical run on the context-dependent structure (Table 1.1). In the left matrix, the rows index the input cue, in the order I, J, A, B, C, and D, as indicated along the left edge of the matrix. The columns index the hidden node, in the same order, as indicated at the bottom edge of the matrix. Notice that the weights from input node I (lowest row) are positive (2.86 and 2.44) to hidden nodes A and B, but negative (−3.74 and −3.08) to hidden nodes C and D. The weights from input node J show the opposite pattern. These weights indicate that the network has learned to pay attention to A and B in context I, but to pay attention to C and D in context J. The RMSD across 80 training trials and 50 simulated subjects was 0.250.

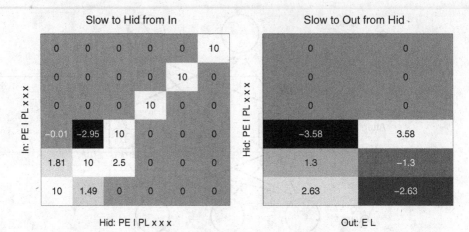

Figure 1.4 Results from test of highlighting, using the same architecture and parameter values as in Figure 1.3. These weights result in a strong preference for outcome E when tested with cue I, and a strong preference for outcome L when tested with cues PE.PL. Notice in the left matrix that there is a strong inhibitory weight (−2.95) from cue PL to hidden node I, indicating that the network has learned to suppress cue I when cue PL is present. The right matrix shows that the weights from hidden node I to the outcomes are not symmetric; they excite outcome E (+1.3) but inhibit outcome L (−1.3).

cues. The pattern of results for the optimal learning rates was the same, but the RMSD decreased to 0.233, and the magnitude of highlighting increased.

These simulations establish examples of what we mean by learned attention: individual cue activations are amplified or attenuated depending on which other cues are present. The networks have learned to selectively enhance or suppress particular cues, in a context-dependent manner. It is this sort of context-dependent, learned modulation that we call "selective attention" when analyzed at the level of hidden network activations. At the behavioral level, attention can only be assayed by overt outcome-activation patterns without reference to hidden internal activations. We use the highlighting effect as a behavioral-level signature of selective attention.

In the final discussion we shall return to these explorations in the design of network architectures but with other training environments. Before those explorations, we will describe the more thorough search of design space that is possible via genetic algorithms.

Evolution: genetic algorithms discover fast learners

Human designers cannot manually explore the myriad (indeed infinite) combinations in the design space. It could well be that there are unforeseen combinations of design options that learn even better than those discovered by hill climbing on learning rates in pre-set architectures. In this section we report the results of extensive searches of the design space by simulated evolution, i.e., genetic algorithms (e.g., Goldberg, 1989). An advantage of a genetic algorithm (GA) is that it can explore a wide range of architectural combinations and learning rates simultaneously, unlike the hill-climbing searches that were restricted to a particular architecture. To simulate the evolution of attention in learning we follow the approach presented in Miller and Todd's (1990) and Todd and Miller's (1991) work on evolving networks (agents) that learn. We use a genetic algorithm to evolve populations of agents in the context-dependent-relevance structure of Table 1.1, and we look for signs of attention shifting (i.e., highlighting) in the best-performing agents.

Overview

Agents

Each agent in the simulation consists of a connection matrix that describes each node in the network, the type of connection between each of the nodes (no connection, fixed connections, slow-learning, or first-fast connections), and the initial strength of each of the connections. Additionally, each agent contains a structure that specifies the learning rates to be used for back-propagation of error at each layer of the network and other learning-related details such as whether the agent implements multiplication of hidden activations by cue activations.

This genetic structure can be used to specify an infinite space of backpropagation networks with different numbers of input, hidden, and output nodes, different connection architectures, learning rates, and error propagation methods. In our simulations, the "genome" explicitly specifies various weights and learning rates, which might not be very biologically plausible, but nevertheless serve our purpose of thoroughly searching the space of design possibilities. More biologically plausible specifications may be possible; see, for example, the work of Burgos (2007). In order to keep the evolutionary process tractable and to make comparison with the hill-climbing simulations straightforward, the networks are constrained as follows: each network has six input nodes (one for each of the binary cue values I, J, A, B, C, and D), six hidden nodes, and a single output node. The single output node represents outcome X by an activation of 1, and outcome Y by an activation of 0. Its threshold is fixed at zero, so the outcome node's baseline activation is 0.5, the neutral value between X and Y. Each input node is constrained to have a fixed 1-to-1 connection weight of 10, and the hidden nodes' thresholds for the sigmoid functions were fixed at 10.

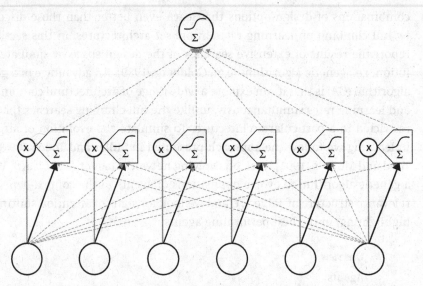

Figure 1.5 An architecture showing potential connections for an evolved network. The faint dotted lines indicate connections that may be fixed (non-learning), slow-learning, or first-fast connections. The faint lines to multiplication nodes indicate that a particular agent may or may not evolve attentional multiplication. Note that for simplicity not all of the possible connections from the input to the hidden layer were included in the diagram.

Each network is trained in an environment that has a random assignment of abstract cues (i.e., I, J, A, B, C, and D) to physical input nodes. Because no individual agent knows which cues will play which role, the best evolved initial weights should be symmetric across input cues. To simplify the simulations, we enforced this logical symmetry rather than let it noisily evolve. This symmetry is produced in a three-step process when birthing a network. First, as noted above, each input node will have a fixed 1-to-1 connection. Second, the connection type and initial weight for the connection between the first input node and its adjacent hidden node is copied identically for each input-to-adjacent-hidden node connection. Third, the connection type and initial weight for the connection between the first hidden node and the output node is replicated to each hidden-to-output connection. Figure 1.5 shows a simplified diagram of the possible network architectures. Figure 1.5 is much like Figure 1.2 except that all six cues are explicitly indicated, and there is only a single outcome node, as described above.

Environment and fitness

The scenario under which our agents are evolving is a very simple context environment. The agents do not have to move, they do not have to actively seek out stimuli, and they do not have to interact with, or face competition from, other agents or any other outside factors. As with Todd and Miller's

(1991) simulations, it may be helpful to think of the agents as being born in an aquatic world where they are attached to the sea floor, passively watching potentially edible stimuli float by. Each passing stimulus has a set of distinctive cues and based on those cues the agent must decide whether the stimulus is edible or inedible. The agent's fitness is increased when it makes a correct decision, to eat something that is edible or to avoid something that is not, and the agent's fitness is identically decreased when it makes an incorrect decision. After each trial, the agent receives feedback on the correct eat/avoid response for the just-seen stimulus, thereby allowing the agent to learn the regularities of the environment throughout its lifetime.

In this environment of the passive learner, temporal changes in contextual cues are generated by the environment. In the sea-floor scenario, context cues might change with daylight, tides, or seasons. For example, what indicates food at high tide might be irrelevant at low tide. Context could also be the presence or absence of schools of fish, which may occur more randomly and not at fixed intervals. For example, what indicates food when schools of jellyfish are around might be irrelevant when the waters are clear.

Reproduction

Each agent sees a fixed number of stimuli during its lifetime and its total fitness level is the sum of the trial-by-trial fitness that it has accumulated across all learning trials. Agents for the next generation are selected (on the basis of the current agents' fitnesses) in one of three ways. First, the next generation can be generated using crossover and mutation. In crossover, two agents are selected from the current population, with the probability of selection directly related to the relative fitness. The genetic specifications of the two agents are spliced together and a small degree of random mutation is applied to generate an agent to be used in the next population. A second method of reproduction is by mutation only. Again, agents with higher relative fitness have higher probability of being chosen as progenitors of mutated offspring, but there is no crossover with other agents. Finally, the third method of reproduction ensures that the best current solution is not wiped out by a mutation or ill-advised mating. The genetic specification of the highest-fitness agent in the population is simply copied into the next generation. Over time, this random but fitness-driven selection process should result in populations of networks that are very good at performing in a context environment.

Assessing selective attention by highlighting

As with the hill-climbing simulations, a highlighting task was used to determine whether the evolved agents were exhibiting signs of selective

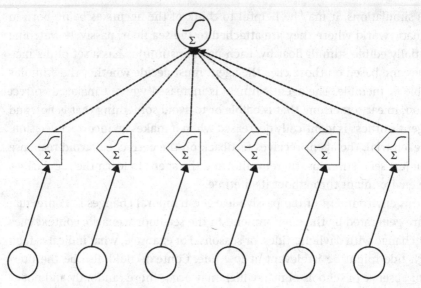

Figure 1.6 The architecture of the initial population of agents for all evolutionary simulations. The input and hidden layers are connected through non-learning 1-to-1 connections and the hidden and output layers are connected through slow-learning connections. Multiplicative attention is not active.

attention. At the end of each agent's lifetime its learned connection weights were reset to 0 and it was subjected to a highlighting task, as described previously for the hill-climbing simulations. The agent's responses during both the learning and testing phases of the highlighting task were recorded for analysis but played no role in the agent's fitness and thus the highlighting task performance had no effect on the evolutionary trajectory. An agent was labeled as "highlighting" if the ordinality of its responses to the ambiguous I and PE.PL cues showed the signature torsion in preferences described previously, i.e., if its output activation preferred E to L for input I and its output activation preferred L to E for input PE.PL.

Simulation parameters

For the results reported below, the GA was run with the following parameters: each simulated population ran for 4000 generations and each generation consisted of 100 agents. The initial population was seeded with the "base" agents shown in Figure 1.6. Each agent had fixed 1-to-1 connections with a weight of 10 between each input node and its direct hidden node. Initially there were no other connections between the input and hidden layer. Each hidden node was connected to the output node with a slow learning connection with an initial weight of 0 and a slow learning rate selected from a Gaussian distribution centered on 0.05 with a standard deviation of 0.04. If the selected learning rate was negative, the absolute value of the rate was used, ensuring that all initial learning rates were small positive values. It should be noted that this base agent behaves as a single-layer network and cannot perform perfectly in a non-linear discrimination such as the context-dependent-relevance environment.

At the end of each generation the parents for the next generation were selected. The first step of this process was to copy the most fit agent from the current generation into the new generation without any crossover or mutation (elitist selection with $N = 1$). This step ensured that the best-performing agent's genetic structure was not corrupted by a non-adaptive mutation or crossover.

After the best creature had been copied the rest of the parents were selected using fitness proportionate selection. In order to provide the maximum differentiation between agents even when the population was converging on similar solutions, the agents' actual fitness values were modified before the selection process. Each agent's fitness was reduced by a value slightly less than the worst-performing agent's fitness. This subtraction had the effect of stretching the fitness values so that the worst agents had a "relative fitness" value of near zero while the best agent's relative fitness values was equal to the difference in fitness between the best and worst agents in the population. All agents were then subjected to roulette-wheel selection based on their relative fitness values. Each agent that was selected as a parent had a 50% chance of creating offspring via sexual reproduction and a 50% chance of asexual reproduction.

Agents selected for asexual reproduction were subjected to a mutation process where each gene (connection types, learning rates, etc.) had a small chance of being mutated. The exact mutation rate was selected so that there would be approximately one mutation that was expressed in the symmetric agent's phenotype per generation. Once a particular gene was selected for mutation, the new value for that gene was drawn from a Gaussian distribution centered on the gene's current value and with a standard deviation proportional to the gene's current value. This process ensured that small values underwent small changes while larger values could change more drastically in a given mutation.

Agents selected for sexual reproduction underwent a crossover process to generate an offspring. Once the two parents were selected, two distinct crossover operations were performed. First, the matrix of connection information was crossed over, creating an architecture that was a hybrid of the architectures from the two parents. Instead of the classic technique of treating the matrix as a single long vector and selecting a crossover point (or points), the crossover operation acted on the level of entire rows and/or columns of the matrix. The first step of this process was to set the offspring's connection matrix to be an exact copy of the first parent's matrix. Then specific rows/columns from the second parent's connection matrix were copied into the corresponding rows/columns of the offspring. Transplanting an entire row of the connection matrix from a parent had the effect of copying all of the "outgoing" connection information – connection types and connection weights – from a particular node in the architecture. For example, if the third row of a parent's matrix was crossed over to the offspring, then all of the parent network's connections from node three to other nodes in the network would be copied into the offspring. Similarly, transplanting an entire column of the connection matrix had the effect of copying all of the "incoming" connection information. The particular rows and columns that were crossed over were selected randomly, and the crossover could select a single row and/or column, multiple contiguous rows and/or columns, or multiple non-contiguous rows and/or columns.

Once the connection matrix crossover operation was complete, the second crossover operation was performed. In this procedure the genetic material specifying the agent's learning rates was crossed over. In the agents the learning rate settings were stored as a vector of floating point values specifying the slow and fast learning rates for each layer of the network. As with the connection matrix, the first step of the process was to make an exact copy of the first parent's learning rate settings in the offspring. Next, a standard version of crossover was implemented. A single crossover point was randomly selected in the offspring's learning rate vector and the learning rate settings from the second parent were spliced into the offspring from that point forward. Following crossover, the resulting agent underwent the same mutation process described for asexual reproduction.

At the beginning of each generation a randomly selected context environment was created and all agents were trained in the same type of environment. Agents were exposed to a randomized block of the four stimuli from one context, then the context was switched and the four trials from the second context were randomly presented. This continued for a total of 80 learning trials. Within each generation, all agents were presented with the same sequence of training trials: the mapping of the context and focal cues, the context switches, and the specific trial order was identical across agents. To monitor the overall accuracy of the evolving agents, at the end of an agent's lifetime it was presented with a randomized block of the eight stimuli from the environment and its responses to those stimuli were recorded. As with the highlighting test, these trials had no bearing on the agent's fitness. The agent was labeled as "successful" in the context environment if it made ordinally correct decisions across all eight of these test trials.

Results: evolved learners exhibit highlighting

Because evolution via a genetic algorithm is an inherently probabilistic and noisy process, data must be collected from large numbers of simulations and then analyzed both aggregately and as independent evolutionary runs before strong conclusions can be drawn. In the first set we ran 50 different populations for 4000 generations each, tracking for each generation the agent's fitness, accuracy, highlighting status, successfulness, and details about their architectures and learning rates.

Across the 50 populations, the evolved networks diverged into two distinct architectural solutions, shown in Figure 1.7. There was a local maximum in the fitness landscape not far from where the populations began. Populations quickly evolved to have fixed-weight connections between the input and hidden layers and with learning connections from the hidden layer to the output node. This solution cannot achieve 100% accuracy in the context environment, but it can make correct eat/avoid decisions on 7 of the 8 stimuli, which is better accuracy than many other potential architectures. Almost all of the simulated populations converged on this architecture in their early generations, but the vast majority eventually evolved away from this sub-optimal solution. Only 3 of the 50 simulations reached 4000 generations without moving away from this architecture.

The remaining 47 populations evolved to a higher-accuracy architecture marked by learning connections on both the hidden and output levels. Not surprisingly, these populations performed well in the context environment, with nearly all of the agents in each population achieving perfect ordinal accuracy on the final eight testing trials. Within this architecture, two distinct solutions were found by the simulations. In 43 of the 47 successful runs, a matched-rate solution evolved. These populations converged on a solution where the learning rate on the hidden layer and the learning rate on the output layer evolved to be similar values (typically around 30). In the other four runs, the populations converged on a solution with a high output learning rate. These agents evolved a learning rate to the output layer that was 40 to 50 times higher than the learning rate on the hidden layer (with rates between 70 and 100 on the output layer and 1 to 2 on the hidden layer).

Both the matched-rate solution and the high output-rate solution learned the environment quickly, and the evolved agents were not making any *ordinal* mistakes on the learning trials at the end of their lives. However, only the matched-rate agents showed signs of attentional learning as tested with the highlighting task. After the highlighting training, the matched-rate agents showed a moderate preference for response E when probed with cue I $(E \approx 0.6, L \approx 0.4)$ and a similar preference for response L when probed with cue PE.PL $(E \approx 0.4, L \approx 0.6)$. Overall the

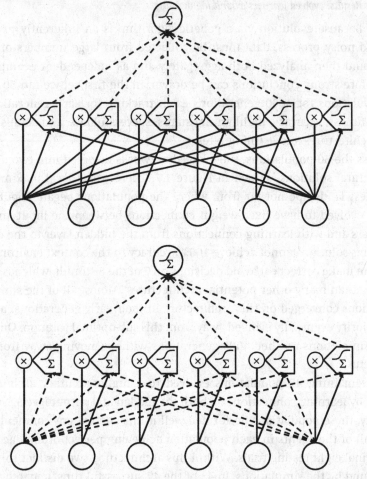

Figure 1.7 Two classes of evolved architectures. The top architecture has all fixed-weight (non-learning) connections from the input to the hidden layer and learning connections to the output layer. These agents can only perform a linear division of the solution space and as a result can respond correctly on up to 7 of the 8 distinct learning trials. The bottom architecture has fixed 1-to-1 weights on the direct input connections and first-fast learning connections between input nodes as the adjacent hidden nodes. The connections between the hidden nodes and the output nodes were learning connections; slow learning in some agents and first-fast learning in others. As a result of learning connections on the lower layer, the agents in this class of architectures are not limited to a linear discrimination of the solution space. Therefore, these agents can learn to respond correctly on all 8 of the distinct learning trials.

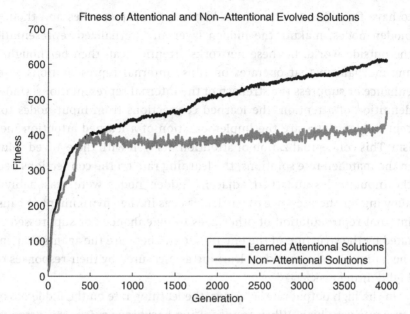

Figure 1.8 A comparison of the average fitness of the best-performing agents that exhibit learned attention (i.e., showed signs of highlighting) vs. agents that learned the correct responses to all 8 training items in the context environment but did not exhibit signs of attention. Attentional mechanisms clearly confer a fitness benefit in the context environment.

torsion of preference is not quite as strong as that seen in the hill-climbing simulations, but it does demonstrate clear highlighting effects. The high output-rate solutions showed no preference for E or L when presented with either of the critical test items. Therefore, it appears as though the matched-rate agents were solving the context environment through the use of learned attentional mechanisms while the high output-rate agents were using a non-attentional solution.

This distinction between the attentional and non-attentional solutions allows us to look at whether or not an attentional mechanism is truly adaptive in the context environment. If attention is one of many equivalent ways to learn quickly and perform well in the environment, then we should not see any clear difference between the overall fitness of the attentional creatures when compared with those that do not exhibit signs of learned attention. Figure 1.8 shows that this is not the case. If we plot the average fitness levels of the best-performing 10% of the agents in both the attentional and non-attentional solutions, we see that the agents with learned attention are clearly outperforming the agents that have not evolved an attention-based solution.

Analysis of the architectures shows that the evolved agents match our interpretation of learned attention. Recall that the evolved agents are constrained to have fixed 1-to-1 connections between the input nodes and their direct hidden nodes, making the hidden layer an internalized representation of the outside world. In these networks attention can then be thought of as any mechanism that operates on those internal representations to either enhance or suppress the strength of the internal representations. Under this definition of attention, the learned connections from input nodes to adjacent hidden notes are the implementation of a learned attention mechanism. This conceptualization of attention fits well with the evolved solutions. In the matched-rate solutions, the learning rate on the connections between the input nodes and their adjacent hidden nodes were reasonably high, allowing for the presence of particular cues in the environment to cause the internal representation of other cues to be enhanced or suppressed as dictated by the structure of the environment. These are the agents that showed the hallmarks of attentional learning as measured by their responses on the highlighting task.

In the high output-rate solutions, the learning rate on the hidden-to-output layer was very high. When trained using backpropagation, this arrangement means that most of the error-driven weight changes happen at the output level, and little error signal is propagated to the lower level. The small error that is propagated has even less influence because of very low learning rates between the input and hidden nodes. Therefore, the high output-rate solutions do not learn to effectively enhance or suppress the critical internal representations and do not show the corresponding signs of learned attention.

Further evidence that learned attention (as represented by fast learning of activation or suppression of internal representations based on input cues) does confer an adaptive benefit can be seen in the evolution of the learning rates and fitness for single populations. Figure 1.9 shows plots from a population that eventually evolved attentional agents. While this plot is the clearest example of the connection between the learning rates and fitness, nearly all of the 43 runs that evolved attentional mechanisms show the same basic relationship between the learning rates and fitness.

Early in the simulated evolution, the agents evolve fixed-weight connections between the input and hidden layers and learning connections from the hidden layer to the output node, allowing them to learn correct responses to 7 of the 8 stimuli. In Figure 1.9, the result of this architectural improvement can be seen by the plateau in average fitness that begins around generation 300, where the fixed-weight architecture takes over the population. The fixed-weight architecture dominates the population until generation 1800, when the population's average fitness moves to a slightly higher plateau. This new architecture is the high output-rate architecture described above. The learning rate

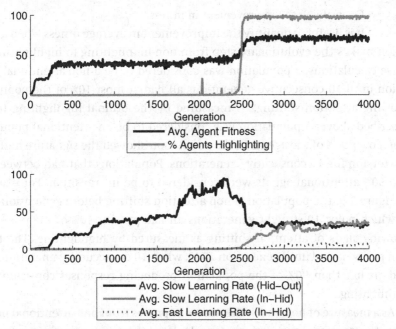

Figure 1.9 Data from a single population showing the relationship between learning rates, fitness, and highlighting across generations. The top graph shows the average agent fitness and the percentage of the agents in the population that show highlighting effects. Fitness has been scaled so that a fitness level of 100 indicates perfect performance across all learning trials. The lower graph displays the average learning rates for the same population.

for the hidden-to-output layer is at its highest levels during this period of evolution. Simultaneously at the beginning of this period, the connections on the input-to-hidden layer make the switch to learning connections, but with very low learning rates. This solution offers a slight improvement, but it does not yet maximize performance.

Around generation 2400, the population shows a dramatic improvement in fitness. It is only when the learning rates (both slow and first-fast) at the input-to-hidden level increase, and the learning rates on the hidden-to-output level decrease, that the fitness is maximized. The increase in the input-to-hidden layer learning rate allows an agent to shift attention towards or away from focal cues based on the context cues. The decrease in the hidden-to-output learning rate allows more of the error signal to be propagated to the lower layer, creating more efficient error-driven attentional shifts. These changes, which can be seen occurring between generations 2400 and 2700 in Figure 1.9, coincide with the population's transition from non-highlighting agents to highlighting agents, as shown in the upper panel.

Quantifying the improvement in fitness

It is useful to quantify the improvement in average fitness when a population makes the evolutionary step from non-highlighting to highlighting. For these calculations, a population was considered to be a non-attentional population until 10 consecutive generations all had at most 10% of the population showing attention shifting, as measured by the ordinal highlighting torsion described above. A population was considered to be an attentional population when over 90% of the agents in the population showed the signature highlighting torsion for 10 consecutive generations. Populations that had between 10% and 90% attentional agents were considered to be in transition. For example, in Figure 1.9, the population is non-attention shifting before generation 2471, at which point 10 straight generations all had at least 10% of the population showing signs of attention shifting as measured by highlighting. The transition period lasted until generation 2530, when 10 consecutive generations each had greater than 90% of the population producing responses consistent with highlighting.

As a measure of how much the fitness improves from non-attentional populations to attentional populations, we calculated the difference of mean fitnesses across phases relative to the standard deviation of fitnesses within phases. This measure is analogous to "effect size" in statistics and d' in signal detection theory. To calculate the effect size, the average fitness of the final 100 generations of the non-attentional population (generations 2371–2470 in the simulation shown in Figure 1.9) was subtracted from the average fitness of the first 100 generations of the attentional population (generations 2530–2629 in Figure 1.9), and the difference of the two means was divided by the average standard deviation within the two windows. For Figure 1.9, this yields an effect size of 5.5. In other words, when the population changes from non-attentional to attentional, the fitness improves by more than 5 standard deviations of ordinary generation-to-generation variation.

The dynamics of context duration

We have shown that attentional mechanisms provide learning benefits in a cue–outcome structure where there are context-dependent relevances of cues, when the context switches at a particular rate. In this section we explore the robustness of the attentional advantage as a function of the rate of context switches. We find that the attentional advantage is robust across different rates of context switching, but is strongest at an intermediate rate. We explain the reasons for this "sweet spot" in the rate of context switches, and gain some additional insight into why attention can help learning.

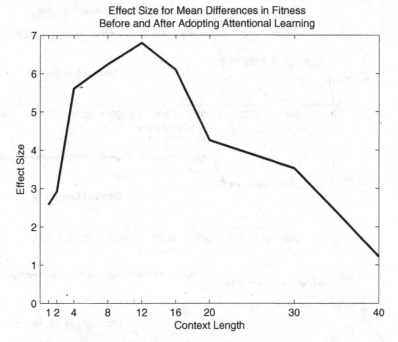

Figure 1.10 Effect size for the improvement in fitness from non-attentional to attentional populations as a function of number of trials between context shifts.

We ran simulations that were identical to the simulations described above except that the number of trials between context shifts was changed. In the first simulation, the agents saw a single trial in the first context before switching to the next context for one trial, then back to the first context. In the second simulation, the agents saw two trials from a particular context before a switch, and so on. In total, we tested context durations of 1, 2, 4, 8, 12, 16, 20, 30, and 40 trials. In these runs, the agent's lifetime was always set to 80 trials; consequently, in the fastest-shifting environment the agent would experience 79 context shifts and in the slowest-shifting environment the agent would only experience a single context shift.

Figure 1.10 shows the benefit of adopting an attentional architecture as a function of the number of trials between context shifts. Each data point on the graph represents the average effect size across 50 simulations for each context length. The graph of effect sizes shows an inverted U-shaped relationship between the relative benefit provided by the evolution of attentional mechanisms and the context length. While the populations all benefited from the evolution of attentional mechanisms, the shortest and longest context lengths exhibited smaller gains in fitness than the populations evolved in moderate-length contexts.

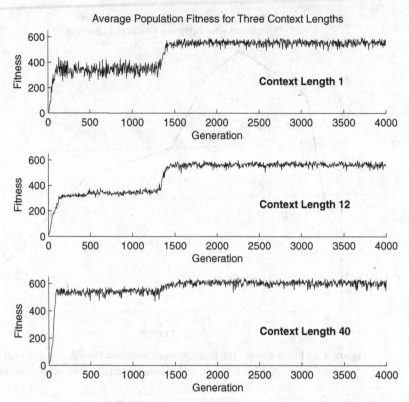

Figure 1.11 Average population fitness for three simulations run with differing context lengths. From top to bottom the three graphs show the fitness across generations for populations that experienced context shifts after every trial, after every 12 trials, and after 40 trials, respectively. In all three simulations, the populations made the transition to attention-shifting architectures around generation 1400.

Figure 1.11 helps to interpret this result. When the context duration is brief, and context is changing very frequently, the context cues vary as frequently as the outcomes and the focal cues. Consequently, the associations from context cues to outcomes can track spurious short-term covariation, leading to difficulty in discovering a stable solution. Without sustained time in a given context to learn which cues are focal and which are context, building the right associations is a challenging task. Therefore, in the generations before the population makes the shift to architectures with learned attention, there is considerable variation in individual agents' success, and large variance in the average population fitness. This variability can be seen in the upper panel of Figure 1.11 as the large variation in fitness for generations 200–1300, as if a seismograph were recording a large and sustained earthquake. Nevertheless, attentional learning was still highly beneficial. When the populations made the transition to attentional mechanisms, at around generation 1400, the average fitness increased drastically. In fact, the mean increase in fitness from pre-attentional to attentional populations is approximately the same for the short-duration contexts as it is for the moderate-duration contexts, as can be seen by comparing the top and middle panels of Figure 1.11. But the effect size is smaller for the short-duration context because of the larger variability from one generation to the next. For moderate context durations, the context was changing far less frequently than the focal cues, making the environmental regularities easier to learn. However, across the agent's lifetime, there were still a large number of context shifts, so in order to perform well the agents must not only have reacted quickly at the context boundaries, but must also have preserved the associations from the previous context, so that those associations did not have to be learned again when the context recurs. The attentional mechanism promotes fast learning of new associations by shunting attention away from previously learned associations that are causing errors in the new context. This allows for the rapid acquisition of new associations on the most diagnostic cues, and it allows for preservation of previous associations on the cues that are no longer relevant in the new context. As a result, when an agent evolves an attention-shifting architecture, it rapidly dominates the population and the population's average fitness drastically increases.

As the context duration extends, the few errors produced in the first few trials of a new context become less costly to the agents, so fast learning becomes less of a priority. At the extreme, where agents experience only a single context shift, we see only a small improvement in fitness for the evolution of attentional mechanisms. The bottom panel of Figure 1.11 shows that when there is only a single context shift in an agent's lifetime (i.e., context length 40), the pre-attentional agents were already performing very well. With only one context shift to contend with, the networks rapidly evolved architectures like those of the non-successful, non-highlighting, relatively poor solutions from the original 4-trial context simulations. In the 40-trial context environment, the best pre-attentional agents had fixed weights across all connections between the input and hidden layer, and learning connections with moderately high learning rates connecting the hidden and output layers. Analysis of these networks shows that the high learning rates allow them to quickly and accurately learn the regularities of the context into which they are born. They perform well for 40 learning trials, and then switch contexts. In the first few trials of the new context they make a few errors, but the high learning rates of the output connections quickly learn associations for the mappings of the new context. Since the agents will never return to the original context it is of little consequence that the originally learned associations are overwritten at the context boundary. In this environment attention does not provide a strong adaptive benefit because fast learning rates alone are enough to perform nearly optimally.

In summary, attentional mechanisms can be especially beneficial when stable and useful associations should be retained for future re-use, despite a temporary change to a new context in which the associations are not useful. When the changes of context are very frequent, there is a benefit from attentional mechanisms, but the frequent changes of context cause learning to be noisy within a context, and therefore cause the relative benefit of attention to be diluted. When the changes in context are rare, then only rarely are there costs incurred from the context change, and therefore only little advantage is gained by attentional mechanisms.

Discussion

Our simulations have demonstrated that selection of fast learners at the behavioral level, as measured by high accuracy over the course of learning, also favors attentional learning at the behavioral level, as measured by exhibition of highlighting. We have shown that the fastest learning at the behavioral level is instantiated at the mechanistic level by particular backprop architectures that include learnable, contextual modulation of cue activations. These demonstrations explored a delimited space of possible mechanistic instantiations. Future work will explore a wider range of possible learning architectures and mechanisms. Our demonstrations also explored a limited range of learning environments. The next section reports results from additional variations in environments to bolster our suggestion that attentional learning may facilitate overall accuracy in a wide array of situations.

Environments that encourage attentional learning

We have emphasized a particular environmental structure for which learned selective attention is adaptive, namely, the structure in Table 1.1 that expresses context-dependent cue relevance. Presumably, there are variations of this environment that would also engender attentional learning. We believe that a key motivator for the evolution of attentional learning is the combination of an environmental contingency structure in which cue relevance varies according to context, with a reproductive advantage given to fast learners. The structure in Table 1.1 (illustrated in Figure 1.1) was our attempt to distill the essence of such an environment.

We speculate that environments with more contextual dependencies would produce even stronger benefits for attentional learning. For such environments,

Table 1.2 *A linearly separable training environment that has context-dependent relevancies and four outcomes. See corresponding illustration in Figure 1.12.*

Context Cues		Focal Cues				Outcomes			
I	J	A	B	C	D	X	Y	V	W
1	0	1	0	1	0	1	0	0	0
1	0	1	0	0	1	1	0	0	0
1	0	0	1	1	0	0	1	0	0
1	0	0	1	0	1	0	1	0	0
0	1	1	0	1	0	0	0	1	0
0	1	1	0	0	1	0	0	0	1
0	1	0	1	1	0	0	0	1	0
0	1	0	1	0	1	0	0	0	1

Note: Presence of a cue or outcome is denoted by a 1, and absence is denoted by a 0.

most cues would be irrelevant in most contexts. Environments in which there is massive irrelevance can be very costly to learning agents, because learning will track the irrelevant variation and cause error on subsequent occasions, or at least be costly metabolically. These costs can be mitigated by learning to suppress attention to irrelevant cues, according to context. Therefore, one goal for future research is to simulate environments that expand the basic structure shown in Table 1.1 across many more cues.

In the remainder of this section we describe two other environments that also yield an advantage for attentional learners. In both environments, the cue–outcome mapping is linearly separable, unlike the structure of Table 1.1. Because the structures are linearly separable, perfect accuracy can be achieved with only a single layer of connections, and there is no structural necessity to evolve an attentional layer in the network. Nevertheless, when fitness is based on speed of learning, not just eventual accuracy, attentional architectures do evolve.

Linearly separable, four outcomes, with contextual dependency

Table 1.2 and Figure 1.12 show a training environment in which both the relevant cues and the outcomes depend on the context. Notice that in this structure there are four outcomes instead of only two. Like the training environment previously studied in Table 1.1, when context cue I is present, focal cues A and B are relevant, but when context cue J is present, focal cues C and D are relevant. This new structure has different outcomes in the two contexts. Specifically, outcomes X and Y occur in context I, but outcomes V and W occur in context J.

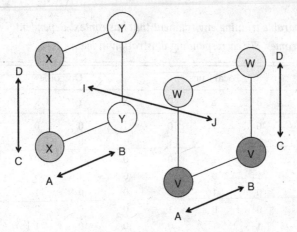

Figure 1.12 Spatial representation of the training structure in Table 1.2. Each circle represents a combination of cues A, B, C, D, I, and J. The letter in the circle, V, W, X, or Y, represents the correct outcome for that cue combination. The rhombus on the left has a letter I in its center to indicate that cue I is present, while the rhombus on the right has a letter J in its center to indicate that cue J is present. The upper circles have cue D present, while the lower circles have cue C present. The remaining dimension marks whether cue A or cue B is present. Although this diagram represents A–B, C–D, and I–J as if on dimensions, the basic structure does *not* encode or assume any dimensional relationship among the cues.

The reason this structure in Table 1.2 is interesting is that it is linearly separable, unlike the previous structure. This linear separability means that the mapping can be solved merely by learning the connections fanning into the outcome nodes, and there is no need to learn any "lateral" connections to the hidden nodes. In other words, the cue–outcome contingencies by themselves do not demand any learned attention.

Despite not needing attentional learning to correctly solve the mapping, the solution can be learned more quickly when attentional learning is available. This claim is confirmed through hill-climbing optimizations. Consider first a restricted architecture in which there is no multiplicative gating and in which the learning rates on the connections fanning into the hidden nodes are set to *zero*. This is like the "base-agent" architecture shown in Figure 1.6. We use hill-climbing optimization to find the optimal learning rate for the outcome nodes. In this case, the accuracy of prediction gets fairly good, with RMSD = 0.211, because the outcome layer alone can solve the mapping. A representative run for the best outcome-learning rate is shown in the upper panels of Figure 1.13. In the subsequent highlighting test, however, *no* highlighting is exhibited. No highlighting occurs because there is no attentional shifting at the hidden nodes.

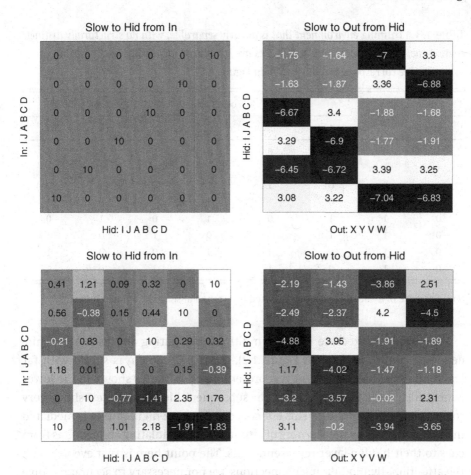

Figure 1.13 Examples of learned weights when trained on the linearly separable, four-outcome structure shown in Table 1.2 and Figure 1.12. The upper panels show a typical run when using the best learning rate on the output nodes and *when there is zero learning of connections fanning into the hidden nodes*, resulting in RMSD = 0.211. Notice that the weights to the hidden nodes from the input nodes, shown in the upper left matrix, remain fixed at their starting values of zero (except for the diagonal weights, which are fixed at 10). The lower panels show a typical run when using the best learning rates when there *is* learning allowed for connections fanning into the hidden nodes, resulting in RMSD = 0.174. Notice that the weights to hidden nodes from input nodes, in the lower left matrix, have mostly learned non-zero values. The model has learned that when cue I is present, attend to cues A and B and suppress cues C and D (and the opposite for when cue J is present). The learning rates for the lower panels *do* produce highlighting, but the learning rates for the upper panels do *not* produce highlighting.

Table 1.3 *A training environment that is linearly separable, with no structurally distinct context cue. The "context" and "focal" cues are structured identically, so the labeling is arbitrary. See corresponding illustration in Figure 1.14.*

Context Cues		Focal Cues				Outcomes	
I	J	A	B	C	D	X	Y
1	0	1	0	1	0	1	0
1	0	1	0	0	1	1	0
1	0	0	1	1	0	1	0
1	0	0	1	0	1	0	1
0	1	1	0	1	0	1	0
0	1	1	0	0	1	0	1
0	1	0	1	1	0	0	1
0	1	0	1	0	1	0	1

Note: Presence of a cue or outcome is denoted by a 1, and absence is denoted by a 0.

When the architecture includes multiplicative gating and learning of hidden-node connections (as in Figure 1.2), then the problem is solved with far less total error (RMSD = 0.174). A representative solution is shown in the lower panels of Figure 1.13. Importantly, the subsequent highlighting test shows very robust highlighting effects. This effect occurs because highlighting is mediated in these networks by the learning of attentionally modulating connections from cues to their hidden-layer representations. The point here is that even though the attentionally modulating connections are not necessary to accurately solve the cue–outcome mapping, those learnable connections do improve the speed of learning. Those learnable connections also, as a side effect, engender highlighting. Again, this result supports our general claim that faster learning can be accomplished by attentional learning, in this case even when attentional learning is not necessary to solve the task.

Linearly separable with no contextual dependency

Table 1.3 and Figure 1.14 show a training environment in which the cue–outcome mapping is linearly separable, and the cues are structurally equivalent to each other. In other words, the labeling of one cue as "context" is completely arbitrary. (This structure corresponds to what Shepard *et al.* [1961] called Type IV if the cues are represented on dimensions as shown in Figure 1.14.)

Consider first what happens when the 8 training items are randomly intermixed, such that each 8-trial block of training contains an independently permuted order of the 8 training items. For this training regime, there is no

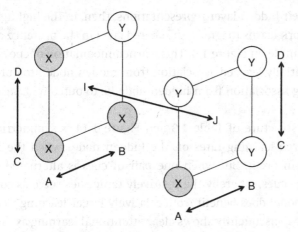

Figure 1.14 Spatial representation of the training structure in Table 1.3. Although this diagram represents A–B, C–D, and I–J as if on dimensions, the basic structure does *not* encode or assume any dimensional relationship among the cues.

structural or temporal distinction whatsoever between context and focal cues. When all the learning rates are freely optimized the weights fanning into the hidden nodes have only small learning rates. Consequently, when tested on highlighting, the optimal-learning network does not show highlighting. This makes intuitive sense: when the training structure is completely symmetric and provides little benefit from attentional learning, then little, if any, highlighting will be exhibited.

Consider what happens, however, if we make one of the cues relatively stable across trials during training, such that the cue behaves as a temporal context cue. For this simulation, we blocked together the four trials with cue I, and alternated them with blocks of four trials with cue J. Otherwise the training was the same as before. For this blocked-context training procedure the best learning rates on the hidden nodes were reasonably high. Examination of the learned weights revealed why the attentional learning was beneficial. The model learned that when (context) cue I was present, cues A and C should be attended while cues B and D should be suppressed, but when (context) cue J was present, cues B and D should be attended but cues A and C should be suppressed. Moreover, these attentional weights were symmetric in sign, such that, for example, when cues A or C were present, they gave attention to cue I but suppressed cue J. Importantly, when subsequently tested in the highlighting procedure, the network showed robust highlighting effects.

The reason the network exhibited highlighting is the same as explained for previous simulations: when there is significant learnability of connections between cues and their hidden-layer representations, then, in the highlighting procedure, the network learns to ignore the shared cue I in the presence of cue PL, as shown, for example, in Figure 1.4. This learned modulation of cue activations protects the initially learned association from hidden node I to outcome E, and yields a strong association from hidden node PL to outcome L, again as shown in Figure 1.4.

In summary, the structure of Table 1.3 and Figure 1.14 is symmetric and does not demand large learning rates on the hidden nodes when the items are trained in random order. But when one pair of cues is alternated more slowly than the other cues, whereby the relatively tonic cues serve as context for the others, the model does benefit from relatively larger learning rates on the hidden layer, and consequently shows clear attentional learning as assayed by highlighting.

Summary: environments that encourage attentional learning

The training structure in Table 1.1 and Figure 1.1 was designed to embody two key qualities that might encourage attentional learning. The structure incorporated cues that were individually uncorrelated with the outcomes, but which indicated what other cues were predictive of the correct outcomes. The indirectly relevant "context" cues were also held relatively constant across training trials. We showed that the structure did indeed encourage learning architectures and learning rates that exhibited attentional effects when the goal was to maximize total accuracy across the lifetime of training.

The structures of the present section (Table 1.2 and Table 1.3) begin to expand and delimit the range of environments in which attentional learning improves overall accuracy. We showed that even when hidden-layer learning is not necessary for eventual perfect accuracy, attentional learning can still be beneficial for acquiring the mapping quickly. This benefit of attentional learning for overall accuracy is especially strong when there are contextual cues to relevance, as exemplified for structural context cues by Tables 1.1 and 1.2, and for temporal context cues by Table 1.3. In the latter case, even when the mapping is linearly separable and perfectly symmetric, if one cue merely alternates more slowly than the others, and thereby may serve as a context cue, then attentional learning is adaptive. Importantly, we also showed that attentional learning is not merely trivially *always* adaptive. Specifically, when the structure is symmetric and training is ordered randomly then the best hidden-layer learning rates are weak and little, if any, highlighting occurs. Another case in which attentional learning had little benefit was when training with the original structure of Table 1.1 but alternating the context only once; recall that in this case the evolved architecture settled on no learning of hidden-layer weights because the cost of the single context switch could be absorbed by fast outcome-weight learning alone.

Costs and benefits of selective attention

When considering selective attention, many people think of it as a necessary evil caused by limited-capacity processing in the brain and body. In a review of the causes and consequences of limited attention, Dukas (2004, p. 107) defined limited attention as a "restricted rate of information processing by the brain" and he focused on the costs of limited attention, such as hindering foragers' probability of detecting cryptic food items, and failing to notice an approaching predator while engaged in an attention-demanding task. Clark and Dukas (2003) developed a detailed model of foraging while avoiding predators. They analyzed the optimal width of the focus of attention, and optimal processing capacity. They also assumed an accelerating metabolic cost of increased processing capacity. From the model, they concluded that the use of selective attention was an optimal solution to the trade-offs between foraging for cryptic food, avoiding predators, and sustaining a high-demand processing system.

In our approach, however, we have not had to assume an increased metabolic cost for higher learning rates. We have not had to assume any additional cost for inclusion of additional learnable connections. Instead, selective attention emerged as an optimal solution to an informational problem, not as a compromise conceded to physical shackles. In environments with context-dependent cue relevance learnable allocation of attention can improve speed of learning.

Moore (2004) provided an extensive review of types of learning, including habituation, sensitization, discrimination learning, imprinting, navigation, mimicry, instrumental learning, language acquisition, etc. He suggested a large cladogram indicating possible evolutionary relationships among the various forms of learning. But nowhere in the catalog did there appear the notion of learning to attend. We believe, on the contrary, that learning what to attend to is a critical aspect of learning well.

Author note

For helpful discussion and comments, we thank José Burgos, Nestor Schmajuk, and Peter M. Todd. Correspondence can be addressed to John K. Kruschke, Department of Psychological and Brain Sciences, Indiana University, 1101 E. 10th St., Bloomington IN 47405–7007, or via electronic mail to kruschke@indiana.edu. Supplementary information can be found at http://www.indiana.edu/~kruschke/

References

Burgos, J. E. (2007). Evolving artificial neural networks in Pavlovian environments. In J. W. Donahoe and V. Packard-Dorsel, eds., *Neural-Network Models of Cognition: Biobehavioral Foundations*. The Netherlands: North-Holland Elsevier, pp. 58–80.

Chun, M. M. (2000). Contextual cueing of visual attention. *Trends in Cognitive Sciences*, **4**(5), 170–178.

Clark, C. W. & Dukas, R. (2003). The behavioral ecology of a cognitive constraint: limited attention. *Behavioral Ecology*, **14**(2), 151–156.

Dibbets, P., Maes, J. H. R., Boermans, K. & Vossen, J. M. H. (2001). Contextual dependencies in predictive learning. *Memory*, **9**(1), 29–38.

Dukas, R. (2004). Causes and consequences of limited attention. *Brain, Behavior and Evolution*, **63**, 197–210.

Edmonds, B. & Norling, E. (2007). Integrating learning and inference in multi-agent systems using cognitive context. *Lecture Notes in Computer Science*, **4442**, 142.

Goldberg, D. E. (1989). *Genetic Algorithms in Search, Optimization, and Machine Learning*. Reading, MA: Addison–Wesley.

Goodman, N. D., Tenenbaum, J. B., Feldman, J. & Griffiths, T. L. (2008). A rational analysis of rule-based concept learning. *Cognitive Science*, **32**(1), 108–154.

Hall, G. & Channell, S. (1985). A comparison of intradimensional and extradimensional shift learning in pigeons. *Behavioural Processes*, **10**, 285–295.

Hinton, G. E. & Plaut, D. C. (1987). Using fast weights to deblur old memories. In *Proceedings of the 9th Annual Conference of the Cognitive Science Society*. Hillsdale, NJ: Erlbaum, pp. 177–186.

Johnston, T. D. (1982). Selective costs and benefits in the evolution of learning. *Advances in the Study of Behavior*, **12**, 65–106.

Kamin, L. J. (1969). Predictability, surprise, attention, and conditioning. In B. A. Campbell and R. M. Church, eds., *Punishment*. New York: Appleton–Century-Crofts, pp. 279–296.

Kruschke, J. K. (1992). ALCOVE: an exemplar-based connectionist model of category learning. *Psychological Review*, **99**, 22–44.

Kruschke, J. K. (1996a). Base rates in category learning. *Journal of Experimental Psychology: Learning, Memory, and Cognition*, **22**, 3–26.

Kruschke, J. K. (1996b). Dimensional relevance shifts in category learning. *Connection Science*, **8**, 201–223.

Kruschke, J. K. (2001). Toward a unified model of attention in associative learning. *Journal of Mathematical Psychology*, **45**, 812–863.

Kruschke, J. K. (2003). Attentional theory is a viable explanation of the inverse base rate effect: a reply to Winman, Wennerholm, and Juslin (2003). *Journal of Experimental Psychology: Learning, Memory, and Cognition*, **29**, 1396–1400.

Kruschke, J. K. (2009). Highlighting: a canonical experiment. In B. Ross, ed., *The Psychology of Learning and Motivation, vol. 51*. Illinois: Elsevier, pp. 153–185.

Kruschke, J. K. & Blair, N. J. (2000). Blocking and backward blocking involve learned inattention. *Psychonomic Bulletin and Review*, **7**, 636–645.

Kruschke, J. K., Kappenman, E. S. & Hetrick, W. P. (2005). Eye gaze and individual differences consistent with learned attention in associative blocking and highlighting. *Journal of Experimental Psychology: Learning, Memory, and Cognition,* **31**, 830–845.

Little, D. R. & Lewandowsky, S. (2009). Beyond non-utilization: irrelevant cues can gate learning in probabilistic categorization. *Journal of Experimental Psychology: Human Perception and Performance,* **35**(2), 530–550.

Lubow, R. E. (1989). *Latent Inhibition and Conditioned Attention Theory.* Cambridge, UK: Cambridge University Press.

Mackintosh, N. J. (1975). A theory of attention: variations in the associability of stimuli with reinforcement. *Psychological Review,* **82**, 276–298.

McCloskey, M. & Cohen, N. J. (1989). Catastrophic interference in connectionist networks: the sequential learning problem. In G. Bower, ed., *The Psychology of Learning and Motivation, vol. 24.* New York: Academic Press, pp. 109–165.

Medin, D. L. & Edelson, S. M. (1988). Problem structure and the use of base-rate information from experience. *Journal of Experimental Psychology: General,* **117**, 68–85.

Mery, F. & Kawecki, T. J. (2003). A fitness cost of learning ability in Drosophila melanogaster. *Proceedings of the Royal Society B: Biological Sciences,* **270**(1532), 2465–2469.

Miller, G. F. & Todd, P. M. (1990). Exploring adaptive agency i: theory and methods for simulating evolution of learning. In D. S. Touretzky, J. L. Elman, T. J. Sejnowski, and G. E. Hinton, eds., *Proceedings of the 1990 Connectionist Models Summer School.* San Mateo, CA: Morgan Kaufmann, pp. 65–80.

Miller, R. R. & Matzel, L. D. (1988). The comparator hypothesis: a response rule for the expression of associations. In G. H. Bower, ed., *The Psychology of Learning and Motivation: Advances in Research and Theory, vol. 22.* San Diego, CA: Academic Press, pp. 51–92.

Moore, B. R. (2004). The evolution of learning. *Biological Review,* **79**, 301–335.

Nelson, J. B. & Sanjuan, M. (2006). A context-specific latent inhibition effect in a human conditioned suppression task. *The Quarterly Journal of Experimental Psychology,* **59**(6), 1003–1020.

Nosofsky, R. M., Gluck, M. A., Palmeri, T. J., McKinley, S. C. & Glauthier, P. (1994). Comparing models of rule-based classification learning: a replication of Shepard, Hovland, and Jenkins (1961). *Memory and Cognition,* **22**, 352–369.

Nosofsky, R. M., Palmeri, T. J. & McKinley, S. C. (1994). Rule-plus-exception model of classification learning. *Psychological Review,* **101**, 53–79.

Raine, N. E. & Chittka, L. (2008). The correlation of learning speed and natural foraging success in bumble-bees. *Proceedings of the Royal Society B: Biological Sciences,* **275**(1636), 803–808.

Rescorla, R. A. & Wagner, A. R. (1972). A theory of Pavlovian conditioning: variations in the effectiveness of reinforcement and non-reinforcement. In A. H. Black and W. F. Prokasy, eds., *Classical Conditioning ii: Current Research and Theory.* New York: Appleton–Century–Crofts, pp. 64–99.

Rosas, J. M. & Callejas-Aguilera, J. E. (2006). Context switch effects on acquisition and extinction in human predictive learning. *Journal of Experimental Psychology: Learning, Memory, and Cognition*, **32**(3), 461–474.

Rumelhart, D. E., Hinton, G. E. & Williams, R. J. (1986). Learning internal representations by back-propagating errors. In D. E. Rumelhart and J. L. McClelland, eds., *Parallel Distributed Processing, vol. 1*. Cambridge, MA: MIT Press.

Schmajuk, N. A. (2002). *Latent Inhibition and Its Neural Substrates: From Animal Experiments to Schizophrenia*. Norwell, MA: Kluwer Academic.

Schmajuk, N. A., Lam, Y. W. & Gray, J. A. (1996). Latent inhibition: a neural network approach. *Journal of Experimental Psychology: Animal Behavior Processes*, **22**, 321–349.

Shepard, R. N., Hovland, C. L. & Jenkins, H. M. (1961). Learning and memorization of classifications. *Psychological Monographs*, **75**(13). (Whole No. 517.)

Slamecka, N. J. (1968). A methodological analysis of shift paradigms in human discrimination learning. *Psychological Bulletin*, **69**, 423–438.

Todd, P. M. & Miller, G. F. (1991). Exploring adaptive agency II: simulating the evolution of adaptive learning. In J.-A. Meyer and S. W. Wilson, eds., *From Animals to Animats: Proceedings of the First International Conference on Simulation of Adaptive Behavior*. Cambridge, MA: MIT Press, pp. 306–315.

Yang, L.-X. & Lewandowsky, S. (2003). Context-gated knowledge partitioning in categorization. *Learning and Memory*, **29**(4), 663–679.

2

The arguments of associations

JUSTIN A. HARRIS

Abstract

This chapter considers associative solutions to "non-linear" discrimination problems, such as negative patterning (A+ and B+ vs. AB−) and the biconditional discrimination (AB+ and CD+ vs. AC− and BD−). It is commonly assumed that the solution to these discriminations requires "configural" elements that are *added* to the compound of two stimuli. However, these discriminations can be solved by assuming that some elements of each stimulus are *suppressed* when two stimuli are presented in compound. Each of these approaches can solve patterning and biconditional discriminations because they allow some elements, as the arguments of associations, to have differential "presence" on reinforced versus non-reinforced trials, and thus differential associability and control over responding. The chapter then presents a more specific version of one of these models, describing how interactions between stimuli, particularly the competition for attention, provide a mechanism whereby some elements are more suppressed than others when stimuli are presented simultaneously as a compound.

Most computational models of conditioning adopt associative strength (V) as the variable that tracks learning about the association between a conditioned stimulus (CS) or action and the reinforcing unconditioned stimulus (US). Many of these models make very simple assumptions about the arguments of associations – the CSs and USs themselves. For example, the Rescorla–Wagner model treats these stimuli as singular units such that, during learning, a single connection strengthens between the CS unit and US unit (Rescorla & Wagner, 1972; Wagner & Rescorla, 1972). While the Rescorla–Wagner model has proved a successful account of the algorithms that underlie many aspects of learning, its simple treatment of the stimuli involved in conditioning has not equipped it to explain a number of important findings. Two particular pieces of evidence that will be considered here are the demonstrations that animals can learn, albeit with difficulty, to master negative patterning and biconditional discriminations. In the simplest case of a negative patterning discrimination, two distinct CSs, A and B, are each individually paired with reinforcement (+), and these trials are intermixed among trials in which the compound of the same two CSs, AB, is presented without reinforcement (−). Many different species in many different paradigms have successfully learned this discrimination, responding more on A+ and B+ trials than on AB− trials (Kehoe & Graham, 1988; Pavlov, 1927; Rescorla, 1972, 1973; Whitlow & Wagner, 1972). The biconditional discrimination represents an even more difficult task in which four CSs are combined as two compounds (AB and CD) that are both reinforced, while on intermixed trials the same four stimuli are presented as different pairwise combinations (AC and BD) but these compounds are not reinforced. Again, there are demonstrations that animals can learn this discrimination, responding more on AB+ and CD+ trials than on AC− and BD− trials (Rescorla, Grau, & Durlach, 1985; Saavedra, 1975), although this appears to pose even greater difficulty than the negative patterning discrimination (Harris & Livesey, 2008; Harris, Livesey, Gharaei, & Westbrook, 2008).

The difficulty for models like Rescorla–Wagner derives from the way they treat the generalization of associative strength between single CSs and their compounds, or, in the case of the biconditional discrimination, between different compounds composed of the same stimuli. The Rescorla–Wagner model makes the simple assumption that associative strengths are additive between CSs; an assumption at the heart of its common-error term that has been instrumental in providing an account of many conditioning phenomena, from blocking and overshadowing to conditioned inhibition (see Le Pelley, 2010, Chapter 3 in current volume). Indeed, the numerous demonstrations of response summation (e.g., Kehoe, 1982, 1986; Rescorla, 1997; Thein, Westbrook, & Harris, 2008) support the assumption that most of the associative strength of two CSs generalizes to their combined presentation as a compound. However, if associative strength reliably generalizes between CSs and their compounds, there will always be a consistent ordering in the level of responding shown to single CSs and their compounds. Typically, responding to the compound will be greater than that to the single CSs because the summed associative strengths of the CSs in the compound will be greater than the strength of either individual CS. As such, animals could never learn to respond less to a compound than to its individual CS components in a negative patterning discrimination, or could never learn to respond differentially to the different compounds in a biconditional discrimination.

Configural solutions to non-linear discriminations

The solution to negative patterning and biconditional discriminations requires non-symmetrical generalization of associative change between single CS and compound trials, or between compounds composed of common stimulus components. For example, an animal learning a negative patterning discrimination must acquire associative strength during A+ and B+ trials that does not generalize to the AB compound, or else it must acquire inhibitory strength on AB– trials that does not generalize to A and B individually. In the biconditional case, some excitatory associative strength acquired on AB+ and CD+ trials must not generalize to AC and BD, or inhibitory strength acquired on AC– and BD– trials must not generalize to AB and CD. A computationally expedient way to achieve this is to allow an associative unit to be present during reinforced but not non-reinforced trials, or vice versa. Spence (1952) pointed out that this could be achieved by assuming that a compound of two CSs is more than the sum of the individual stimuli, in that the *configuration* of the two stimuli is itself represented as an added element (i.e., there is a computational unit that stands for the conjunction of two or more stimuli). Rescorla (1972, 1973) and Whitlow and Wagner (1972) showed how these added configural units can be incorporated into the Rescorla–Wagner model to provide a ready solution to negative patterning and biconditional discriminations. In negative patterning, the compound configural unit acquires inhibitory strength that suppresses responding on AB– trials, but this inhibition does not generalize to A+ and B+ trials because the configural unit is absent on those trials. Similarly, in a biconditional discrimination, configural units for AB and CD acquire excitatory associative strength on reinforced trials that does not generalize to AC and BD, whereas configural units for AC and BD acquire inhibitory strength on non-reinforced trials that does not generalize to AB and CD (Saavedra, 1975).

The configural hypothesis described above does not successfully accommodate findings from a number of more recent experiments on negative patterning discriminations (see Pearce, 1994, for review). Such evidence has informed alternative descriptions of configural representations. For example, Wagner and Brandon (2001) have proposed that compound configural units are not simply added to the arguments of associations, but that these units *replace* some elements of the component stimuli. Therefore, in negative patterning, some units are present in the compound but absent from single-CS trials, whereas other units are present on single-CS trials but absent from the compound. This facilitates learning because associative strength acquired to the latter units during A+ and B+ trials does not generalize to AB– trials, as well as allowing inhibitory strength to be acquired by the compound configural unit that does not generalize to A+ and B+ trials.

The configural approach has been incorporated in layered network models which place configural units within a hidden layer between input and output layers (e.g., Kehoe, 1988; Schmajuk & Di Carlo, 1992). The behavior of these hidden configural units differs from that of traditional models in which configural units are added to the representation of stimuli. In the earlier models, configural units have a fixed and predefined relation to the stimulus inputs (configural unit AB is necessarily activated by A and B in compound), whereas hidden configural units have adaptive relationships to the sensory input, allowing them to be "tuned" to specific combinations of inputs. This provides the hidden configural units with greater flexibility, allowing them to contribute to learning phenomena beyond solving non-linear discriminations, such a learning-to-learning (Kehoe, 1988) and occasion-setting (Schmajuk, Lamoureux, & Holland, 1998).

A quite different approach has been described by Pearce (1987, 1994). He has argued that all CSs, be they single stimuli or compounds, are represented by a single configural unit that codes for the entire pattern of sensory input. This model assumes that only one configural unit undergoes associative change on a given trial, and therefore one configural unit acquires excitatory associative strength on reinforced trials, whereas a different configural unit acquires inhibitory strength on non-reinforced trials. Since the strength of activation of each configural unit on a given trial is proportional to the overlap between the current pattern of sensory input and the pattern of input coded by that unit, the associative strength acquired on reinforced trials generalizes only partially to non-reinforced trials and the inhibition acquired on non-reinforced trials generalizes only partially to reinforced trials.

The models described above have, in common, their use of configural representations to solve negative patterning and biconditional discriminations. Indeed, it has become common for students of associative learning to consider these discriminations as "proof" of the existence of configural representations because it is assumed that a solution to these discriminations can only be achieved by configural units. A key objective of this chapter is to show that this assumption is false. As described earlier, the solution to negative patterning and biconditional discriminations requires asymmetrical generalization of excitatory and inhibitory associative strength between reinforced and non-reinforced trials. For negative patterning, this can be achieved by assuming that some elements, such as configural representations, are present on compound trials but not on single-stimulus trials. However, it can also be achieved by assuming that some elements are present on single-stimulus trials but not on compound trials. Similarly, the biconditional discrimination can be solved if different configural units are present for each different compound, but it can also be solved if different stimulus elements are lost (or reduced) for the different compounds. Thus, each approach can provide a successful computational solution to these discriminations. The remainder of this chapter will be given over to describing computational models that do not involve configural representations.

Elemental solutions to non-linear discriminations

Two formal computational models have been proposed that can solve negative patterning and biconditional discriminations without invoking configural representations. Both assume that the arguments of associations are arrays of elemental units that represent the multiple features of a given stimulus or stimuli. One of these models, proposed by McLaren and Mackintosh (2000, 2002), assumes that all stimuli share a large proportion (at least 50%) of their elements in common, and it is these common elements that provide the solution to negative patterning and biconditional discriminations. An important feature of this model is the non-linear relationship between elemental activation strength and the input strength of the corresponding feature (the relationship is modeled as a steep sigmoid or even step function; see Figure 2.1). The nature of this function means that features that are weakly present in both stimuli may become strongly represented in the compound, even though they are virtually absent from the representation of each stimulus individually. Consider, for example, a feature, X, with weak input in stimulus A and stimulus B, shown as points X_A and X_B in Figure 2.1. The element corresponding to X will be virtually inactive when either A or B is present on its own. However, when both stimuli are presented together, the inputs from each stimulus will sum, reaching point X_{AB} which is located on the ascending part of the function and thus achieves a significant level of activation of that element. This constitutes a mechanism whereby arguments of associations may be present during a compound but effectively absent during the individual stimuli. (Note that while this mechanism does not describe these elements as configural, in that they do not specifically code for the conjunction of two or more stimuli, their computational behavior is equivalent to that of added configural units in the Rescorla–Wagner model.)

The McLaren–Mackintosh model has a second means for solving patterning and biconditional discriminations. Any element whose feature is strongly present in both individual stimuli will be activated during presentations of each individual stimulus and will also be activated during presentations of the compound. However, if the input in each case falls on the upper, flat portion of the curve, the strength of the element's activation will be the same for each

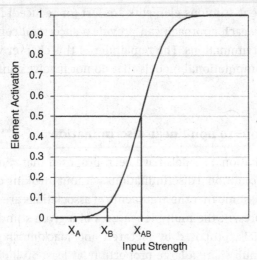

Figure 2.1 The sigmoidal relationship between the input (the physical intensity of a stimulus feature) and the resultant strength of activation of the corresponding elemental unit, as assumed in the McLaren–Mackintosh model (2002). Note that a feature (X) with low input strength in each of two stimuli (X_A and X_B in this example) provokes very little activation of the corresponding element when either stimulus is present alone. However, when the same two stimuli are presented together, the sum of those physical inputs (X_{AB}) can provoke strong activation of that element, far exceeding the simple sum of the activations from each single stimulus.

single stimulus and for the compound. When associative strength of each element is updated using a common delta-rule, such as that proposed by Rescorla and Wagner (1972), such elements can contribute to solving patterning and biconditional discriminations because they have a higher rate of reinforcement than do other elements (those present in one stimulus but not in the other). For example, in a negative patterning schedule with equal numbers of A+, B+, and AB– trials, any element, X, that is common to both A and B will be present on all trials and reinforced on 2/3rds of those trials. By contrast, any element, Y, that is present in only one of the two stimuli will be present on 2/3rds of all trials but reinforced on only half of these trials. Consequently, because X has a higher reinforcement rate than Y, it will acquire greater excitatory associative strength and Y will eventually acquire inhibitory strength. Errorless performance is achieved on the discrimination when the associative strength of X elements is 2λ and the associative strength of Y elements equals –λ.

The second computational model that does not invoke configural representations was proposed by Harris (2006). At the heart of this model, non-linear activation of stimulus elements is created by a limited-capacity attention mechanism that boosts the activation strength of those elements that have successfully entered attention. The multiple elements within and between stimuli compete for access to attention, with the more salient elements (those with high input) winning over the less salient elements. This competition for attention means that some elements in each individual stimulus lose activation strength when the stimulus is presented as part of a compound. Specifically, some elements benefit from the attention boost when their stimulus is present on its own, but lose that boost when the same stimulus is presented as part of a compound because the increase in total number of elements increases competition for attention.

The decline in activation of some elements when a stimulus is presented in a compound provides a mechanism for a variety of cue interaction effects, such as one-trial overshadowing (James & Wagner, 1980; Mackintosh & Reese, 1979), external inhibition (Brimer, 1970; Pavlov, 1927), and incomplete summation between CSs (Thein et al., 2008). In the latter two cases, the decrease in responding is attributed to a decline in activation of some elements because responding is modeled as the sum of each element's activation multiplied by its associative strength. Of course, in many such cases, decrements in responding could reflect performance interactions, such as when the orienting response to a novel stimulus interferes with performance of conditioned responses (CRs) to a CS. However, there is evidence that one CS may reduce the CR produced by another CS even when the CRs themselves do not compete for expression in behavior. A particularly clear illustration is provided in an unpublished experiment by Robert Polewan (2006). In an eyelid conditioning experiment, rabbits were trained with two CSs, a light and tone, at different CS–US intervals: 300 ms for the light, 700 ms for the tone. Conditioning at these different latencies gave rise to temporally distinct CR waveforms, with the conditioned eyeblink response developing earlier after onset of the 300 ms CS than the 700 ms CS. After such CRs were established to the two CSs, the rabbits were given probe tests in which the light and tone were presented together as a compound. If the associative strength of each CS were effectively expressed on these compound trials, the waveform of the eyeblink CR should have two peaks, corresponding to the two original CR waveforms from each individual CS. However, Polewan found that the waveform on these compound probe trials showed only a single peak that was closer to the peak response to the tone, and in general the early CR (to the light) was suppressed. The is not due to a limitation in the temporal dynamics of the eyeblink response, because other experiments have shown that rabbits can produce bimodal CR waveforms, with both early and late peaks, when trained with a mixture of two CS–US intervals (Choi & Moore, 2003; Millenson, Kehoe, & Gormezano, 1977), including a mixture of 300 and

700 ms intervals (Polewan, 2006). As Polewan suggested, it was as if the "rabbits ignored the light and focused their attention to the tone on compound trials, resulting in TL– waveforms that resembled T– waveforms" (pp. 90–91). This specific direction of this interaction is likely due to the greater salience of the tone than the light. The fact that one CS can interfere with the CR to another CS, even when the CRs to each CS do not themselves interfere with one another, is consistent with the model proposed by Harris (2006), in that the presence of the more salient tone would steal attention from the light, thereby reducing activation of the light elements and, in turn, reducing the ability of those light elements to associatively activate the US elements at the appropriate time.

The difference in activation strength of certain elements when a stimulus is presented alone versus as a part of a compound, combined with a common-error-term learning rule, allows these elements to solve negative patterning. That is, because these elements are strongly activated on reinforced trials but weakly activated on non-reinforced trials, they ultimately acquire most of the associative strength, while the elements that receive attention on both single-CS and compound trials become inhibitory. However, this mechanism is less readily equipped to solve the biconditional discrimination. To do so, it must assume there are some differences between the different compounds in the level of competition for attention. Such differences can arise from differences in the salience of the different stimuli themselves: even differences that are idiosyncratic to individual subjects due to variations in their sensitivity to the different stimuli. For example, if stimulus A is less salient than stimulus D, B will have steeper competition for attention on BD– trials than on AB+ trials. Therefore, some elements of B will receive the attention boost in activation on AB+ trials but will not receive this boost on BD– trials. As a result, these elements will acquire excitatory associative strength that will produce greater responding on AB+ trials than BD– trials. At the same time, C will have steeper competition for attention on CD+ trials than on AC– trials, and therefore some elements of C will receive boosted activation on AC– trials but not on CD+ trials. Thus, these elements will acquire inhibitory strength that will reduce responding on AC– trials relative to CD+ trials. While such differences are sufficient for the model to solve the biconditional discrimination, it solves it much more slowly than a negative patterning discrimination. It is worth pointing out that humans and rats also find the biconditional discrimination more difficult than negative patterning (Harris & Livesey, 2008; Harris et al., 2008).

The model proposed by Harris (2006) relies on an attention system that is selective in its action. That is, more salient elements selectively enter attention and thereby receive a multiplicative boost to their activation, while less salient elements that do not compete effectively for attention receive no boost.

In the rest of this chapter, I will describe an alternative formulation of the way that attention can modulate the activation of elements. Rather than assuming that attention selectively exerts its effect on some elements and not others, I propose that the elements vary in their sensitivity to attention as an inherent property of their own activation function. The theoretical processes underlying this are ones that have been developed already in the psychophysical and sensory neuroscience literatures. They capture the way that stimuli interact within sensory systems and how attention influences this interaction. Thus, the formulation presented here has the advantage of being better grounded in sensory–perceptual research. It also specifies in greater detail the mechanism by which attention operates on the elemental network to create non-linear changes in element activation.

One crucial feature of the operations I describe below is the non-linear relationship between the input strength of a stimulus and the response of the sensory–perceptual system. It has been long known that the rate of change in perceived magnitude of a stimulus decreases as the absolute magnitude of the stimulus increases, as captured by the Weber–Fechner law and Stevens' power law (Stevens, 1962). While this relationship holds for most of any stimulus dimension, the opposite relation has also been observed frequently for the lowest end of many stimulus dimensions. That is, for stimuli near detection threshold, observers become more sensitive in discriminating the relative magnitudes of stimuli as their absolute magnitude increases (Arabzadeh, Clifford, & Harris, 2008; Solomon, 2009). The two contrasting psychophysical effects indicate that the relationship between the physical intensity of a stimulus and its perceived intensity is sigmoid. This relationship has been confirmed in numerous experiments using electrophysiological recordings in cats or primates to determine the relationship between the intensity of a stimulus (e.g., the contrast of a visual grating) and the response magnitude of neurons tuned to that stimulus (Crowder, Price, Hietanen, Dreher, Clifford, and Ibbotson, 2006). As mentioned earlier, this sigmoid relationship has already been used by McLaren and Mackintosh (2002) to predict non-linear summation between element input strengths and thereby provide a solution to non-linear problems such as negative patterning and biconditional discriminations. Here, however, I explore a very different means by which this relationship can affect the type of interstimulus interactions that are required to solve non-linear discriminations.

The formulation I present below derives in large part from computational models of sensory systems that incorporate a normalization model of gain control (Heeger, 1992; Reynolds & Chelazzi, 2004; Reynolds & Heeger, 2009). The approach used here is similar to the network normalization rules used by Grossberg's (1975) model of attention and associative learning, which uses on-centre, off-surround shunting inhibition to constrain entire network activity at an upper bound, and to quench noise in the network (see also Schmajuk & Di Carlo, 1992). Such normalization also has the advantage that it allows the number of elements (or stimuli) to be increased indefinitely without saturating the network. The present model achieves normalization by defining the activation strength, R, of a given element as equal to the strength of the sensory input to which that element is tuned, S, subjected to a divisive normalization (or "gain control") that sums across all sensory inputs weighted according to a suppressive field, z. This relationship between S and R for element x is shown in Equation 2.1.

$$R_x = \frac{S_x}{\sum_{i=1}^{n} z_j S_i} \tag{2.1}$$

The properties of the suppressive field are similar to those of the receptive field to which an element is tuned, in that some inputs have a greater effect than others on the normalization of S_x depending on how close they are to X in topographic and featural space. Inputs that are close to X have greater weighting in the inhibitory field, such that $z_x = 1$, and for any input Y, $z_y < 1$. The greater the difference between X and Y, the smaller z_y becomes, and if X and Y are very different sensory inputs (e.g., from different sensory modalities), $z_y = 0$. If all inputs apart from X are held constant, the summed weighted value for all inputs other than X is constant (C). Therefore, to describe how R_x changes across variations in S_x, we can simplify Equation 2.1 as:

$$R_x = \frac{S_x}{S_x + C} \tag{2.2}$$

Equation 2.2 is a monotonically increasing function with an asymptote of 1. It represents a specific instance of a more general relationship expressed in Equation 2.3, which, as shown in Figure 2.2, describes a sigmoid function between R_x and S_x, again with an asymptote of 1. The power, p, determines the slope of the curve, and C determines the position of the curve such that R_x equals half its maximum height (0.5) when S_x^p equals C.

$$R_x = \frac{S_x^p}{S_x^p + C} \tag{2.3}$$

In Equation 2.3, increasing the amount of sensory input by, for example, adding a new stimulus, will increase the value of C. This will shift to the right the function relation R_x to S_x, as shown in Figure 2.3. The consequence of this will be a reduction in activation of each element, as per the normalization effect.

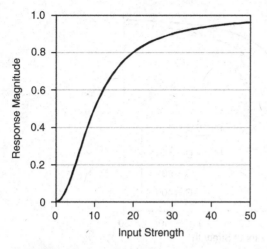

Figure 2.2 The function relating the strength of a sensory input (S) to the magnitude of the sensory response (R) as described in Equation 2.3. In this example, p = 2 and C = 100.

But more specifically, the amount that R_x decreases will depend on S_x, with the greatest drop in R_x for values of S_x^p close to C. Therefore, some elements with strong input will suffer relatively little change in their activation, whereas other elements with intermediate input will suffer a substantial decrease in activation strength. It is this differential effect, whereby some elements suffer greater loss of activation than others when their stimulus is presented as part of a compound, which provides a solution to non-linear discriminations such as negative paternnning.

The normalization process described above captures how stimuli can affect the activation of one another's elements in such a way as to provide a solution to non-linear discriminations. As described, this process relies on the features of each stimulus acting within the supressive field of the other, but this presents a limitation. The mechanism can operate for stimuli from the same modality, but it is less plausible that stimuli from different modalities should act to affect one another in this way. Attention, as an amodal mechanism, provides a means to explain how stimuli from different modalities can affect one another's activation. Attention is modeled as a spatially and featurally selective field that multiplicatively increases the input strength, S, of a stimulus. Thus, if a stimulus or feature, X, captures (or receives) attention, its input strength is increased by a gain factor, γ. The consequence of this for R is shown in Equation 2.4.

$$R_x = \frac{\gamma S_x^p}{\gamma S_x^p + C} \tag{2.4}$$

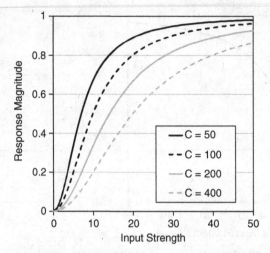

Figure 2.3 The relationship between the physical intensity of sensory input (S) and the magnitude of the sensory response (R) as described in Equation 2.3. In each of these examples, p = 2. Note how increasing C shifts the function to the right, and in each case R_x equals 0.5 when S_x^p equals C.

This shows the attention gain exclusively applied to S_x. In practice, it is likely to affect some other elements close to X, and therefore have some effect on C. However, as long as the attention field is smaller (more selective) than the suppressive field, most elements in the suppressive field for X will not be in the attention field, and therefore C will increase less than S_x. Therefore, for simplicity, I will allow attention to increase S_x but not C. As such, we can re write Equation 2.4 by dividing through by γ to give Equation 2.5.

$$R_x = \frac{S_x^p}{S_x^p + \dfrac{C}{\gamma}}$$
(2.5)

Equation 2.5 makes it clear that attention directed to S_x will effectively reduce C, and therefore shift to the left the function relating S_x to R_x. Conversely, a decrease in attention to S_x will result in the opposite shift.

The operations just described represent the key ingredients of the current proposal. Whenever two stimuli are presented as a simultaneous compound, attention directed to the features of one stimulus reduces (or removes) attention to the features of the other. In effect, attention is simply divided equally among all the stimuli that are present. As a result, the function relating R_x and S_x is effectively shifted to the right, resulting in an overall decrease in their activation strength (R). More importantly, because of the non-linear nature of this

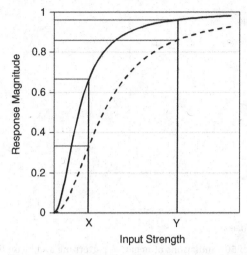

Figure 2.4 A rightward shift in the function relating S to R produces a large drop in R for values of S close to X (at which S^p is close to C), but produces only a small change in R for high values of S (such as at Y), or for very low values of S. For points X and Y, the shift from the solid curve to the dashed curve corresponds to a decrease in R of 0.33 and 0.10, respectively. These represent 50% versus 10% reductions.

function, the rightward shift will have much greater impact on some elements (those for which S^p is close to C) than on others (those with higher values for S). Figure 2.4 illustrates this point, showing how a rightward shift effected by a decrease in attention can differentially reduce R_x depending on the magnitude of S_x. Thus, one stimulus changes the pattern of element activation of another stimulus, rather than simply scaling the activity uniformly across elements, making a compound qualitatively distinct from its component stimuli.

To confirm that this model can solve negative patterning and biconditional discriminations, Figure 2.5 plots the average of 50 simulations for both types of discrimination. In these simulations, all stimuli had 10 elements and the activation strength (R) for each element was calculated using Equation 2.5. The sensory input, S_x, was a random number between 1 and 10, the power, p, was set at 2, and the constant, C, was 4. The loss of attention when any stimulus was combined with a second stimulus was simulated by defining γ in proportion to the sum of the initial (pre-normalized) values of the second stimulus. This is specified below in Equation 2.6 for a stimulus, X, when compounded with a stimulus Y containing 10 elements.

$$\gamma_x = \frac{20}{\sum_{i=1}^{10} S_{i,y}}$$

(2.6)

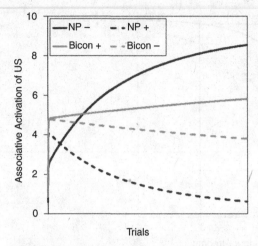

Figure 2.5 The average of 50 simulations of negative patterning and biconditional discriminations, showing the sum of the products of associative strength and activation strength (R) for each element (the maximum value is 10). Bicon+ and Bicon− refer to reinforced and non-reinforced trials, respectively, of the biconditional discrimination (i.e., the mean of AB+ and CD+ versus the mean of AC− and BD− trials). NP+ and NP− refer to reinforced (A+ and B+) and non-reinforced (AB−) trials of the negative patterning discrimination, respectively.

This simulates a process in which attention is shared between stimuli in proportion to the salience of their elements. Figure 2.5 shows the predicted conditioned response strength across all 10 elements for each single CS, or 20 elements of each compound. The term R'_y, defined below in Equation 2.7, is the activation strength of a US element, y, in response to the summed "internal" input from every other element. As such, the aggregate of R'_ys for all US elements gives the estimated conditioned response strength. On each trial, the associative strength (V) between each CS element (x) and each US element (y) is updated according to a modified version of the Rescorla–Wagner (1972) rule, as defined in Equation 2.8 with β set at 0.02. It is worth noting that, by incorporating this learning rule, the model is equipped to deal with the range of empirical findings, such as cue-competition effects like blocking, that are explained by the Rescorla–Wagner model.

$$R'_y = \sum_{i=1}^{n} R_j \cdot V_{i-y} \tag{2.7}$$

$$\Delta V_{x-y} = R_x \cdot \beta \cdot (R_y - R'_y) \tag{2.8}$$

The operations described above produce differential changes in the activation of elements depending on whether they are part of a single CS or compound.

The proposal uses attention because this is a plausible mechanism by which one stimulus could influence the sensory response to another even when those stimuli are very different, such as from different sensory modalities. However, the model does predict an even greater interaction between stimuli that are more similar due to the fact that such stimuli would not only compete for attention, but could also fall within the suppressive field, and thus contribute directly to the normalization process. That is, for two similar stimuli, the value of C may increase for each stimulus, shifting to the right the function relating S to R.

In conclusion, this chapter considers the nature of stimulus interactions that are required to explain how animals can solve non-linear discriminations such as negative patterning and the biconditional discrimination. While some researchers (e.g., Melchers, Shanks, & Lachnit, 2008) have assumed that these discrimination problems can only be solved by recourse to configural representations that uniquely code stimulus conjunctions, the modeling discussed in the present chapter shows that this is not correct. Non-linear discriminations are intractable to those associative models that assume a 1-to-1 relationship between the representation of an event and the separate components of that event (e.g., between a compound of two stimuli and the individual stimuli themselves), because these models predict effective generalization of associative change between reinforced and non-reinforced trials. Viable models of associative learning must assume that stimulus representations involve a non-linear combination of stimulus elements. This can be achieved by adding configural elements to the representation of each compound, or by suppressing the activation of some stimulus elements when stimuli are presented in compound. As such, the most complex discriminations can be solved relying solely on elemental representations. Of course the model formulated here was designed with the express purpose of solving those non-linear discriminations. The mechanisms proposed do not equip the model with the means to explain a range of phenomena that extend beyond the scope of this chapter. Perhaps relevant among these phenomena are learning-to-learn and occasion-setting, given that these can be accounted for by layered network models that incorporate configural representations (Kehoe, 1988; Schmajuk & Di Carlo, 1992).

Acknowledgments

The author thanks Nestor Schmajuk, Mike Le Pelley, and an anonymous reviewer for comments on an earlier draft of this chapter. He also thanks John Moore for discussions and for providing the PhD dissertation of Robert Polewan.

References

Arabzadeh, E., Clifford, C. W. G. & Harris, J. A. (2008). Vision merges with touch in a purely tactile discrimination. *Psychological Science, 19*, 635–641.

Brimer, C. J. (1970). Disinhibition of an operant response. *Learning and Motivation, 1*, 346–371.

Choi, J.-S. & Moore, J. W. (2003). Cerebellar neuronal activity expresses the complex topography of conditioned eyeblink responses. *Behavioral Neuroscience, 117*, 1211–1219.

Crowder, N. A., Price, N. S. C., Hietanen, M. A., Dreher, B., Clifford, C. W. G. & Ibbotson, M. R. (2006). Relationship between contrast adaptation and orientation tuning in V1 and V2 of cat visual cortex. *Journal of Neurophysiology, 95*, 271–283.

Grossberg, S. (1975). A neural model of attention, reinforcement, and discrimination learning. *International Review of Neurobiology, 18*, 263–327.

Harris, J. A. (2006). Elemental representations of stimuli in associative learning. *Psychological Review, 113*, 584–605. 10.1037/0033-295X.113.3.584.

Harris, J. A. & Livesey, E. J. (2008). Comparing patterning and biconditional discriminations in humans. *Journal of Experimental Psychology: Animal Behavior Processes, 34*, 144–154.

Harris, J. A., Livesey, E. J., Gharaei, S. & Westbrook, R. F. (2008). Negative patterning is easier than a biconditional discrimination. *Journal of Experimental Psychology: Animal Behavior Processes, 34*, 494–500. 10.1037/0097-7403.34.4.494.

Heeger, D. J. (1992). Normalization of cell responses in cat striate cortex. *Visual Neuroscience, 9*, 181–197.

James, J. H. & Wagner, A. R. (1980). One-trial overshadowing: evidence of distributive processing. *Journal of Experimental Psychology: Animal Behavior Processes, 6*(2), 188–205.

Kehoe, E. J. (1982). Overshadowing and summation in compound stimulus conditioning of the rabbit's nictitating membrane response. *Journal of Experimental Psychology: Animal Behavior Processes, 8*, 313–328.

Kehoe, E. J. (1986). Summation and configuration in conditioning of the rabbit's nictitating membrane response to compound stimuli. *Journal of Experimental Psychology: Animal Behavior Processes, 12*, 186–195.

Kehoe, E. J. (1988). A layered network model of associative learning: learning-to-learn and configuration. *Psychological Review, 95*, 411–433.

Kehoe, E. J. & Graham, P. (1988). Summation and configuration: stimulus compounding and negative patterning in the rabbit. *Journal of Experimental Psychology: Animal Behavior Processes, 14*, 320–333.

Le Pelley, M. E. (2010). The hybrid modeling approach to conditioning. In N. A. Schmajuk, ed., *Computational Models of Conditioning*. Cambridge, UK: Cambridge University Press.

Mackintosh, N. J. & Reese, B. (1979). One-trial overshadowing. *Quarterly Journal of Experimental Psychology, 31*, 519–526.

McLaren, I. P. L. & Mackintosh, N. J. (2000). An elemental model of associative learning I: latent Inhibition and perceptual learning. *Animal Learning and Behavior,* **28**(3), 211–246.

McLaren, I. P. L. & Mackintosh, N. J. (2002). Associative learning and elemental representation ii: generalization and discrimination. *Animal Learning and Behavior,* **30**, 177–200.

Melchers, K. G., Shanks, D. R. & Lachnit, H. (2008). Stimulus coding in human associative learning: flexible representations of parts and wholes. *Behavioural Processes,* **77**(3), 413–427.

Millenson, J. R., Kehoe, E. J. & Gormezano, I. (1977). Classical conditioning of the rabbit's nictitating membrane response under fixed and mixed CS–US intervals. *Learning and Motivation,* **8**, 351–366.

Pavlov, I. P. (1927). *Conditioned Reflexes: An Investigation of the Physiological Activity of the Cerebral Cortex.* (G. V. Anrep, Trans.). New York: Dover.

Pearce, J. M. (1987). A model for stimulus generalization in Pavlovian conditioning. *Psychological Review,* **94**(1), 61–73. 10.1037/0033-295X.94.1.61.

Pearce, J. M. (1994). Similarity and discrimination: a selective review and a connectionist model. *Psychological Review,* **101**(4), 587–607. 10.1037/0033-295X.101.4.587.

Polewan, R. J. (2006). Physiological and behavioral studies of rabbit eyeblink conditioning under temporal uncertainty: Purkinje cell response and compound conditioning. Unpublished doctoral dissertation, University of Massachusetts.

Rescorla, R. A. (1972). "Configural" conditioning in discrete-trial bar pressing. *Journal of Comparative and Physiological Psychology,* **79**(2), 307–317. 10.1037/h0032553.

Rescorla, R. A. (1973). Evidence for a unique stimulus interpretation of configural conditioning. *Journal of Comparative and Physiological Psychology,* **85**, 331–338.

Rescorla, R. A. (1997). Summation: assessment of a configural theory. *Animal Learning and Behavior,* **25**(2), 200–209.

Rescorla, R. A. & Wagner, A. R. (1972). A theory of Pavlovian conditioning: variations in the effectiveness of reinforcement and nonreinforcement. In A. H. Black and W. F. Prokasy, eds., *Classical Conditioning II: Current Research and Theory.* New York: Appleton–Century–Crofts, pp. 64–99.

Rescorla, R. A., Grau, J. W. & Durlach, P. J. (1985). Analysis of the unique cue in configural discriminations. *Journal of Experimental Psychology: Animal Behavior Processes,* **11**, 356–366.

Reynolds, J. H. & Chelazzi, L. (2004). Attentional modulation of visual processing. *Annual Review of Neuroscience,* **27**, 611–647.

Reynolds, J. H. & Heeger, D. J. (2009). The normalization model of attention. *Neuron,* **61**, 168–185.

Saavedra, M. A. (1975). Pavlovian compound conditioning in the rabbit. *Learning and Motivation,* **6**, 314–326.

Schmajuk, N. A. & Di Carlo, J. J. (1992). A neural network approach to hippocampal functioning in classical conditioning. *Behavioral Neuroscience, 105*, 82–110.

Schmajuk, N. A., Lamoureux, J. A. & Holland, P. C. (1998). Occasion setting: a neural network approach. *Psychological Review, 105*(1), 3–32.

Solomon, J. A. (2009). The history of dipper functions. *Attention, Perception, and Psychophysics, 71*, 435–443.

Spence, K. W. (1952). The nature of the response in discrimination learning in animals. *Psychological Review, 59*, 89–93. 10.1037/h0063067.

Stevens, S. S. (1962). The surprising simplicity of sensory metrics. *American Psychologist, 17*, 29–39.

Thein, T., Westbrook, R. F. & Harris, J. A. (2008). How the associative strengths of stimuli combine in compound: summation and overshadowing. *Journal of Experimental Psychology: Animal Behavior Processes, 34*, 155–166. 10.1037/0097-7403.34.1.155.

Wagner, A. R. & Brandon, S. E. (2001). A componential theory of Pavlovian conditioning. In R. R. Mowrer and S. B. Klein, eds., *Handbook of Contemporary Learning Theories*. Mahwah NJ, USA: Lawrence Erlbaum Associates, Inc., pp. 23–64.

Wagner, A. R. & Rescorla, R. A. (1972). Inhibition in Pavlovian conditioning: application of a theory. In M. S. Halliday and R. A. Boakes, eds., *Inhibition and Learning*. San Diego, CA: Academic Press, pp. 301–336.

Whitlow, J. W. & Wagner, A. R. (1972). Negative patterning in classical conditioning: summation of response tendencies to isolable and configural components. *Psychonomic Science, 27*(5), 299–301.

3

The hybrid modeling approach to conditioning

M. E. LE PELLEY

Abstract

Broadly, models of conditioning and associative learning have two main goals: (1) to describe the way in which stimuli are represented in the learning system (see Harris, 2010, this volume), and (2) to describe the mechanics of the learning process itself, that is to say, the factors that determine the amount of learning that a given stimulus will undergo on a given learning episode. Clearly these two issues are not perfectly separable: as Harris demonstrates, the nature of stimulus representation used by a learning system can influence the type of associative process that must be assumed in order for that system to learn in a similar manner to animals or humans. Nevertheless, the focus of the current chapter will be almost exclusively on the second of these issues. More specifically, this chapter will consider the various ways in which an organism's prior experience of stimuli, and prior learning about their consequences (the "associative history" of those stimuli), influences the amount that the organism will learn about those stimuli in future.

Over a century's worth of research on animal conditioning has generated a wealth of empirical evidence relating to the influence of associative history on future learning. Historically, in developing models of learning, theorists have tended to concentrate on one such influence and build a model centered on that aspect. For example (and to anticipate), the model developed by Mackintosh (1975) deals exclusively with examples of positive transfer of the processing of cues; Pearce and Hall's (1980) model was developed purely on the basis of examples of negative transfer of cue processing; and Rescorla and Wagner's (1972) model deals with competition between cues on the basis of the surprisingness of the outcome.

In reviewing a wide range of empirical studies of the influence of associative history, Le Pelley (2004) argued that these models, while able to provide an account of phenomena within their relatively narrow scope of expertise, fail to provide a full and satisfactory account of the varying effects of associative history on the learning undergone by cues on a given learning episode. This led to the suggestion that it was perhaps time to move on from the extreme position offered by these single-process models, and instead accept that the influence of prior learning on future learning might be multiply determined. Le Pelley suggested combining the properties of several single-process models to yield a "hybrid" model of the influence of associative history that aimed to account for a wider range of data than any of its individual components.

This chapter will review the evidence supporting the suggestion that multiple processes might contribute to the influence of associative history on the conditioning undergone by a given cue on a given learning episode. I will then go on to discuss whether these ideas are confined to animal conditioning, or whether they can be extended to the case of human contingency learning.

CS processing and US processing

Single-process models of associative learning can broadly be divided into two categories, based on the way in which they view prior learning as influencing future learning. The first class of models appeals to changes in the effectiveness of the unconditioned stimulus (US, or "outcome"; the terms will be used interchangeably) as being the crucial determinant of learning, and hence can be termed US-processing theories (e.g., Bush & Mosteller, 1951; Estes, 1950; Pearce, 1987, 1994; Rescorla & Wagner, 1972). According to such models, the amount of learning that a US can support on a given learning episode is determined by how surprising that US is: a surprising US can support more new learning than an unsurprising (well-predicted) US.

The second class of models instead sees changes in the effectiveness of the conditioned stimulus (CS, or "cue"; the terms will again be used interchangeably) as being the crucial determinant of learning, and hence can be termed CS-processing theories (e.g., Mackintosh, 1975; Pearce & Hall, 1980; Sutherland & Mackintosh, 1971). These models assume that the readiness with which a given CS will engage the learning process and undergo changes in associative strength – the "associability" of the CS – can vary as a product of the CS's training history.

The distinction between these two classes of theories is neatly illustrated in the accounts they offer of "blocking." In a blocking experiment, animals first receive training in which an individual cue, A, is paired with an outcome (denoted A+). Subsequently, animals experience trials in which a compound of A with another stimulus is paired with the same outcome (AB+). Typically, responding on test trials with B by itself is weaker than if the initial training with A is omitted (Kamin, 1969). Thus, prior learning about A is said to block learning about the redundant cue B on AB+ compound trials.

The US-processing account of blocking sees A+ pretraining as rendering the outcome unsurprising on AB+ trials, since it is already predicted by the presence of A. Hence, this expected outcome will be less able to support learning about the added cue, B, than if pretraining with A had been omitted (such that the outcome on AB+ trials would be surprising and hence able to support learning).

In contrast, CS-processing theories state that blocking results from a reduction in the effectiveness of the added cue, B, on AB+ trials. Essentially this approach suggests that, because the outcome occurring on AB+ trials is already well predicted by the presence of A, the associability of the redundant cue B will rapidly decline. Since the associability of a cue determines its ability to enter into associations, this decline means that B will be less able to enter into association with the outcome on AB+ trials, and blocking will be the result.

Consistent with the general thesis of the hybrid model, that multiple mechanisms might combine to influence the learning about a cue, there exists evidence to suggest that blocking is multiply determined, involving both CS- and US-processing mechanisms.

In support of a CS-processing contribution to blocking, studies indicate that previously blocked cues are slower to enter into novel associations, consistent with the suggestion that blocking treatment has caused these cues to undergo a reduction in associability. Mackintosh (1978; see also Mackintosh & Turner, 1971) administered a blocking procedure to rats using a weak shock (denoted sh) as the US. The AB compound was then paired with a strong shock (denoted SH). Thus, these rats received A–sh, AB–sh, AB–SH training. Subsequent test trials with B alone revealed weaker responding than in a group of animals for which the AB–sh trials were omitted, such that B was not blocked with respect to the weak shock prior to training with the strong shock.

An interesting case is provided by Baxter, Gallagher, and Holland (1999). Table 3.1 shows the essential parts of the design of their Experiment 2. Half of the rats in this study had lesions of the cholinergic input to the hippocampus; the other half were sham-lesioned animals. Rats in experimental conditions (BLK-E and BLK-I in Table 3.1) received A+, AB+ blocking training, while rats in a control condition received AB+ training without prior conditioning of A alone. Blocking was observed, in that in a subsequent test in extinction, conditioned responding to B was significantly lower in the experimental conditions than

Table 3.1 *Design of experiment by Baxter, Gallagher, and Holland (1999)*

Condition	Stage 1	Stage 2	Blocking Test	Savings Test
BLK-E	A+	AB+	B−	B+
BLK-I	A+	AB+	B−	A+, AB−
CON		AB+	B−	

Note: This experiment was run on a between-subjects basis; the three conditions in the above table were each implemented in a different group of rats. BLK = blocking treatment; CON = behavioral control treatment; E = excitatory savings test; I = inhibitory savings test.

in the control condition. Importantly, the magnitude of this blocking effect did not differ between lesioned and sham-lesioned rats; both groups showed equivalent blocking.

Following this test for blocking, animals in condition BLK-E received an excitatory savings test in which B was paired individually with the US (B+). Conditioned responding to B in condition BLK-E developed significantly more rapidly in lesioned animals than in shams. Rats in condition BLK-I instead received an inhibitory savings test, which involved A+, AB− training such that B should become a conditioned inhibitor of the US, signaling the omission of an otherwise-expected outcome (conditioned inhibition is discussed in more detail in the next section). Inhibitory learning about B, measured as the difference in conditioned responding on reinforced A+ trials and non-reinforced AB− trials, once again proceeded more rapidly in lesioned rats than in shams.

The fact that both excitatory *and* inhibitory conditioning of B was more rapid in lesioned rats than in shams indicates that the associability of B was higher in the former group, the implication being that lesioning the cholinergic input to the hippocampus has prevented the decline in associability (i.e., CS-processing) that a blocked cue would otherwise undergo. So B did not seem to have undergone a reduction in associability in lesioned rats, but puzzlingly (as noted above) these rats still demonstrated a blocking effect that was of equal magnitude to that observed in shams. Holland and Fox (2003) found similar results following ibotenic acid lesions of the hippocampus.

The implication of the results of these studies is that, while blocking produces a decrement in associability, the phenomenon of blocking itself is not necessarily a product of this decrement. Having taken CS-processing mechanisms out of the picture, the implication is that US-processing mechanisms must have been responsible for the blocking observed in lesioned animals. If prior training of A renders the US occurring on AB+ trials unsurprising and hence unable to support learning (as anticipated by the US-processing approach), then little learning about B will occur regardless of its associability. Thus, even if the associability of B remains at a high level in lesioned animals, the low effectiveness of the outcome will still ensure that blocking occurs.

This example thus supports the fundamental idea of the hybrid modeling approach that multiple mechanisms might contribute to conditioning. In this case the evidence indicates that both CS- and US-processing might have a part to play. In the remainder of this chapter we shall see that perhaps the evidence warrants even finer-grained distinctions than this.

US processing

Summed error

US-processing mechanisms are based on the surprisingness of the US occurring on a given trial. This surprisingness can be quantified as the discrepancy between the observed magnitude of the US on that trial, and the expected (or predicted) magnitude of that US. This discrepancy is also known as the *error* in the prediction of the US, and learning will proceed so as to reduce the size of this error.

The question now becomes one of how we should define the expected magnitude of the US. One approach is to sum the expectancy of the US across all presented cues. For example, if two cues A and B are presented, and cue A predicts a US magnitude of 10 units while B predicts a US magnitude of 20 units, then the summed expectancy would be for a magnitude of 30 units. This approach is implicit in the US-processing account of blocking discussed above, wherein the effectiveness of the US for entering into association with B on AB+ trials is reduced because that US is already predicted by the presence of A. The suggestion is that learning about one cue (B) is influenced by the prediction made by other cues with which it is paired (A).

The single best piece of evidence in support of the idea that a summed error contributes to learning (and of the importance of US-processing mechanisms in general) is the phenomenon of conditioned inhibition (Pavlov, 1927; Rescorla, 1969). As an example, in the first stage of an experiment by Pearce, Nicholas, and Dickinson (1982), rats experienced trials on which a clicker signaled shock (C+) in a conditioned suppression procedure. In the second stage, trials on which the clicker was followed by shock were intermixed with trials on which a compound of the clicker and a light was not followed by shock (CL−). Thus the light signaled the absence of a shock that was otherwise predicted by the presence of the clicker. Following this training, presentation of the clicker suppressed lever-pressing for food, indicating that rats had learnt the clicker→shock association. In contrast, the clicker–light compound produced considerably less suppression of lever-pressing, indicating that the rats had learnt that the light signaled the absence of shock, and that this learning opposed the excitatory learning about the clicker. In support of the idea that the light had acquired inhibitory potential as a result of this training, Pearce *et al.* found that when the light was subsequently paired with shock, conditioning proceeded more slowly than for a cue that had not previously received this inhibitory training (the retardation test for conditioned inhibition). Furthermore, they demonstrated that following conditioned inhibition training, the light would also counteract the conditioned suppression produced by a CS that was trained separately, i.e., it was able to transfer its inhibitory potential to a novel excitor (the summation test for conditioned inhibition).

Conditioned inhibition provides an absolutely compelling case for the influence of a US-processing mechanism based on summed error. The drive to develop inhibition to L on CL– trials comes from the prediction of the outcome made by C. Thus, learning about L is clearly influenced by the expectancy of the outcome generated by a separate cue with which it is paired. If this were not the case, then there would be no difference between C+, CL– training, and X+, CL– training (where X is some other cue) in terms of learning about L. And yet there clearly is a difference, in that C+, CL– training endows L with the properties of a conditioned inhibitor, while X+, CL– training does not (Pearce, Nicholas *et al.*, 1982). Moreover, it is very hard to see how a CS-processing mechanism alone could ever produce conditioned inhibition. In essence, CS-processing mechanisms can control the *rate* of learning about a cue, but do not control the *sign* of that learning (excitatory or inhibitory). This latter factor must be determined by the processing of the US: whether it is currently under-predicted (the expected magnitude is less than the observed magnitude, so learning should be excitatory) or over-predicted (expected magnitude greater than observed magnitude, so learning should be inhibitory).

Individual error

However, it is possible that outcome expectancy based on a sum across all presented cues may not be the whole story. Evidence from a series of studies by Rescorla (2000, 2001, 2002; see also Leung & Westbrook, 2008) suggests that learning might also be influenced by the prediction of US magnitude made by each cue considered individually.

In a typical experiment (Rescorla, 2000), cues A and C were initially trained to be excitatory through direct pairings with the US (A+ and C+), while cues B and D were trained as conditioned inhibitors through non-reinforced pairings with an excitatory CS (X+, BX–, DX–). In a subsequent phase, A and B were reinforced in compound (AB+). On these latter trials, the summed error that applies to learning about A and B would be identical, since the overall US expectancy on these trials would be generated by summing across the expectancies produced by A and B[1]. Consequently, if learning about a given cue were determined solely by a summed-error term, then we would expect both A and B to undergo an equal-sized increment in associative strength on each AB+ trial. Rescorla tested this prediction by examining conditioned responding to compounds AD and BC in a final test. If these compounds were compared in the absence of AB+ training, they should yield equal responding, since each consists of one excitatory cue (A or C) and one inhibitory cue (B or D). If AB+ trials led to equal-sized increments in the strengths of A and B, then responding to the AD and BC compounds would remain equal (as each begins AB+ training at the same level and undergoes the same change). Contrary to this idea, Rescorla found greater responding to BC than to AD, indicating that B had undergone a greater increment in associative strength than had A over AB+ training.

As noted earlier, conditioned inhibition clearly indicates that learning about a given cue is influenced by a summed-error term. However, Rescorla argued that his findings of differential learning about the elements of a cue compound demonstrated that learning about a cue was also influenced by the discrepancy between the observed outcome magnitude and the outcome expectancy generated by each cue individually – the "individual error" of each cue. With regard to the experiment described above, prior A+ training will ensure that the discrepancy between the observed outcome on AB+ trials and that predicted by A alone will be small, i.e., A will have a small individual error. In contrast, prior inhibitory conditioning to B will ensure that the discrepancy between the observed outcome on AB+ trials and that predicted by B alone (namely, the absence of the outcome) will be very large; B will have a large individual error. Thus, if it is assumed that learning about cues is also fuelled by their individual error, then it is possible to anticipate that B will undergo a greater increment than will A on AB+ trials.

The data discussed in this section thus point to the idea that learning about a cue on a given trial is influenced by prior learning about that cue considered alone (which determines the cue's individual error), and also by prior learning about other cues with which it is simultaneously presented (which contribute to the summed error). Hence, it seems that, consistent with the hybrid modeling approach, more than one US-processing mechanism might combine to determine the learning undergone by a given cue on a given trial. Brandon,

---

[1] For this reason, a summed-error term is sometimes also referred to as a "common-error" term, since exactly the same error will apply to all cues that are presented on the same trial.

Vogel, and Wagner (2003) have presented a model based on just such a combination of US-processing mechanisms, and have demonstrated that it is able to account for the results of many of Rescorla's studies.

That said, however, the case for an influence of individual error is not quite as clear-cut as that for summed error. For example, Harris (2006) has demonstrated that a system in which learning is based solely on summed error can model Rescorla's data, as long as a particular system of stimulus representation is assumed. Similarly, Schmajuk (2009) has demonstrated that CS-processing mechanisms could contribute to the advantage in responding for BC over AD observed in Rescorla's (2000) study described above (and many of the other findings presented by Rescorla, 2000, 2001, 2002). Essentially, this account suggests that, as a consequence of repeated exposure to A and B during AB+ training, responding to these cues habituates. As a result, responding to AD on test will be dominated by the influence of the non-habituated D (which is inhibitory), while responding to BC will be dominated by the non-habituated C (which is excitatory); the result will be greater responding to BC than to AD. Rescorla (2000) himself has noted that AB+ training might not influence the strength of just A–US and B–US associations, but might also promote the formation of an A–B within-compound association. The formation of such an association might be expected to reduce responding to the excitatory A and enhance responding to the inhibitory B, and hence, even if the A–US and B–US associations underwent equal increments (as anticipated by a summed-error view), AB+ training could augment total responding to B more than to A. While further experiments aimed to reduce the possible impact of these within-compound associations (e.g., Rescorla, 2000, Experiments 5 and 6), they cannot rule out this influence entirely.

Hence while Rescorla's data certainly provide persuasive evidence for an influence of individual error, they do not necessarily force us to take this step. The extent to which these "alternative accounts" are able to provide a full account of the data indicating differential learning about the elements of a stimulus compound remains to be seen. For example, in an elegant series of experiments on extinction, Leung and Westbrook (2008) came to the conclusion that this aspect of learning was also influenced by both summed and individual error. The extent to which Harris's representational account or Schmajuk's attentional account are also able to account for the findings adduced by Leung and Westbrook as evidence for individual error has yet to be established – it does, however, seem that these data might be open to interpretation in terms of the formation of within-compound associations, much as suggested above.

CS processing

Earlier, blocking was used to demonstrate that both CS- and US-processing mechanisms might influence the learning about a given stimulus on a given trial. It was then noted that it is possible to distinguish between different types of US-processing mechanism (based on summed versus individual error), and that, once again, both might contribute to learning. In this section we will see that a similar argument can be applied to CS-processing mechanisms.

Two theoretical perspectives have dominated the study of CS-processing mechanisms. The first, associated most strongly with Mackintosh's (1975) theory (but see also Kruschke, 2001; Lovejoy, 1968; Sutherland & Mackintosh, 1971; Zeaman & House, 1963), suggests that a CS will maintain a high associability to the extent that it is the best available predictor of the outcome with which it is paired. Consider Mackintosh and Turner's (1971) blocking study described earlier, in which demonstrated that a blocked cue undergoes a decrement in associability. Pretraining of A will ensure that, on AB+ trials, B is a poorer predictor of the US than is A. Hence, Mackintosh's theory correctly predicts that the associability of B will decline.

Mackintosh's approach makes intuitive sense; it seems sensible to devote processing resources to cues that have been useful in predicting things in the past, since these cues are likely to be useful in predicting things in the future. In a testament to the danger of relying on intuition, however, a directly opposing account can also be made to sound intuitively plausible. Pearce and Hall (1980) argued that it makes little sense to devote learning resources to those cues whose consequences are already well established, i.e., those cues that predict well the outcome with which they are paired. Instead, Pearce and Hall suggested that processing resources should be devoted to cues to the extent that the outcome with which they are paired is surprising, such that animals will tend to learn more rapidly about the true significance of those cues. Let us consider again Mackintosh and Turner's (1971) blocking study. Pretraining of A will ensure that the outcome occurring on AB+ trials is unsurprising, and hence the Pearce–Hall model suggests that there will be a decline in the associability of the cues, A and B, which are followed by this unsurprising outcome.

Rather bizarrely, then, given that the Mackintosh theory (which suggests that high associability will be maintained by cues that are consistently followed by the same outcome), and the Pearce–Hall theory (which suggests that associability will decline for cues that are consistently followed by the same outcome) are essentially opposites of one another, both are able to account for the observed decline in associability of a blocked cue. Other phenomena of learning, however, do have the potential to discriminate between these theories.

Evidence for the Mackintosh model: positive transfer

Some of the most powerful evidence in support of Mackintosh's theory comes from studies of dimensional shifts in discrimination learning. Many of these studies have used instrumental choice procedures (Dias, Robbins, & Roberts, 1996; Mackintosh, 1969; Shepp & Eimas, 1964; Shepp & Schrier, 1969). Given the title of this book, however, I will focus on a study by George and Pearce (1999), which used classical conditioning. Pigeons were trained in a successive discrimination using stimuli that could vary on two dimensions. These stimuli were squares that were divided in half. One half was filled with a particular color (red or green) while the other half contained black and white lines at a certain orientation (+45° or −45° to the vertical). During a first stage, pigeons were trained on a successive discrimination in which one dimension was relevant to the solution of the discrimination, with food being delivered after every stimulus that contained one value on this dimension, and food never being delivered after any stimulus that contained the other value on this dimension. The other dimension was irrelevant, with each value on this dimension being followed by food on half of the trials. Figure 3.1 shows an example set of rewarded and unrewarded stimuli with color relevant (and red being the rewarded value on that dimension).

Following training on this first discrimination, pigeons were shifted to a new discrimination in which the stimuli contained new values on each dimension (colors were now blue and yellow, orientations were vertical and horizontal). As before, one dimension was relevant to the solution of the new discrimination and the other was irrelevant. For group IDS, the dimension that was relevant in this latter discrimination (color or orientation) was the same as that which was relevant in the first discrimination; these pigeons experienced an "intradimensional" shift. For group EDS, the dimension that was relevant in the latter dimension was that which had been irrelevant to the first discrimination; these pigeons experienced an "extradimensional" shift. George and Pearce observed significantly faster learning of this second discrimination by group IDS than group EDS. This constitutes an example of positive transfer, in that it demonstrates an advantage in learning for cues (here dimensions) that have high prior predictive value.

Mackintosh's theory correctly anticipates this finding. During training on the initial discrimination, the associability of values on the relevant dimension will increase (since these values are the best available predictors of the outcome that occurs on each trial), while the associability of values on the

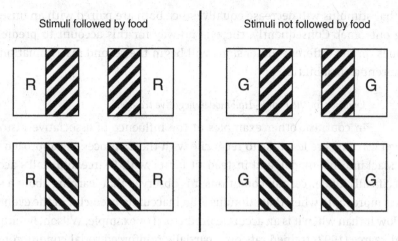

Figure 3.1 An example set of stimuli from the experiment by George and Pearce (1999). "R" indicates that the rectangle was colored red; "G" indicates that it was colored green. In this case, color is the relevant dimension, with red being the rewarded value on that dimension (such that any stimulus containing red is paired with delivery of food), and green being the nonrewarded value (such that any stimulus containing green is not paired with food). The orientation of the black and white lines is irrelevant to the solution of this discrimination. For other subjects, orientation would be relevant and color irrelevant (likewise, across participants each value could appear as the rewarded or nonrewarded value of the relevant dimension).

irrelevant dimension will decline (as these values are poor predictors of the outcome that will occur). If it is assumed that these changes in associability will generalize to other values on the same dimension (by virtue of their similarity), then this approach correctly predicts that the test discrimination will be learnt more rapidly by group IDS than by group EDS. For example, for a pigeon for whom color was relevant during the initial discrimination (such that values on the color dimension will maintain higher associability than will values on the orientation dimension), the values "blue" and "yellow" will begin the second discrimination with higher associability than will the values "vertical" and "horizontal." This will aid solution of an intradimensional shift, since blue and yellow are the values that must be learnt about to solve this discrimination, but will hinder solution of an extradimensional shift, since vertical and horizontal are the values that must be learnt about in this case.

In contrast, the Pearce–Hall model is unable to account for the advantage shown by group IDS. The outcome occurring on each trial of the initial discrimination is well predicted by the compound stimulus that is presented, and hence the Pearce–Hall model states that the associability of both components of that stimulus will decrease equally (since both are paired with an unsurprising outcome). Consequently, there is no way for this account to predict that values on the different dimensions will begin the second discrimination with different associabilities.[2]

Evidence for the Pearce–Hall model: negative transfer

In contrast, other examples of the influence of associative history on novel learning are less easy to reconcile with the CS-processing approach taken by Mackintosh's model, and instead fit better with Pearce and Hall's account. Specifically, under certain conditions it is observed that learning about a stimulus is more rapid when that stimulus is an inaccurate predictor of the events that follow it than when it is an accurate predictor. For example, Wilson, Boumphrey, and Pearce (1992) trained rats on a partially reinforced serial conditioning procedure. A light was followed by a tone; on half of the trials this tone terminated with delivery of a food US, on the other half no food US was provided (i.e., training was with L→T→US and L→T→Ø trials). This procedure resulted in only minimal conditioned responding (magazine orienting) to the light. These rats were then divided into two groups. For Group Consistent training continued as before. For Group Shift, the tone was omitted on all non-reinforced trials (i.e., trials were L→T→US and L→Ø→Ø). Hence, while the relation between the light CS and the food US was maintained for Group Shift, its relation to the tone was changed from 100% to 50%. According to the Pearce–Hall model, this will result in a higher associability for the light in Group Shift, for which the event following the light (the tone) is unpredictable, as compared with Group Consistent, for which the tone consistently followed the light. In line with this idea Wilson *et al.* (1992) found that, when the light was subsequently paired directly with food, conditioning to the light occurred more rapidly in Group Shift than in Group Consistent. This is an example of negative transfer, in that there is an advantage in learning for a cue that has lower prior predictive value.

This demonstration of negative transfer runs against the principles of the Mackintosh model. In both Group Shift and Group Consistent, the light is the

---

[2] This is a consequence of the fact that the Pearce–Hall model uses a summed-error term to determine the associability of each cue; given that this error term will be equal for both components of the same stimulus, these components must therefore have the same associability. An alternative would be to allow the associability of each component to be determined by the individual predictiveness of that stimulus. However, this makes the situation worse: this discrepancy will be larger for irrelevant components (and hence these cues will maintain a higher associability) than for relevant components during the initial discrimination. Hence, this account predicts that, if anything, an EDS will be solved more rapidly than an IDS, the opposite of the result observed empirically.

best available predictor of the tone throughout serial conditioning training; even during L→T→US and L→∅→∅ for Group Shift, the tone never occurs in the absence of the light. Hence, this model predicts that the light will maintain a high associability in both groups (if anything, the associability of the light will be higher in Group Consistent, given that the light is a more accurate predictor of the tone in this group than it is in Group Shift). Consequently, during the final L→US pairings, the Mackintosh model incorrectly anticipates either equally rapid conditioning to the light in both groups, or more rapid conditioning in Group Consistent.

A reconciliation: two CS-processing mechanisms

In general, the Mackintosh model tends to predict positive transfer of CS processing, while the Pearce–Hall model predicts negative transfer. The problem for modelers is that both positive and negative transfer effects are observed in different studies. While we have focused on the IDS/EDS effect and Wilson et al.'s (1992) "inconsistency advantage" effect here, there exist several other examples of both positive (e.g., Baker & Mackintosh, 1977, 1979; Bennett, Wills, Oakeshott, & Mackintosh, 2000; Lawrence, 1952; Mackintosh, 1969, 1973; Reid, 1953) and negative (e.g., Hall & Pearce, 1979; 1982; Kaye & Pearce, 1984; Pearce, Kaye, & Hall, 1982; Swan & Pearce, 1988) transfer effects in animal conditioning.

So we have, on the face of it, reliable and independent support for two opposing models of CS-processing effects. What are we to make of this? One solution is to acknowledge that there is an element of truth to both theories, and hence that two different CS-processing mechanisms interact to determine the overall rate of learning about a given cue. Let us refer to the associability controlled by the Mackintosh model as α and that controlled by the Pearce–Hall model as σ, and let us suppose that both mechanisms operate independently, with the overall learning rate for a stimulus being determined by $\alpha \times \sigma$. The problem then is to explain why certain studies reveal evidence consistent with α, while other studies reveal evidence consistent with σ.

In fact, a subtle distinction between the Mackintosh and Pearce–Hall models suggests a potential resolution. The Mackintosh model, as originally framed, is based on a comparison of the *relative* predictiveness of different cues. That is, a cue maintains a high α according to the extent to which it is a better predictor of the outcome of the current trial *than are other presented cues*. The model achieves this by having α changes based on a comparison of the individual error terms of different, simultaneously presented cues. The cue with the smallest error term is the best individual predictor of the outcome, and so, according to the model, will maintain a high α, while that of other cues will fall.

In contrast, the original formulation of the Pearce–Hall model makes use of the *absolute* predictiveness of cues: how well a given cue (or compound of cues) predicts the current outcome, regardless of whether that cue is a better or worse predictor of the outcome than are others. The model achieves this by having σ changes based on the error term itself, rather than on a comparison of the error terms of different cues. If a cue is associated with a large error term (i.e., it has low absolute predictiveness), it will have a high σ; if it is associated with a small error term (it has high absolute predictiveness), it will have a low σ.

Given that the two theories are based on different properties of a cue (its relative versus its absolute predictiveness), they may not be as incompatible as first appears. This encourages the possibility that the two mechanisms might be made to work side by side. Indeed, the relative versus absolute distinction makes a clear prediction as to when each mechanism might be expected to dominate. Specifically, the Mackintosh α mechanism should dominate when predictiveness is established during a pretraining phase that involves multiple, simultaneously presented stimuli, some of which are more predictive than others, since these are the circumstances under which a comparison of the relative predictiveness of these cues will produce a differential change in α. This is clearly the case in the IDS/EDS study described above: the stimulus presented on each trial is made up of two components, one of which is more predictive than the other. Hence, a comparison of the relative predictiveness of these components will yield a higher α for the relevant component than for the irrelevant component. Meanwhile, the absolute predictiveness mechanism of the Pearce–Hall model will not differentiate between these components; since they are both part of the same compound stimulus, the common-error term of this mechanism will ensure that σ falls at the same rate for both components as the outcome comes to be predicted by the stimulus. The upshot is that $\alpha \times \sigma$ will be greater for relevant cues than for irrelevant cues, and hence a positive transfer effect is correctly predicted.

Conversely, the hybrid approach anticipates that σ will dominate when two cues do not differ in their relative predictiveness, but do differ in terms of absolute predictiveness. Wilson *et al.*'s (1992) study provides a clear illustration. As noted earlier, in both Group Consistent and Group Shift, the light is the best available predictor of the tone (since the light is the only punctate cue presented prior to the tone on each trial), and hence α_{LIGHT} will be equal in both groups. The absolute predictiveness of the light with respect to the tone will be higher in Group Consistent than in Group Shift, and hence σ_{LIGHT} will be lower in Group Consistent than in Group Shift. Consequently $\alpha_{LIGHT} \times \sigma_{LIGHT}$ will be greater for Group Shift than for Group Consistent, and a negative transfer effect is correctly predicted.

Consistent with this account, it is exactly those experiments involving pretraining in which the critical cues are presented simultaneously and differ in relative predictiveness that demonstrate positive transfer and hence provide support for a dominance of the α mechanism (e.g., Baker & Mackintosh, 1977, 1979; Bennett *et al.*, 2000; Lawrence, 1952; Mackintosh, 1969, 1973; Reid, 1953).[3] Similarly, all of the studies demonstrating negative transfer have involved separate training of cues that differ in their absolute predictiveness, but with each being the best available predictor of the outcome with which it is paired (Hall & Pearce, 1979, 1982; Kaye & Pearce, 1984; Pearce, Kaye *et al.*, 1982; Swan & Pearce, 1988).

A particularly neat example of the distinction between relative and absolute predictiveness is provided by recent experiments conducted in Pearce and Haselgrove's labs (Dopson, Esber, & Pearce, 2010; Haselgrove, Esber, Pearce, & Jones, in press). Dopson *et al.* trained pigeons with a set of true discriminations, such as AX+, CX−, and BW+, DW−, in which one cue of each compound is relevant (A and B consistently signal reinforcement, C and D consistently signal non-reinforcement), while the other cue is irrelevant (W and X are reinforced on half of trials and non-reinforced on the other half); the full design is shown in Table 3.2. This training is with multiple, simultaneously presented cues which differ in their relative predictiveness, and consequently the argument presented above anticipates that Mackintosh-type associability processes will dominate, such that the relevant cues (A, B, C, and D) should subsequently be learnt about more rapidly than the irrelevant cues (W and X). A subsequent test phase involved training with AW+, AX−, BW− trials. Learning to discriminate successfully between AW+ and BW− relies on learning about the previously relevant cues A and B (which are the relevant cues in this test phase discrimination), and hence should occur relatively quickly. In contrast, learning to discriminate between AW+ and AX− relies on learning about the previously

---

[3] In demonstrations of "simple" learned irrelevance, prior experience of an individual CS as being uncorrelated with a US leads to a retardation in subsequent learning about that CS (e.g., Baker & Mackintosh, 1977, 1979; Bennett *et al.*, 2000; Mackintosh, 1973; but see Bonardi & Hall, 1996; Bonardi & Ong, 2003). As in Wilson *et al.*'s (1992) study, the single CS is the only punctate cue presented on each trial. Crucially, however, in the case of learned irrelevance training the CS is a poorer predictor of the US than is the experimental context: the US can occur in the absence of the CS, but never in the absence of the context. Consequently, a relative predictiveness mechanism will discriminate against the CS. Indeed, the "standard" analysis of learned irrelevance in terms of attentional theories such as the Mackintosh model relies on a comparison of relative predictiveness between CS and context. In contrast, in studies supporting the Pearce–Hall model (e.g., Wilson *et al.*, 1992), the individually pretrained CS is a better predictor of the US than is the context, so there is no scope for a comparison of relative predictiveness to lead to a detriment in learning about that CS.

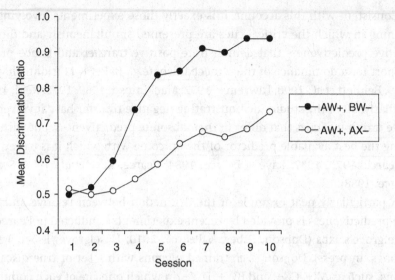

Figure 3.2 Mean discrimination ratios across the 10 sessions of test discrimination training in Experiment 1 of Dopson, *et al.* (2010). Discrimination ratios are calculated as CS+/(CS+ + CS−), where CS+ represents conditioned responding during the reinforced stimulus compound, and CS− represents responding during the non-reinforced compound.

irrelevant cues W and X (which are the relevant cues in this test discrimination), and hence should occur more slowly. Dopson *et al.*'s empirical data confirmed this prediction; the AW+, BW− discrimination was learnt significantly more rapidly than the AW+, AX− discrimination (Figure 3.2).

Haselgrove *et al.* (in press), ran a conceptually similar experiment using rats, but in which pretraining was with A+, B+, W+/−, X+/− trials. Thus A and B were consistently reinforced (as they were in Dopson *et al.*'s study), while W and X were partially reinforced (again, as they were in Dopson *et al.*'s study). The important difference between these two studies is that in Haselgrove *et al.*'s experiment, pretraining was with individual cues, each of which is the best available predictor of the outcome with which it is paired. Thus even on X+ trials, X is the best available predictor of reinforcement (it is a better predictor than the experimental context). Hence in this study, all cues will be more equal in relative predictiveness, such that the Pearce–Hall mechanism, based on absolute predictiveness, should dominate. One group of rats was subsequently trained with an AW+, BW− discrimination, the solution of which relies on learning about the high absolute predictiveness cues A and B, and hence should be learnt relatively slowly. A second group was trained with an AW+, AX− solution, which relies on learning about the low absolute predictiveness cues W

Table 3.2 *Design of experiment by Dopson,* et al. *(2010)*

Training Discriminations		Test Discrimination
AX+ CX−	AW+ CW−	
BW+ DW−	BX+ DX−	AW+ AX− BW−
AZ+ CZ−	AY+ CY−	
BY+ DY−	BZ+ DZ−	

Note: This experiment was run on a within-subjects basis; in each phase of training, all pigeons experienced all trial types indicated in the table.

and X, and which should therefore be learnt more rapidly. Again Haselgrove *et al.*'s empirical data confirmed this prediction: the AW+, AX− discrimination was learnt significantly more rapidly than the AW+, BW− discrimination (Figure 3.3).[4]

Thus, despite the initial training of these two experiments involving fundamentally the same cue–outcome relationships, diametrically opposite results were observed in each. This implies that the *form* of the initial training was the critical determinant of the overall associability of each of the cues involved, with multiple cue pretraining emphasizing the contribution of a Mackintosh-type process based on relative predictiveness, while individual cue pretraining emphasizes the contribution of a Pearce–Hall-type process based on absolute predictiveness. (That said, of course, we must acknowledge that these two studies were run in different species, using correspondingly different procedures. An even stronger case would be made if such opposing effects could be observed within a single species using one experimental procedure; this remains for the future.)

---

[4] Haselgrove *et al.*'s (in press) experiment is also noteworthy in that it provides, to the best of my knowledge, the only demonstration of a negative transfer associability effect in which predictiveness is established on a withinsubjects basis. Wilson *et al.*'s (1992) Experiment 3 also manipulated predictiveness within subjects but, in contrast to Experiments 1 and 2, only examined the influence of this manipulation on the magnitude of the orienting response elicited by the cues involved, and not on the rate of novel learning about these cues. Consequently, this study reveals nothing about how this within-subjects manipulation of predictiveness influenced the associability of the cues. Given the possibility that between-subjects training with differently predictive cues might induce motivational differences between the groups involved that could exert a general influence on the learning rate of those groups, Haselgrove *et al.*'s within-subjects demonstration is particularly important. The corresponding concern, however, is that considerable weight is being placed on a single, currently unpublished study; hopefully future studies will replicate this effect.

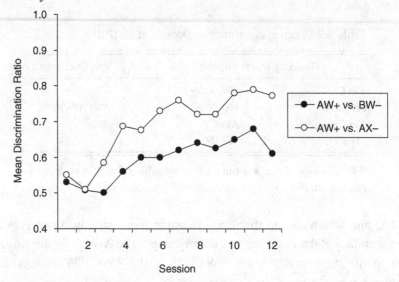

Figure 3.3 Mean discrimination ratios across the 12 sessions of test discrimination training in Experiment 1 of Haselgrove, Esber, Pearce, and Jones (in press). Discrimination ratios are calculated as described in the legend for Figure 3.2.

A hybrid model

The evidence regarding US- and CS-processing mechanisms reviewed above suggests that multiple processes might interact to determine how much is learnt about a given cue on a given trial. The implication is that the early "single-process" models of learning (Bush & Mosteller, 1951; Mackintosh, 1975; Pearce, 1987; Pearce & Hall, 1980; Rescorla & Wagner, 1972) are unable to provide a full account of the influence of associative history on future learning. This is not hugely surprising, given that these models have generally been developed to account for experimental effects within a fairly restricted domain.

Clearly, a more general model that is able to account for a wider range of effects of associative history must go beyond these single-process accounts. But the successes of certain models in their (restricted) domains mean that to abandon them entirely would be a case of throwing the baby out with the bathwater. An alternative approach is to combine the properties of several single-process models to yield a "hybrid" model of the influence of associative history that can account for a wider range of data than any of its individual components. One such model has been proposed by Le Pelley (2004). This was not the first model to bring multiple mechanisms together in order to better describe a range of data (e.g., Brandon *et al.*, 2003; Pearce, George, & Redhead, 1998; Schmajuk, Lam, & Gray, 1996), nor will it be the last (e.g., Pearce & Mackintosh, in press).

Here Le Pelley's (2004) model is merely used as an illustration of one way in which such a hybrid model may be built. Indeed, I am not particularly wedded to any specific formalization of such a model; my wider aim in this chapter is to demonstrate that multiple factors may contribute to the influence of associative history on future learning, and hence to provide support for the hybrid modeling approach in general.

The hybrid model has four component processes, each supported by the experimental evidence reviewed above:

Component 1: individual error term (US-processing)

Allows the model to account for unequal learning about the elements of a reinforced or non-reinforced compound (e.g., Leung & Westbrook, 2008; Rescorla, 2000, 2001, 2002). As noted earlier, these are the *only* effects that require this component; the model cannot explain such findings if this component is removed, but its account of other effects of associative history is essentially unchanged. Given recently suggested alternative accounts of Rescorla's findings (e.g., Harris, 2006; Schmajuk, 2009), the necessity of this component is not as clear as it perhaps first appeared.

Component 2: summed-error term (US-processing)

Allows the model to account for conditioned inhibition.

Component 3: "attentional associability," α (CS-processing)

Based on Mackintosh (1975) and determined by relative predictiveness; the best available predictor of the outcome on each trial maintains high α, while the α of other cues falls. Allows the model to account for demonstrations of positive transfer of associability.

Component 4: "salience associability," σ (CS-processing)

Based on Pearce–Hall (1980) and determined by absolute predictiveness; cues belonging to compounds with high absolute predictiveness will tend to have lower σ than cues belonging to compounds with low absolute predictiveness. Allows the model to account for demonstrations of negative transfer of associability.

Following Konorski (1967; see also Pearce & Hall, 1980; Schmajuk & Moore, 1985), the hybrid model draws a qualitative distinction between the associations on which excitatory and inhibitory conditioning are based. Excitatory associations are modeled as links between a representation of a CS and a representation of a US; inhibitory associations are modeled as links between a representation of the CS and a "no-US" representation ($\overline{US}$). It is assumed that there exists an inhibitory relationship between US and $\overline{US}$ representations such that if both are activated simultaneously, activity in the $\overline{US}$ representation will inhibit activity in the US representation. Hence, greater activation of the $\overline{US}$ representation will tend (other things being equal) to produce a reduction in conditioned responding.

Of course, a given CS might be followed by the US on some trials and by its absence on others, and as such might develop both excitatory and inhibitory associations. If we label the strength of the excitatory CS–US association for a given CS, A, as V_A, and the strength of the inhibitory CS–$\overline{US}$ association for this same cue as $\overline{V}_A$, then conditioned responding to A will be proportional to V_A^{NET}, where:

$$V_A^{NET} = V_A - \overline{V}_A \tag{3.1}$$

V_A^{NET} specifies the net extent to which the US is predicted by the presence of cue A. If several cues are presented simultaneously on a trial, then the overall expectancy of the US given the presence of all of these cues is calculated by summing V^{NET} across all presented cues. If we label the magnitude of the observed outcome on this trial as λ, then the summed error is given by R, where:

$$R = \lambda - \sum V^{NET} \tag{3.2}$$

If R is positive, then the expected magnitude of the outcome given the presence of these cues should increase, i.e., this is a trial that will support excitatory learning, so the value of V for each of the presented cues should increase. The equation determining this change for each cue, A, (labeled ΔV_A) on trials with R > 0 is:

$$\Delta V_A = \alpha_A \sigma_A \beta_E \cdot \left(1 - V_A^{NET}\right) \cdot R \tag{3.3}$$

where β_E is a learning-rate parameter for excitatory learning, and α_A and σ_A are CS-processing parameters that are discussed further below.

If, instead, R is negative, then the expected magnitude of the outcome given the presence of these cues should decrease, i.e., this is a trial that will support inhibitory learning, so the value of $\overline{V}$ for each of the presented cues should increase. The equation determining this change for each cue, A, on trials with R < 0 is:

$$\Delta \overline{V}_A = \alpha_A \sigma_A \beta_I \cdot \left(1 + V_A^{NET}\right) \cdot |R| \tag{3.4}$$

where β_I is a learning-rate parameter for inhibitory learning.

Note that each of Equations 3.3 and 3.4 contains a term relating to the individual prediction made by each cue $[(1-V_A^{NET})$ and $(1+V_A^{NET})$ respectively], and a summed-error term, R, both of which directly modulate the amount of learning that is undergone by that cue. These are the Components 1 and 2 mentioned above. Le Pelley (2004) demonstrated by simulation that these individual and summed-error terms allow the model to account for conditioned inhibition, and also Rescorla's demonstrations of unequal learning about the elements of a reinforced stimulus compound.

The α and σ terms relate to the CS-processing Components 3 and 4, respectively. α is determined following the framework suggested by Mackintosh (1975), wherein a cue maintains a high α to the extent that it is the best available predictor of the current outcome. The extent to which the outcome is predicted by cue A is represented by the absolute value of the individual error term relating to A on that trial, and consequently changes in α are determined by a comparison of the individual error term for A with that for all other presented cues, labeled X here. So on trials with $R > 0$, we have:

$$\Delta \alpha_A = \theta_E \cdot \left(\left| \lambda - V_X^{NET} \right| - \left| \lambda - V_A^{NET} \right| \right) \tag{3.5}$$

Thus, if the error term for A is smaller than that for all other cues, α_A will rise. When $R < 0$ the change in α is given by:

$$\Delta \alpha_A = \theta_I \cdot \left(\left| R + V_X^{NET} \right| - \left| \lambda + V_A^{NET} \right| \right) \tag{3.6}$$

So if A does a better job than X of predicting the absence of an absent-but-expected outcome, α_A will rise. θ_E and θ_I are learning-rate parameters for changes in α on excitatory and inhibitory trials, respectively.

The Pearce–Hall component determines σ on the basis of absolute predictiveness; cues belonging to compounds with high absolute predictiveness will have lower σ than those belonging to compounds with low absolute predictiveness. The hybrid model uses the equation suggested by Pearce, Kaye, and Hall (1982) in their amendment of the original Pearce–Hall model to determine σ_A on each trial n:

$$\sigma_A^n = \gamma \left| \lambda - \sum V^{NET} \right| + (1-\gamma) \sigma_A^{n-1} \tag{3.7}$$

Here the n and $n-1$ superscripts indicate that the value of σ_A on trial n is influenced by its former value on trial $n-1$, with the strength of this influence being determined by the parameter γ. If $\gamma \approx 1$ then σ is determined almost solely by the events of the immediately preceding trial, with earlier trials having little effect. Conversely, if $\gamma \approx 0$ then σ is determined largely by earlier trials, with the immediately preceding trial having little effect.

As shown in Equations 3.3 and 3.4, the overall CS-processing of cue A is determined by $\alpha_A \sigma_A$. The higher the value of $\alpha_A \sigma_A$, the more rapidly cue A will be learnt about. In order to account for certain empirical CS-processing effects, Le Pelley (2004) assumed that α operated over a wider range than did σ: here these values are restricted such that $0.01 \leq \alpha \leq 1$, while $0.3 \leq \sigma \leq 1$. This means that reductions in α can effectively halt learning about a cue regardless of its σ value (if $\alpha_A = 0.01$ then $\alpha_A \sigma_A$ will be small, even if $\sigma_A = 1$). Reductions in σ, while attenuating the rate of learning about a stimulus, will not prevent that learning to nearly the same extent (if $\sigma_A = 0.3$ then A can still undergo relatively large changes in associative strength if α_A is high).

These constraints mean that, in psychological terms, α (which is based on relative predictiveness) can be seen as a "selection" mechanism: *of the available stimuli, which is the best predictor of the outcome, i.e., which is the best candidate on which to focus processing resources?* In contrast, σ (which is based on absolute predictiveness) addresses the question: *given that a particular stimulus has been selected by the α mechanism, how much is there left to learn about this stimulus?* A stimulus that is not selected by the "attentional" α mechanism (i.e., a stimulus for which α is low) should receive little overall processing regardless of the accuracy of the predictions that it makes, and this is ensured because $\alpha \cdot \sigma$ will be low for such a stimulus.

As an illustration of how this hybrid model works, we can see how it applies to some of the studies that were discussed earlier.

Simulation 1: Baxter, et al. (1999, Experiment 2)

The design of Baxter *et al.*'s study of blocking is shown in Table 3.1. To recap, while lesions of the cholinergic input to the hippocampus had no effect on the magnitude of blocking observed in the test of B alone following AB+ training (defined as the difference in conditioned responding to B in experimental [BLK-E and BLK-I] versus control [CON] conditions), in the subsequent savings tests for excitatory (condition BLK-E) and inhibitory (condition BLK-I) conditioning, lesioned animals showed significantly more rapid learning than did sham-operated controls.

Figures 3.4 and 3.5 show simulation results for this study, using Le Pelley's (2004) hybrid model with the same set of parameters as used for simulations reported in that article ($\beta_E = 0.5$, $\beta_I = 0.1$, $\theta_E = 0.8$, $\theta_I = 0.1$, $\gamma = 0.1$, starting value of $\alpha = 0.9$, starting value of $\sigma = 0.9$, λ [US present] = 0.8, λ [US absent] = 0). Following Baxter *et al.*'s suggestion that lesioning the cholinergic input to the hippocampus prevents cues from undergoing a reduction in associability, for all simulations involving lesioned rats both α and σ were not permitted to decrease. All other simulation details were identical for lesioned and sham animals.

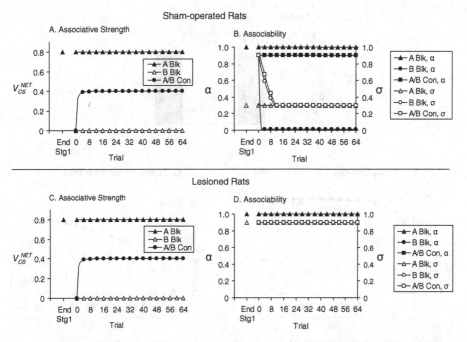

Figure 3.4 Results of a simulation of Baxter, *et al.*'s (1999) Experiment 2, using Le Pelley's (2004) hybrid model. Data are shown separately for cues A and B in the conditions given blocking treatment ("A Blk" and "B Blk"; results are averaged over conditions BLK-E and BLK-I), and as a mean for A and B in the control condition ("A/B Con", since A and B are equivalent in this condition). Data are shown for the final presentation in Stage 1, and across Stage 2 training. Panel A: Net associative strength of each cue for shams. Panel B: Associability (α and σ) of each cue for shams. Panel C: Net associative strength of each cue for lesioned rats. Panel D: Associability (α and σ) of each cue for lesioned rats. Simulation used the same number of presentations of each cue/compound as Baxter *et al.*'s empirical study (96 presentations in Stage 1; 64 in Stage 2; 4 test presentations of B− in extinction; then 64 presentations of the appropriate stimuli in either the excitatory or inhibitory savings test; see Table 3.1).

Blocking is clearly demonstrated in the simulations for sham-lesioned rats: in the test of B following AB+ training, V_B^{NET} is considerably lower in experimental conditions (that have received A+, AB+ blocking training) than in the control condition (that has received only AB+ training). According to the hybrid model, blocking training influences both US- and CS-processing mechanisms in these animals. In terms of US-processing, prior A+ training ensures that the US occurring on AB+ trials is already well predicted (i.e., the summed-error term $\left(\lambda - \left[V_A^{NET} + V_B^{NET}\right]\right)$ is small), and hence this US is able to support very little additional learning about B. In terms of CS-processing, on

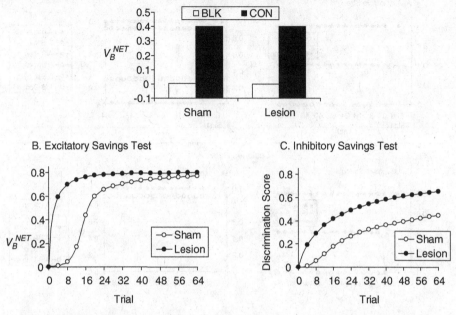

Figure 3.5 Test phase results of a simulation of Baxter, *et al.*'s (1999) Experiment 2, using Le Pelley's (2004) hybrid model. Panel A: Mean net associative strength of cue B during the four blocking test trials in extinction immediately following Stage 2 training. Results have been averaged for conditions BLK-E and BLK-I. The magnitude of the predicted blocking effect is very similar for shams and lesioned rats. Panel B: Net associative strength of B during the excitatory savings test for condition BLK-E. Conditioned responding to B develops more rapidly in lesioned rats than shams. Panel C: Discrimination performance during the inhibitory savings test for condition BLK-I. Discrimination score is the difference between responding on reinforced A+ trials and non-reinforced AB− trials. Discrimination is learnt more rapidly in lesioned rats than shams.

AB+ trials there will be a reduction in both α_B (since B is a poorer predictor of the US on AB+ trials than is A) and σ_B (since the US on AB+ trials is well predicted by the presence of A). Hence, both of these CS-processing components will produce a reduction in the associability of B, reducing the rate of any subsequent learning about B. One consequence of this reduction in the associability of B will be that conditioning (either excitatory or inhibitory) to B in the subsequent savings tests will be retarded relative to lesioned rats, for which B has been prevented from undergoing this reduction in associability; see Figures 3.5B and 3.5C. This is, of course, the pattern observed in Baxter *et al.*'s empirical data.

Crucially, however, despite the fact that blocking treatment has not produced a reduction in the associability of B for lesioned rats, the hybrid model correctly predicts that the magnitude of blocking in these animals will be very similar to that in shams (Figure 3.5A). This is because the US-processing component based on a summed-error term remains intact in lesioned rats: if the US on AB+ trials can support very little additional learning, then very little will be learnt about B regardless of its associability.

So the hybrid model is able to provide a good account of the key findings of Baxter *et al.*'s study (see also Holland & Fox, 2003), and it is able to do so precisely because it implicates both CS- and US-processing mechanisms in blocking.

Simulation 2: Dopson, et al. (2010, Experiment 1)

Table 3.2 shows the design of this study. Recall that pigeons were originally trained with a set of true discriminations, in which one cue of each compound (A, B, C, or D) was relevant to the solution, while the other (V, W, X, or Y) was irrelevant. In a subsequent test, these pigeons learnt a discrimination between AW+ and BW− (the solution of which relies on learning about previously relevant cues A and B) more rapidly than a discrimination between AW+ and AX− (the solution of which relies on learning about previously irrelevant cues W and X).

Figure 3.6 shows simulation results for this study. The empirical data revealed that learning was rather slow in this study, and quite extensive training was used. Hence, to more accurately model these data all rate parameters were reduced by a factor of 10, giving $\beta_E = 0.05$, $\beta_I = 0.01$, $\theta_E = 0.08$, $\theta_I = 0.01$, $\gamma = 0.01$.

The hybrid model anticipates that, during initial training, the α value of relevant cues A–D will increase, while that of irrelevant cues V–Y will decrease, since the relevant cues have higher relative predictiveness on each trial. The σ values of all cues will fall at a similar rate, however, since all *compounds* are equally predictive of the outcome with which they are paired (and σ is calculated using a summed error; see Equation 3.7). Consequently, following training, the overall associability $\alpha \times \sigma$ of relevant cues will be greater than that of irrelevant cues, and hence the model correctly predicts that learning of a discrimination that relies on these relevant cues (AW+, BW−) will proceed more rapidly than one that relies on irrelevant cues (AW+, AX−).

Simulation 3: Haselgrove, Esber, Pearce, and Jones (in press)

During the training phase of this study A and B were consistently reinforced while W and X were partially reinforced. In a subsequent test phase rats learnt a discrimination between AW+ and AX− more rapidly than a discrimination between AW+ and BW−.

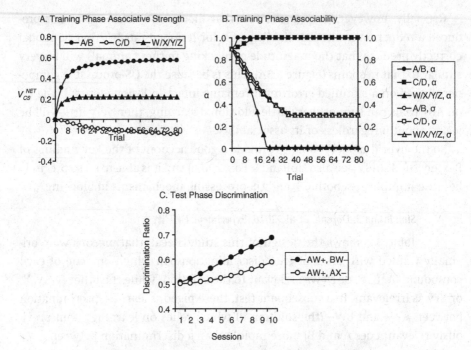

Figure 3.6 Results of a simulation of Dopson, *et al.*'s (2010) Experiment 1, using Le Pelley's (2004) hybrid model. Data have been averaged for cues A and B, for cues C and D, and for cues W, X, Y, and Z. Panel A: net associative strength of cues across training. Panel B: associability (α and σ) of cues across training. Panel C: discrimination performance across the ten 20-trial sessions of the test phase, with discrimination ratios calculated as described in the legend for Figure 3.2. Simulation used the same number of presentations of each compound as Dopson *et al.*'s empirical study (80 presentations during training phase; 200 during test phase). Related empirical data are shown in Figure 3.2.

Figure 3.7 shows simulation results for this study, using the same parameters as for Dopson *et al.*'s study as described above. During the training phase, the α value of all cues rises, since all cues are the best (and only) available predictors of the outcomes with which they are paired.[5] However, the σ values of these cues fall at different rates. Learning about the consistently reinforced cues A and B ensures that they quickly become accurate predictors of the US with which they are paired, and hence σ_A and σ_B will fall rapidly. In contrast,

[5] A more complete simulation of this experiment would include a cue representing the experimental context that is present on each trial. However, continual, non-reinforced exposure to the context during inter-trial intervals ensures that the context will be a poor predictor of the US on any trial on which it occurs, such that inclusion of a context cue will have very little effect on the α values of the punctuate cues (as simulations have confirmed). Consequently, for simplicity, the context is omitted in the simulations reported here.

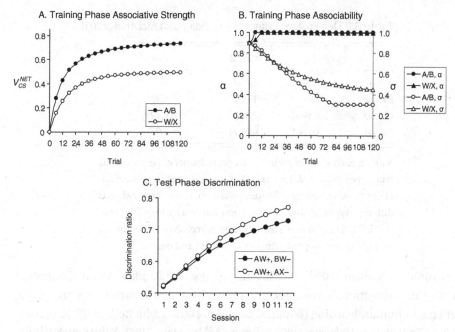

Figure 3.7 Results of a simulation of Haselgrove, Esber, Pearce, and Jones's (submitted) Experiment 1, using Le Pelley's (2004) hybrid model. Data have been averaged for cues A and B, and for cues W and X. Panel A: net associative strength of cues across training. Panel B: associability (α and σ) of cues across training. Panel C: discrimination performance across the twelve 16-trial sessions of the test phase, with discrimination ratios calculated as described in the legend for Figure 3.2. Simulation used the same number of presentations of each compound as Haselgrove *et al.*'s empirical study (240 presentations during training phase [each "trial" of Panels A and B involves two presentations of each compound]; 192 during test phase). Related empirical data are shown in Figure 3.2.

the inconsistency of the outcome following W and X ensures that these cues never become such accurate predictors, and hence σ_W and σ_X fall more slowly. The upshot is that, following training, the overall associability $\alpha \times \sigma$ of W and X will be greater than that of A and B, and hence the model correctly predicts that learning of a discrimination that relies on these relevant cues (AW+, BW−) will proceed more rapidly than one that relies on irrelevant cues (AW+, AX−).

CS-processing mechanisms in human contingency learning

Up to this point we have been considering the impact of associative history on future learning in studies of animal conditioning. It has been suggested, however, that under some circumstances at least, a common associative learning mechanism might underlie animal conditioning and human contingency

Table 3.3 *Design of experiment by Le Pelley and McLaren (2003)*

	Stage 1	Stage 2	Test
AV–o1	AW–o1	AX–o3	AC?
BV–o2	BW–o2	BY–o4	BD?
CX–o2	CY–o2	CV–o3	VX?
DX–o1	DY–o1	DW–o4	WY?

Note: In each stage of training, all participants experienced all trial types indicated. Letters A–Y represent cues to be learned about (foods eaten by a fictitious patient), associated with various different types of allergic reactions (outcomes o1–o4). On test, participants rated how strongly they perceived each of the compounds shown as predicting outcomes o3 and o4.

learning (Dickinson, 2001; Dickinson, Shanks, & Evenden, 1984). Consistent with this suggestion, several recent studies have demonstrated CS-processing effects in human learning (Bonardi, Graham, Hall, & Mitchell, 2005; Kruschke, 1996; Le Pelley & McLaren, 2003; Livesey & McLaren, 2007; Whitney & White, 1993). Notably, all of these studies have demonstrated faster learning about previously predictive cues than previously nonpredictive cues, and hence all are consistent with the Mackintosh model. That said, all of these studies established predictiveness in a pretraining phase involving multiple, simultaneously presented cues, some of which were better predictors than others – exactly the circumstances that, as argued above, would allow the relative predictiveness mechanism of the Mackintosh model to dominate.

As an example, the design of Le Pelley and McLaren's (2003) experiment is shown in Table 3.3. This experiment used an allergy prediction cover story, in which participants had to predict what sort of allergic reaction (outcome) a patient would suffer after eating various foods (cues). Letters A to D and V to Y represent cues and o1–o4 represent outcomes; e.g., "AV–o1" indicates that cues A and V (e.g., apples and ham) were presented together, and were paired with allergic reaction o1 (e.g., headache). During Stage 1, cues A and D were consistently paired with o1, B and C were consistently paired with o2, and V–Y provided no basis for discrimination, being paired with o1 and o2 equally. Hence, cues A–D were better predictors during Stage 1 than were cues V–Y, such that α_{A-D} (used to denote the α values of cues A–D, all of which are equivalent) will be higher than α_{V-Y}. Since all *compounds* are equally predictive of the outcomes with which they are paired, the absolute predictiveness mechanism of the Pearce–Hall model will not differentiate between these cues. The upshot

Table 3.4 *Design of the experiment by Le Pelley et al. (2010)*

Stage 1		Stage 2
A–o1	A–o1	A–o3
B–o2	B–o2	B–o4
C–o2	C–o2	C–o3
D–o1	D–o1	D–o4
X–o1	X–o2	X–o3
Y–o1	Y–o2	Y–o4

Note: In each stage of training, all participants experienced all trial types indicated. Letters A–Y represent cues to be learned about (names of fictional companies), associated in Stage 1 with different colors of business cards (o1 and o2), and in Stage 2 with profit or loss (o3 and o4).

is that $\alpha \times \sigma$ will be greater for relevant cues than for irrelevant cues, and hence a positive transfer effect is predicted.

On each Stage 2 trial a compound of a previously relevant and a previously irrelevant cue was paired with a new outcome (o3 or o4). If the overall associability of previously relevant cues were higher than that of previously irrelevant cues, then we should expect that, for example, on AX–o3 trials participants will learn more about the A–o3 relationship than the X–o3 relationship. To test this idea, in a final test phase, participants were asked to rate various combinations of cues according to how strongly they were perceived as predicting outcomes o3 and o4. A positive transfer effect was demonstrated, in that participants judged compound AC (which comprised cues that were relevant during Stage 1, and which were paired with o3 in Stage 2) as a significantly stronger cause of o3 than was compound VX (which comprised cues that had received identical training to A and C during Stage 2, but which had been irrelevant in Stage 1). Likewise, BD was judged to be a stronger cause of o4 than was WY.

If the mechanisms underlying cue-processing effects in humans and animals are similar, then on the basis of the argument presented earlier, we might expect that pretraining human participants with separately presented, individual cues (thereby minimizing any influence of relative predictiveness) might instead produce results consistent with the Pearce–Hall model; namely, more rapid learning about previously nonpredictive cues than previously predictive cues. This possibility has recently been assessed by Le Pelley, Turnbull, Reimers, and Knipe (2010), using the design shown in Table 3.4.

During Stage 1, participants had to predict the colors of business cards (outcomes) produced by various companies (cues). As in Le Pelley and McLaren's (2003) study, cues A–D were consistently paired with a particular outcome, while cues X and Y were paired with o1 on half of trials and with o2 on the other. But crucially, in this latter experiment training was with individual cues, such that each cue was the best available predictor of the outcome with which it was paired on each trial, and hence, relative predictiveness does not discriminate between cues. The absolute predictiveness of cues A–D will, of course, be greater than that of X and Y, and hence, if cue-processing mechanisms in humans are analogous to those in animals, we would expect subsequent learning to be more rapid for cues X and Y (the previously nonpredictive cues) than for A–D (the previously predictive cues); that is, we should expect negative transfer.

During Stage 2 participants had to learn a discrimination in which the original cues were followed by new outcomes, o3 and o4, as shown in Table 3.4 (in terms of the scenario, subjects had to learn whether investment in a given company would result in a profit [o3] or a loss [o4]). Contrary to the prediction of negative transfer, however, Le Pelley et al. (2010) observed faster learning during Stage 2 for cues A–D than for cues X and Y; just as in Le Pelley and McLaren's (2003) study, positive transfer occurred. Consistent with this finding, Beesley and Le Pelley (2010) have recently provided another example of positive, rather than negative, transfer of associability following individual cue pretraining in an "implicit" learning task.

Unlike in animal studies, where the influence of predictive history on subsequent learning seems to depend on how predictiveness is established (with individual cue training producing more rapid learning about inconsistent predictors than consistent predictors, while training with multiple, simultaneously presented stimuli produces more rapid learning about consistent predictors than inconsistent predictors), these findings imply that in the case of human contingency learning there is always a learning advantage for consistent predictors, regardless of whether cues are trained individually or as part of a compound. Thus, it would seem that the cue-processing mechanisms that operate in animals are not entirely analogous to those that influence human contingency learning.

In fact, the suggestion of a difference between humans and nonhuman animals in tasks involving pretraining with individual cues is not without precedent. It has been noted many times that animals and humans differ in their propensity to show latent inhibition, the detrimental effect of non-reinforced exposure to a CS on the rate of subsequent conditioning of that CS (e.g., Graham & McLaren, 1998; Lubow, 1973; Lubow & Gewirtz, 1995). Latent inhibition is often viewed as reflecting a reduction in the associability of the pre-exposed stimulus during non-reinforced preexposure (which is typically conducted with that stimulus presented in isolation), and follows naturally from the Pearce–Hall model (although alternative accounts have also been advanced, see Hall, 1991). While findings of latent inhibition in animal studies are ubiquitous (see Lubow, 1989), analogous studies with humans have typically failed to reveal a similar effect, and those studies that have claimed to demonstrate "simple" latent inhibition in humans are typically open to alternative explanation (Graham & McLaren, 1998; Le Pelley & Schmidt-Hansen, 2010). Like Le Pelley *et al.*'s (2010) study, then, this interpretation sees latent inhibition as an associability effect arising from single-cue pretraining that differs between humans and nonhuman animals. Moreover, those studies that *have* reported a latent inhibition-like effect in humans have almost invariably used a masking task during pre-exposure, which functions to divert attention away from the pre-exposed stimulus. Consequently, use of a masking task allows relative predictiveness processes to operate, by creating a situation more akin to pretraining with multiple, simultaneously presented cues which differ in their predictiveness (Le Pelley & Schmidt-Hansen, 2010). That is, the pre-exposed stimulus is less predictive of the response to be made on the masking task (being entirely irrelevant to that task) than are the stimuli of the masking task themselves, and hence selective attention (operating on the basis of relative predictiveness much as suggested by Mackintosh, 1975) would tend to move away from the pre-exposed stimulus (a similar analysis is suggested by Graham & McLaren, 1998). Given that, as noted earlier, it is well established that humans and animals alike tend to show a retardation in learning about less predictive cues following multiple-cue pretraining, it is therefore unsurprising that slower learning about the pre-exposed cue is observed under these conditions.

In summary, then, the implication is that while the hybrid model account by Le Pelley (2004) might provide a satisfactory account of associative history effects in animal conditioning, it may not apply equally to related effects in human contingency learning.

Falsifiability and parsimony

Before concluding, I would like to address two criticisms that have sometimes been leveled at the hybrid modeling approach. The first is that the greater complexity of hybrid models as compared with single-process accounts can potentially render the former unfalsifiable. This is certainly a concern; combining multiple components in a model of learning will almost inevitably increase the number of free parameters, and this will potentially increase the model's ability to account for *any* observable pattern of data. Indeed, the model outlined above is specifically designed to be able to account for seemingly opposing phenomena (negative and positive transfer). It is understandable that this ability might raise suspicion amongst theorists.

This criticism is valid only to the extent that a particular hybrid model is underspecified. That is, a hybrid model in which the impact of each of the components, and the parameters determining the operation of each component, are allowed to vary arbitrarily between experiments according to the whim of the modeler is not a useful model. Thus, it is absolutely essential that the model acts in a principled way, and specifies clearly and precisely how the components will interact, and when each might be expected to dominate. For example, the fact that, in Le Pelley's (2004) hybrid model, the Mackintosh-type α mechanism relies on a comparison of relative predictiveness while the Pearce–Hall-type σ mechanism relies on absolute predictiveness means that this model makes clear and testable predictions about the circumstances under which positive transfer versus negative transfer will obtain. Indeed, our recent data (Le Pelley *et al.*, 2010) have falsified this hybrid model as an account of cue-processing mechanisms in human contingency learning. Evidently, this is a falsifiable model!

The other criticism of the hybrid modeling approach is that hybrid models are inherently less parsimonious than the single-process models on which they are based. To make this argument, however, is to confuse "parsimony" and "simplicity". It is certainly true that hybrid models are, by definition, less simple than single-process models. Parsimony, however, refers to the idea that "no more entities, causes, or forces than necessary should be invoked in explaining a set of facts or observations." And, as described at length in this chapter, the set of observations that constitutes empirical evidence relating to the influence of associative history on future learning contains many examples of seemingly contradictory effects which defy explanation in terms of simple, single-process models. While these single-process models certainly provide parsimonious accounts of empirical phenomena *within their own domain*, they do not provide a parsimonious account of the wider range of effects of associative history, as they are unable to explain many of these effects. For example, the Pearce–Hall model provides a parsimonious account of negative transfer effects, but it does not provide a parsimonious account of the whole set of both positive and negative transfer effects, as it is unable to account for the positive transfer effects at all. Given the many, varied, and often seemingly contradictory effects of associative history on future learning, it is quite possible that a hybrid model does provide the most parsimonious account of the full set of effects to which it can be applied.

Conclusion

No model claims to provide a complete account of a whole field of psychology, and models of learning are no exception to this rule. Instead, models are developed to explain findings within a (typically) narrowly circumscribed area. This is a reflection of the scientific approach taken when studying associative learning: experiments are carefully designed so as to isolate the influence of a particular, putative learning mechanism, and to control for (and hence minimize the impact of) other potential influences. But this does not deny the *existence* of these "other influences," whatever they may be.

This is clearly a sensible approach to take if our goal is to understand the workings of a complex and multi-faceted system which underlies learning, just as if our goal were to understand the workings of a car's engine, we should want to understand how each component of that engine works in isolation. The aim of this chapter is not to undermine the work that has been done in establishing the various ways in which the associative history of a stimulus might influence future learning about that stimulus, or to argue that accounts that have previously been offered to explain these phenomena are incorrect. Instead, it is simply to suggest that looking at the individual components of the engine in isolation can take us only so far. If we are to truly understand the engine, at some point we must move on from examining the individual components in isolation, and instead begin to look at how they interact with one another. While the hybrid modeling approach clearly does not yet provide a "grand, unified theory" of learning, it represents an attempt to understand these interactions without throwing out what we already know about the individual components.

References

Baker, A. G. & Mackintosh, N. J. (1977). Excitatory and inhibitory conditioning following uncorrelated presentations of CS and UCS. *Animal Learning and Behavior*, **5**, 315–319.

Baker, A. G. & Mackintosh, N. J. (1979). Preexposure to the CS alone, or CS and US uncorrelated: latent inhibition, blocking by context or learned irrelevance? *Learning and Motivation*, **10**, 278–294.

Baxter, M. G., Gallagher, M. & Holland, P. C. (1999). Blocking can occur without losses in attention in rats with selective removal of hippocampal cholinergic input. *Behavioral Neuroscience*, **113**, 881–890.

Beesley, T. & Le Pelley, M. E. (2010). The effect of predictive history on the learning of sub-sequence contingencies. *Quarterly Journal of Experimental Psychology*, **63**, 108–135.

Bennett, C. H., Wills, S. J., Oakeshott, S. M. & Mackintosh, N. J. (2000). Is the context specificity of latent inhibition a sufficient explanation of learned irrelevance? *Quarterly Journal of Experimental Psychology*, **53B**, 239–253.

Bonardi, C. & Hall, G. (1996). Learned irrelevance: no more than the sum of CS and US preexposure effects? *Journal of Experimental Psychology: Animal Behavior Processes*, **22**, 183–191.

Bonardi, C. & Ong, S. Y. (2003). Learned irrelevance: a contemporary overview. *Quarterly Journal of Experimental Psychology*, **56B**, 80–89.

Bonardi, C., Graham, S., Hall, G. & Mitchell, C. J. (2005). Acquired distinctiveness and equivalence in human discrimination learning: evidence for an attentional process. *Psychonomic Bulletin and Review*, **12**, 88–92.

Brandon, S. E., Vogel, E. H. & Wagner, A. R. (2003). Stimulus representation in SOP i: theoretical rationalization and some implications. *Behavioral Processes*, **62**, 5–25.

Bush, R. R. & Mosteller, F. (1951). A mathematical model for simple learning. *Psychological Review*, **58**, 313–323.

Dias, R., Robbins, T. W. & Roberts, A. C. (1996). Dissociation in prefrontal cortex of affective and attentional shifts. *Nature*, **380**, 69–72.

Dickinson, A. (2001). Causal learning: an associative analysis. *Quarterly Journal of Experimental Psychology Section B: Comparative and Physiological Psychology*, **54**, 3–25.

Dickinson, A., Shanks, D. R. & Evenden, J. L. (1984). Judgement of act-outcome contingency: the role of selective attribution. *Quarterly Journal of Experimental Psychology*, **36A**, 29–50.

Dopson, J., Esber, G. R. & Pearce, J. M. (2010). Differences between the associability of relevant and irrelevant stimuli are not due to acquired equivalence and distinctiveness. *Journal of Experimental Psychology: Animal Behavior Processes*, **36**, 258–267.

Estes, W. K. (1950). Toward a statistical theory of learning. *Psychological Review*, **57**, 94–107.

George, D. N. & Pearce, J. M. (1999). Acquired distinctiveness is controlled by stimulus relevance not correlation with reward. *Journal of Experimental Psychology: Animal Behavior Processes*, **25**, 363–373.

Graham, S. & McLaren, I. P. L. (1998). Retardation in human discrimination learning as a consequence of preexposure: latent inhibition or negative priming? *Quarterly Journal of Experimental Psychology*, **51B**, 155–172.

Hall, G. (1991). *Perceptual and Associative Learning*. Oxford, UK: Oxford University Press.

Hall, G. & Pearce, J. M. (1979). Latent inhibition of a CS during CS-US pairings. *Journal of Experimental Psychology: Animal Behavior Processes*, **3**, 31–42.

Hall, G. & Pearce, J. M. (1982). Restoring the associability of a preexposed CS by a surprising event. *Quarterly Journal of Experimental Psychology*, **34B**, 127–140.

Harris, J. A. (2006). Elemental representations of stimuli in associative learning. *Psychological Review*, **113**, 584–605.

Harris, J. A. (2010). The arguments of associations. In N. A. Schmajuk, ed., *Computational Models of Conditioning*. Cambridge, UK: Cambridge University Press.

Haselgrove, M., Esber, G. R., Pearce, J. M. & Jones, P. M. (in press). Differences in stimulus associability following continuous and partial reinforcement. *Journal of Experimental Psychology: Animal Behavior Processes*.

Holland, P. C. & Fox, G. D. (2003). Effects of hippocampal lesions in overshadowing and blocking procedures. *Behavioral Neuroscience*, **117**, 650–656.

Kamin, L. J. (1969). Predictability, surprise, attention and conditioning. In B. A. Campbell and R. M. Church, eds., *Punishment and Aversive Behavior*. New York: Appleton–Century–Crofts, pp. 279–296.

Kaye, H. & Pearce, J. M. (1984). The strength of the orienting response during Pavlovian conditioning. *Journal of Experimental Psychology: Animal Behavior Processes*, **10**, 90–109.

Konorski, J. (1967). *Integrative Activity of the Brain*. Chicago, Ill: University of Chicago Press.

Kruschke, J. K. (1996). Dimensional relevance shifts in category learning. *Connection Science*, **8**, 225–247.

Kruschke, J. K. (2001). Towards a unified model of attention in associative learning. *Journal of Mathematical Psychology*, **45**, 812–863.

Lawrence, D. H. (1952). The transfer of a discrimination along a continuum. *Journal of Comparative and Physiological Psychology*, **45**, 511–516.

Le Pelley, M. E. (2004). The role of associative history in models of associative learning: a selective review and a hybrid model. *Quarterly Journal of Experimental Psychology*, **57B**, 193–243.

Le Pelley, M. E. & McLaren, I. P. L. (2003). Learned associability and associative change in human causal learning. *Quarterly Journal of Experimental Psychology*, **56B**, 68–79.

Le Pelley, M. E. & Schmidt-Hansen, M. (2010). Latent inhibition and learned irrelevance in human contingency learning. In R. E. Lubow and I. Weiner, eds., *Latent Inhibition: Cognition, Neuroscience, and Applications to Schizophrenia*. Cambridge, UK: Cambridge University Press, pp. 94–113.

Le Pelley, M. E., Turnbull, M. N., Reimers, S. J. & Knipe, R. L. (2010). Learned predictiveness effects following single-cue training in humans. *Learning and Behavior*, **38**, 126–144.

Leung, H. T. & Westbrook, R. F. (2008). Spontaneous recovery of extinguished fear responses deepens their extinction: a role for error-correction mechanisms. *Journal of Experimental Psychology: Animal Behavior Processes*, **34**, 461–474.

Livesey, E. J. & McLaren, I. P. L. (2007). Elemental associability changes in human discrimination learning. *Journal of Experimental Psychology: Animal Behavior Processes*, **33**, 148–159.

Lovejoy, E. (1968). *Attention in Discrimination Learning*. San Francisco, CA: Holden-Day.

Lubow, R. E. (1973). Latent inhibition. *Psychological Bulletin*, **79**, 398–407.

Lubow, R. E. (1989). *Latent Inhibition and Conditioned Attention Theory*. Cambridge, UK: Cambridge University Press.

Lubow, R. E. & Gewirtz, J. C. (1995). Latent inhibition in humans: data, theory, and implications for schizophrenia. *Psychological Bulletin*, **117**, 87–103.

Mackintosh, N. J. (1969). Further analysis of the overtraining reversal effect. *Journal of Comparative and Physiological Psychology,* **67**.

Mackintosh, N. J. (1973). Stimulus selection: learning to ignore stimuli that predict no change in reinforcement. In R. A. Hinde and J. S. Hinde, eds., *Constraints on Learning*. London: Academic Press, pp. 75–96.

Mackintosh, N. J. (1975). A theory of attention: variations in the associability of stimuli with reinforcement. *Psychological Review,* **82**, 276–298.

Mackintosh, N. J. (1978). Cognitive or associative theories of conditioning: implications of an analysis of blocking. In H. Fowler, W. K. Honig and S. H. Pulse, eds., *Cognitive Processes in Animal Behavior*. Hillsdale, NJ: Erlbaum, pp. 155–175.

Mackintosh, N. J. & Turner, C. (1971). Blocking as a function of novelty of CS and predictability of UCS. *Quarterly Journal of Experimental Psychology,* **23**, 359–366.

Pavlov, I. P. (1927). *Conditioned Reflexes*. London: Oxford University Press.

Pearce, J. M. (1987). A model for stimulus generalization in Pavlovian conditioning. *Psychological Review,* **94**, 61–73.

Pearce, J. M. (1994). Similarity and discrimination: a selective review and a connectionist model. *Psychological Review,* **101**, 587–607.

Pearce, J. M. & Hall, G. (1980). A model for Pavlovian conditioning: variations in the effectiveness of conditioned but not of unconditioned stimuli. *Psychological Review,* **87**, 532–552.

Pearce, J. M., George, D. N. & Redhead, E. S. (1998). The role of attention in the solution of conditional discriminations. In N. A. Schmajuk and P. C. Holland, eds., *Occasion Setting: Associative Learning and Cognition in Animals*. Washington, D.C.: American Psychological Association.

Pearce, J. M. Kaye, H. & Hall, G. (1982). Predictive accuracy and stimulus associability: development of a model for Pavlovian conditioning. In M. L. Commons, R. J. Herrnstein and A. R. Wagner, eds., *Quantitative Analyses of Behavior: Acquisition* (Vol. 3). Cambridge, MA: Ballinger.

Pearce, J. M. & Mackintosh, N. J. (in press). Two theories of attention: a review and a possible integration. In C. J. Mitchell and M. E. Le Pelley, eds., *Attention and Associative Learning: From Brain to Behaviour*. Oxford, UK: Oxford University Press.

Pearce, J. M., Nicholas, D. J. & Dickinson, A. (1982). Loss of associability by a conditioned inhibitor. *Quarterly Journal of Experimental Psychology,* **34B**, 149–162.

Reid, L. S. (1953). The development of noncontinuity behavior through continuity learning. *Journal of Experimental Psychology,* **46**, 107–112.

Rescorla, R. A. (1969). Pavlovian conditioned inhibition. *Psychological Bulletin,* **72**, 77–94.

Rescorla, R. A. (2000). Associative changes in excitors and inhibitors differ when they are conditioned in compound. *Journal of Experimental Psychology: Animal Behavior Processes,* **26**, 428–438.

Rescorla, R. A. (2001). Unequal associative changes when excitors and neutral stimuli are conditioned in compound. *Quarterly Journal of Experimental Psychology,* **54B**, 53–68.

Rescorla, R. A. (2002). Effect of following an excitatory-inhibitory compound with an intermediate reinforcer. *Journal of Experimental Psychology: Animal Behavior Processes*, **28**, 163–174.

Rescorla, R. A. & Wagner, A. R. (1972). A theory of Pavlovian conditioning: variations in the effectiveness of reinforcement and non-reinforcement. In A. H. Black and W. F. Prokasy, eds., *Classical Conditioning* II: *Current Research and Theory*. New York: Appleton–Century–Crofts, pp. 64–69.

Schmajuk, N. A. (2009). Attentional and error-correcting associative mechanisms in classical conditioning. *Journal of Experimental Psychology: Animal Behavior Processes*, **35**, 407–418.

Schmajuk, N. A. & Moore, J. W. (1985). Real-time attentional models for classical conditioning and the hippocampus. *Physiological Psychology*, **13**, 278–290.

Schmajuk, N. A., Lam, Y. W. & Gray, J. A. (1996). Latent inhibition: a neural network approach. *Journal of Experimental Psychology: Animal Behavior Processes*, **22**, 321–349.

Shepp, B. E. & Eimas, P. D. (1964). Intradimensional and extradimensional shifts in the rat. *Journal of Comparative and Physiological Psychology*, **57**, 357–361.

Shepp, B. E. & Schrier, A. M. (1969). Consecutive intradimensional and extradimensional shifts in monkeys. *Journal of Comparative and Physiological Psychology*, **67**, 199–203.

Sutherland, N. S. & Mackintosh, N. J. (1971). *Mechanisms of Animal Discrimination Learning*. New York: Academic Press.

Swan, J. A. & Pearce, J. M. (1988). The orienting response as an index of stimulus associability in rats. *Journal of Experimental Psychology: Animal Behavior Processes*, **4**, 292–301.

Whitney, L. & White, K. G. (1993). Dimensional shift and the transfer of attention. *Quarterly Journal of Experimental Psychology*, **46B**, 225–252.

Wilson, P. N., Boumphrey, P. & Pearce, J. M. (1992). Restoration of the orienting response to a light by a change in its predictive accuracy. *Quarterly Journal of Experimental Psychology*, **44B**, 17–36.

Zeaman, D. & House, B. J. (1963). The role of attention in retardate discrimination learning. In N. R. Ellis, ed., *Handbook of Mental Deficiency: Psychological Theory and Research*. New York: McGraw-Hill, pp. 378–418.

4

Within-compound associations:
models and data

JAMES E. WITNAUER AND RALPH R. MILLER

Abstract

During compound conditioning in which two or more cues are paired with an unconditioned stimulus (US), animals form associations between each cue and the US and associations between the cues (the latter of which are called within-compound associations). Most contemporary theories of associative learning assert that summation of cue–US associations drives negative mediation (e.g., blocking, overshadowing, and conditioned inhibition) because of their effects on the processing of the US representation. Using a computational modeling approach, we reviewed and simulated experiments that suggest that within-compound associations are necessary for cue interactions. A mathematical model that attributes all cue interactions to within-compound associations provided a better fit than a model that attributes negative mediation effects to variations in processing of the US. Overall, the results of this analysis suggest that within-compound associations are important for all cue interactions, including cue competition, conditioned inhibition, counteraction effects, retrospective revaluation, and second-order conditioning.

Within-compound associations: models and data

Pavlov (1927) discovered that both positive and negative mediation effects can occur when a target cue (X) is presented during training in conjunction with a nontarget cue (A). Positive mediation effects refer to situations in which the presence of A during training results in more excitatory behavioral control by X than if X was trained elementally. An example of positive mediation is second-order conditioning, which occurs when A–unconditioned stimulus (A–US) pairings (Phase 1) precede X–A pairings (Phase 2, which presumably establishes an X–A within-compound association), resulting in more excitatory conditioned responding to X than in a control condition lacking one or the other phase (Pavlov, 1927). Sensory preconditioning (Brogden, 1939) and potentiation (Rusiniak, Hankins, Garcia, & Brett, 1979) are other examples in which A positively mediates responding to X. In each of these examples, compound (AX) training results in greater responding to X than elemental (X) training. Notably, positive mediation may also be exemplified by decreases in A's behavioral control (e.g., extinction of A), resulting in decreases in responding to X.

In contrast to positive mediation effects, negative mediation effects refer to situations in which training X in the presence of A results in less excitatory behavioral control by X than when X is trained elementally. Negative mediation effects include both cue competition and conditioned inhibition phenomena. An example of cue competition is overshadowing (the simplest of cue competition phenomena), which occurs when the presence of A during X–US trials diminishes X's behavioral control relative to a situation in which X is elementally paired with the US (Pavlov, 1927). Blocking, another example of cue competition, occurs when the administration of A–US pairings prior to AX–US trials disrupts X's response potential more than a control condition in which A–US pairings are replaced with training of an irrelevant control cue (Kamin, 1968). In blocking situations, A is usually of relatively low salience, which minimizes overshadowing in the control condition. Other examples of cue competition include the degraded contingency (Rescorla, 1968) and over-expectation (Rescorla, 1970) effects. Conditioned inhibition effects constitute the second class of negative mediation phenomena. There are numerous means of creating a conditioned inhibitor. Pavlov's procedure involves A–US pairings interspersed among non-reinforced XA– presentations, which results in X acquiring the potential to reduce responding to an independently trained (transfer) excitor and decreases the rate with which X gains excitatory behavioral control during subsequent X–US pairings (i.e., summation and retardation tests, respectively). Other strategies for establishing conditioned inhibition to X include the differential (i.e., A+/X–) and explicitly unpaired (EU; i.e., X–/+) procedures.

Cue interactions, including positive and negative mediation effects, have been observed in a variety of experimental situations and have important implications for theories of learning. In principle, each of these phenomena could be explained in terms of the effect of nontarget cues (e.g., A) on the processing of the US during trials involving the target cue (X). This view has gained widespread attention and acceptance through the model developed by Rescorla and Wagner (1972). An alternative and perhaps less publicized view is that variations in within-compound associations support cue interactions. This view has been widely accepted in select cue interaction situations such as second-order conditioning, but has received little attention with respect to most negative mediation effects.

The Rescorla–Wagner (1972) model (in its original form) ignores positive mediation effects but accounts for most negative mediation effects. The model asserts that two conditions are jointly necessary and sufficient for changes in the strength of an association between the target CS (X) and the US. First, consistent with most models that predated it (e.g., Bush & Mosteller, 1955), the Rescorla–Wagner model asserts that contiguous activation of the mental representations of X and the US is necessary for increments in the strength of the X–US association. Second, the model asserts that total error across a stimulus compound is necessary for, and directly related to, changes in the strength of the X–US association. Total error is determined by the difference between the magnitude of the US expectation based on all cues present (which is determined by the sum of cue–US associations) and the strength of the association supportable by the US received by subjects on that trial. Thus, cue interactions, in this model, are driven by the effect of nontarget cues on processing of the US (i.e., total error). This model successfully explains a variety of cue competition and conditioned inhibition phenomena. For example, the model explains blocking by asserting that the presence of the blocking stimulus (A) during X–US pairings increases expectation of the US, which reduces increments in the X–US association. However, this model fails to account for the overshadowing that occurs on the first acquisition trial because on this trial A evokes no expectation of the US (James & Wagner, 1980), but it can account for overshadowing on subsequent trials by using the same mechanism as that used for blocking. The model also successfully accounts for conditioned inhibition. In Pavlov's procedure for establishing conditioned inhibition, during AX− trials subjects expect the US on the basis of A's strong association with the US (encouraged through A–US pairings). Because the US is not administered on these AX− trials, the difference between the strength of the expected and experienced US is negative (i.e., the US is overexpected). Thus, both X and A are expected to undergo a decrease in associative strength. For X, a decrease from zero produces a negative (i.e., inhibitory) association with the US. After many trials, X is expected to have a strong negative (i.e., inhibitory) association with the US (but A is expected to still have a positive [excitatory] association with the US because it continues to be reinforced elementally, which compensates for the inhibition acquired on AX− trials). As a result of its strong negative association with the US, the model predicts that X's behavioral control should be slower to reach asymptote than a neutral stimulus when it is subsequently paired with the US (i.e., retardation should be observed) and X should reduce the amount of responding to a transfer excitor (that signals the same US) when they are tested in compound (i.e., negative summation should be observed). Thus, the Rescorla–Wagner model accounts for negative mediation including cue competition, and conditioned inhibition.

Despite the considerable success of the Rescorla–Wagner model, it encountered problems such as its inability to explain second-order conditioning. Sutton (1988) addressed some of these problems on developing a temporal difference model of learning. Like the Rescorla–Wagner model, this model asserts that differences in responding to stimuli reflect differences in associative strength, which can be attributed to differences in US processing at the time of training. Unlike the Rescorla–Wagner model, the temporal difference model is a real-time model. Thus, it makes predictions about the temporal distribution of associative strength (and responding) within a single trial, which has allowed the model to explain some important behavioral and neuroscientific phenomena (e.g., Waelti, Dickinson, & Schultz, 2001). According to the model, changes in associative strength are proportional to surprise (i.e., total error), which is negatively related to the predicted outcome at time t and positively related to the magnitude of the outcome plus the magnitude of the predicted outcome at time $t + 1$. That is, Error $(t + 1)$ is proportional to Outcome $(t + 1)$ + Prediction $(t + 1)$ − Prediction (t), where predictions are based on all cues present. Alternatively stated, the presence of a cue that is associated with the US increases the prediction of an outcome, the effect of which depends on the timing of a nontarget cue relative to the target cue. This conceptualization of total error permits the model to explain second-order conditioning. In this framework, the presentation of a first-order CS (which usually occurs after the second-order CS during Phase 2) functions to increase Error $(t + 1)$ by increasing Prediction $(t + 1)$. Hence, the association between the second-order CS and the US increases. Critically, this account of positive mediation asserts that the second-order CS's augmented response potential is attributable to variations in the direct, second-order CS–US association (rather than within-compound associations). Like the original Rescorla–Wagner model, it ignores the potentially important contribution of within-compound associations.

Most models of human (e.g., Gluck & Bower, 1988) and nonhuman animal learning (e.g., Fanselow, 1998) assert that variations in US processing drive many phenomena in associative learning. However, limitations to this view were encountered (e.g., retrospective revaluation) and, consequently, many modern models of associative learning were developed that explicitly assume that within-compound associations are sometimes important determinants of the response potential of the target cue (e.g., Durlach & Rescorla, 1980; Rescorla, 1982; Van Hamme & Wasserman, 1994; Dickinson & Burke, 1996; Wasserman & Castro, 2005; Pineno, 2007). Notably, these models trivialize the role of within-compound associations in most negative mediation situations (maintaining that US processing is the important factor) and relegate the contribution of within-compound associations to only a few phenomena.

Among the first challenges to the view that variations in US processing could provide a complete account of associative learning is the observation that responding to a target stimulus (X) can be affected when associates of X (e.g., an overshadowing cue; A) are manipulated following completion of target training, because the early US-processing models assumed that the associative status of a cue could change only when it is present. In the present chapter, we refer to all instances in which the response potential of a target cue changes as a function of post-target training experience with nontarget associates as retrospective revaluation. The first examples of retrospective revaluation were observed in positive mediation situations. For example, Rizley and Rescorla (1972) demonstrated retrospective revaluation after sensory preconditioning. Sensory preconditioning occurs when X acquires behavioral control as a result of training consisting of Phase 1 AX– trials and Phase 2 A–US trials (relative to subjects that receive either unpaired treatments in Phase 1 or 2; Brogden, 1939). In sensory preconditioning, responding to X seems to depend on the associative status of A at the time of testing (rather than during training of X with A). Rizley and Rescorla showed that, when subjects receive A-alone (extinction) trials subsequent to A–US trials, X's response potential is diminished (i.e., sensory preconditioning is reduced). Similarly, other researchers have reported that second-order conditioning can be reduced when associative deflation through extinction of the first-order stimulus is administered (e.g., Rescorla, 1982). While this finding is not ubiquitous (Rizley & Rescorla, 1972; Holland & Rescorla, 1975), it is well established that under some conditions this type of retrospective revaluation can be observed (e.g., Rashotte, Griffin, & Sisk, 1977; Rescorla, 1982). In the conditioned taste-aversion literature, taste–odor potentiation and augmentation are examples of positive mediation phenomena. Potentiation occurs when the presence of a relatively salient taste during odor–illness pairings results in an increase in the odor's aversive properties (Rusiniak et al., 1979). This finding is rather surprising because most theories anticipate that the taste should overshadow the odor (resulting in less responding). Like other positive mediation phenomena, potentiation is typically reduced by post-training extinction of the mediating stimulus (i.e., the taste; Durlach & Rescorla, 1980). Thus, sensory preconditioning, second-order conditioning, and taste–odor potentiation can be reduced through post-training associative deflation of the mediating stimulus.

So-called retrospective revaluation phenomena are problematic for the view that positive mediation is driven by variations in US processing, which assumes that behavior at test reflects changes in associative strength that occurred during target training. Instead, they imply that a within-compound association between the target cue and the mediating cue (e.g., the first-order CS in second-order conditioning) supports positive mediation.

Retrospective revaluation has also been observed in negative mediation situations. In cue competition, Kaufman and Bolles (1981) observed that responding to X increased (i.e., overshadowing was reduced) when the associative status of the overshadowing cue (A) was deflated through extinction treatment after completion of the AX–US overshadowing trials. Similarly, Blaisdell, Gunther, and Miller (1999, Experiment 3) demonstrated that post-training extinction of the blocking cue attenuates the blocking effect. These results suggest that cue competition phenomena, such as blocking and overshadowing, depend on the associative status of the nontarget cue at the time of testing rather than (or in addition to) during acquisition. Recovery from cue competition achieved through retrospective revaluation is a rather general (but not ubiquitous [e.g., Holland, 1999]) finding, with degraded contingency (Witnauer & Miller, 2007), overexpectation (Blaisdell, Denniston, & Miller, 2001), and relative stimulus validity (Cole, Barnet, & Miller, 1995) effects all being sensitive to post-training extinction of the competing cue.

Retrospective revaluation effects have also been observed to result from post-training inflation; that is, reinforcement of the companion (associated) stimulus attenuates responding to the target (e.g., backward blocking; Shanks, 1985; Urushihara & Miller, 2009a). Together, these retrospective revaluation effects in cue competition (like their counterparts in positive mediation), including inflation and deflation effects, highlight the role of within-compound associations in cue interactions. Moreover, they are seemingly inconsistent with the view that variations in learning about cues are entirely attributable to variations in US processing.

In addition to observations of retrospective revaluation in cue competition, several researchers have also observed retrospective revaluation in conditioned inhibition situations. Lysle and Fowler (1985) conducted the first demonstration of so-called deactivation of conditioned inhibition. In their critical experiment, subjects received Pavlovian conditioned inhibition training in which A was trained as an excitor and X was trained as an inhibitor (i.e., A+/AX–). Following this, massive extinction of A and, to a lesser extent, extinction of the training context, resulted in a decrease in X's inhibitory potential. Recent research has extended these findings in two important ways. First, Amundson, Wheeler, and Miller (2005) demonstrated that associative inflation of the training excitor used to establish inhibition to X (i.e., A–US pairings) enhances conditioned inhibition to X, which is analogous to backward blocking in the cue competition domain. Second, deactivation of conditioned inhibition by post-training extinction of the training excitor can be observed even when inhibition is indirectly assessed through the inhibitor's effect on a separately trained excitor (X) that is associated with the inhibitor. Specifically, McConnell, Wheeler, Urcelay, and Miller (2009) demonstrated that when a neutral target stimulus (X) is pre-exposed (i.e., latent inhibition treatment) in the presence of a Pavlovian conditioned inhibitor (Y), X's response potential increased (protection from latent inhibition) relative to when X was preexposed in the presence of a stimulus that was not an inhibitor. Central to the present discussion, extinction of the training excitor used to establish conditioned inhibition to Y attenuated responding to X (i.e., protection from latent inhibition was reduced, allowing an expression of the latent inhibition effect). Analogous effects have been observed in protection from extinction (McConnell & Miller, 2010) and superconditioning situations (Urushihara, Wheeler, Pineno, & Miller, 2005). Such effects are consistent with the view that conditioned inhibition is (at least in part) driven by a within-compound association between the conditioned inhibitor and the training excitor.

Observations of retrospective revaluation prompted some researchers to consider the role of within-compound associations in models of cue interactions. The first theory that emphasized within-compound associations outside of the positive mediation domain was the comparator hypothesis (Miller & Matzel, 1988; Miller & Schachtman, 1985). This model asserts that contiguity (defined as spatiotemporal proximity) is necessary and sufficient for the formation of associations. However, responding is multiply determined, and notably, it involves more than the direct target stimulus–US association. The comparator hypothesis is depicted in Figure 4.1. According to the model, when a target cue (X) is paired with the US in the presence of another (comparator) stimulus (which might include the conditioning context, overshadowing cues, etc.), subjects learn three associations: (1) an association between X and the US (Link 1), (2) a within-compound association between X and the comparator stimulus (Link 2), and (3) an association between the comparator stimulus and the US (Link 3). Upon testing X, the US representation is retrieved directly through Link 1 and indirectly through the X–comparator (Link 2) and comparator–US (Link 3) associative linkage. Responding to X is determined by a comparison between the directly activated US representation and the indirectly activated US representation, such that the strength of the indirectly activated US representation is inversely related to X's response potential.

The Original Comparator Hypothesis

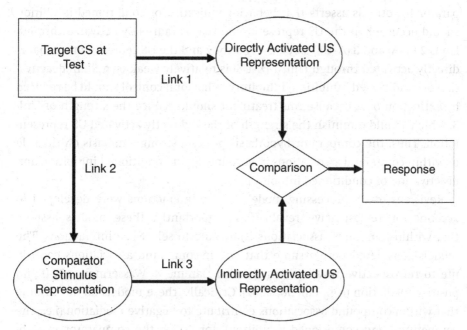

Figure 4.1 The original comparator hypothesis (Miller & Matzel, 1988). Ovals depict stimulus representations; rectangles depict external events; the diamond represents the comparator process. Arrows represent (1) the target CS–US association, (2) the target CS–comparator stimulus within-compound association, and (3) the comparator stimulus–US association. See text for details.

The comparator hypothesis asserts that both cue competition and conditioned inhibition phenomena (including retrospective revaluation) are driven by within-compound associations. Consider the model's account of blocking and recovery from blocking (Blaisdell *et al.*, 1999). When X is paired with the US in the presence of a previously established excitor (A), Link 1 (the X-US association), Link 2 (the X–A within-compound association), and Link 3 (the A–US association) are established (or strengthened if they were previously established, as would be the case for Link 3). In the condition in which A–US trials preceded XA–US trials, Link 3 is expected to be relatively strong, which should (in the absence of posttraining extinction) yield a strong indirectly activated US representation and, consequently, weak responding to X. Extinction of A following blocking should increase responding to X because posttraining extinction of A should decrease the strength of Link 3. A within-compound association (i.e., the X–A association; Link 2) is critical to this account of blocking and retrospective revaluation; otherwise, Link 3 would not be accessed to indirectly activate a representation of the US. Applied to conditioned inhibition, the comparator hypothesis asserts that behavior indicative of conditioned inhibition should occur when the US representation that is indirectly activated through Links 2 (X–A) and 3 (A–US) is relatively strong and the US representation that is directly activated through Link 1 (X–US) is relatively weak or null. In deactivation of conditioned inhibition, inhibitory behavioral control should be reduced by extinction of A because this treatment should reduce the strength of Link 3, which should diminish the strength of the indirectly activated US representation. Thus, the comparator hypothesis places a strong emphasis on the role of within-compound associations in accounting for conditioned inhibition and deactivation of conditioned inhibition.

Revisions of US processing models of cue interactions were developed to account for retrospective revaluation. Importantly, these models assume that within-compound associations contribute to select cue interactions. The models considered here assume that within-compound associations contribute to retrospective revaluation (e.g., Van Hamme & Wasserman, 1994) and positive mediation (e.g., Pineno, 2007). Critically, these models do not assume that within-compound associations contribute to negative mediation (i.e., cue competition and conditioned inhibition), for which the comparator hypothesis assumes that within-compound associations are critical. Instead, they posit that cue competition and conditioned inhibition reflect variations in US processing. The mathematical details of these models are explained below in the "Simulation of models and general modeling methods" section.

Van Hamme and Wasserman's (1994) model extends the Rescorla–Wagner (1972) model and explains retrospective revaluation by asserting that, when a target stimulus is expected (based on within-compound associations) but is omitted, the associability of the target stimulus is proportional to that of the stimulus when physically presented, but negative in value. This modification allows for changes in the associative strength of a cue on trials in which it is absent, thereby permitting the model to account for phenomena like backward blocking and recovery from overshadowing. For example, in the case of recovery from overshadowing, during non-reinforced (Phase 2) presentations of the overshadowing cue (A), the target cue (X) is associatively activated through the A–X within-compound association and, based on X being absent, X's associability should be negative. An increase in the strength of the X–US association is expected during these trials because (1) X's associability is negative and (2) total error is negative in value because of the outcome being expected based on A's presence but not being presented. Similarly, in backward blocking situations a decrease in the strength of the X–US association is expected because (1) X's associability is negative and (2) total error is positive based on the outcome being present and not fully predicted by A. Thus, the model put forth by Van Hamme and Wasserman asserts that within-compound associations drive retrospective revaluation.

Many researchers have asserted that within-compound associations support positive mediation phenomena (e.g., Durlach & Rescorla, 1980; Rescorla, 1982; Pineno, 2007). Within this framework, responding to X can be driven by activation of the US directly through an X–US association and it can also be driven by indirect activation of the US through an X–A–US associative chain. Importantly, the X–A within-compound association contributes to responding. Applied to second-order conditioning, this view asserts that Phase 1 A–US pairings establish an A–US association and Phase 2 X–A pairings establish an X–A association. Presentation of X at test activates a representation of A through the X–A association and A's representation activates a representation of the US through the A–US association (which drives conditioned responding). This view explains the observation that posttraining extinction of A following either second-order conditioning or sensory preconditioning can reduce excitatory responding to X because, within this framework, the A–US association is important at the time of testing. Early research in second-order conditioning revealed results that were interpreted as inconsistent with this view (e.g., Rizley & Rescorla, 1972; Holland & Rescorla, 1975), but subsequent research revealed that second-order conditioning is often supported by within-compound associations (e.g., Rashotte et al., 1977; Rescorla, 1982).

Miller and his colleagues (Miller & Matzel, 1988) have argued that within-compound associations are necessary for all cue interactions. In contrast, the Rescorla–Wagner (1972) model has been repeatedly revised to assign a role to within-compound associations in cue interactions, but these models still assert that variations in US processing (rather than within-compound associations) drive most negative mediation phenomena. For the present simulations, two revisions were considered: Van Hamme & Wasserman's (1994) model of retrospective revaluation and Pineno's (2007) model of positive mediation. These two revisions of the Rescorla–Wagner model were amalgamated, with the resulting model asserting that within-compound associations drive most cue interactions except negative mediation, which is presumed to be largely driven by variations in US processing. By combining these two variants of the Rescorla–Wagner model, we created a single US-processing model that is more powerful than either of the individual models alone. To better appreciate the role of within-compound associations in cue interactions, the following simulations were conducted. In these simulations, we compared this US-processing (USP) model to sometimes competing retrieval (SOCR) because these two models are especially well matched, except with respect to their account of negative mediation (where SOCR uses within-compound associations and the USP model uses a total error-reduction mechanism). If within-compound associations contribute to all cue interactions, the performance of the USP and SOCR models should be equivalent, except when applied to negative mediation phenomena where simulations should reveal an advantage to SOCR based on its consistent use of within-compound associations. The experiments that were simulated in the present chapter were all Pavlovian fear-conditioning experiments with thirsty rats as subjects. The dependent variable was either the time it took subjects to drink for five cumulative seconds in the presence of the CS (lick suppression) or the number of lever presses made for water reinforcement in the presence of the CS (lever-press suppression). The experiments that were simulated were chosen because we considered them to be the most direct tests of the role of within-compound associations across a broad range of cue interactions, including: positive mediation, counteraction, experimental extinction, conditioned inhibition, and cue competition.

Simulation of models and general modeling methods

The sometimes competing retrieval model (SOCR)

The observation that the excitatory response potential of the target cue can increase (decrease) as a function of posttraining associative deflation (inflation) of associates of the target (comparator stimuli) prompted Miller and Matzel (1988) to develop their comparator hypothesis. The extended comparator hypothesis modified the original comparator hypothesis so that it might be applied to situations in which the target stimulus has multiple comparator stimuli (Denniston, Savastano, & Miller, 2001). Recently, Stout and Miller (2007) formalized the extended comparator hypothesis. Their SOCR model of cue interaction makes three critical assumptions: (1) learning is based on a local error-reduction mechanism in which cues do not compete for associative strength; (2) cue interaction, including positive and negative mediation, is driven by within-compound associations between the target and so-called comparator stimuli; and (3) responding to a target stimulus is determined by comparison processes that occur at the time of test. Increases in the strength of the association between two stimuli (Stim1 and Stim2; e.g., X and the US, X and A, etc.) are modeled using the following equation:

$$\Delta V_{Stim1-Stim2} = Salience_{Stim1} \times Salience_{Stim2} \times (\lambda - V_{Stim1-Stim2}) \qquad (4.1)$$

where Salience is a free parameter representing stimulus salience of the cue in question, λ is a fixed parameter (set at 1 by convention) that represents the maximum associative strength supportable by Stim2, and $V_{Stim1-Stim2}$ is the pretrial strength of the Stim1–Stim2 association. The update equation for SOCR (and the USP model) in the present simulations took the form:

$$V_{X^{n+1}} = \Delta V_{X^n} + V_{X^n} \tag{4.2}$$

Decrements in the strength of the Stim1–Stim2 association occur when Stim1 is presented in the absence of the Stim2, and are modeled by the equation:

$$\Delta V_{Stim1-Stim2} = Salience_{Stim1} \times -k1 \times V_{Stim1-Stim2} \tag{4.3}$$

where $k1$ $(0 < k1 < 1)$ is a free parameter representing the rate of extinction. Note that these learning rules are simpler than the Rescorla–Wagner learning rule, because they are insensitive to the associative status of stimuli that are outside of the pair being modeled. SOCR further assumes that responding to X (R_X) is given by the following equation:

$$R_X = V_{X-US} - k2 \times \left(\Sigma Op_{X-i-US} \times rV_{X-i} \times rV_{i-US} \right) \tag{4.4}$$

where $k2$ is a free parameter that weights comparison processes so they have less impact $(0 < k2 < 1)$ than the direct CS–US association (i.e., Link 1), Op_{X-i-US} (termed the operator switch) is a variable that represents the degree of discrimination between directly and indirectly activated US representations (used to model positive mediation effects like second-order conditioning with few trials and negative mediation effects like conditioned inhibition with many trials). rV_{X-i} represents X's potential to activate a representation of a comparator stimulus (i) and rV_{i-US} represents the potential of a comparator stimulus to activate a representation of the US. This response rule captures the psychological intuition that responding to X is determined by a comparison (via subtraction) between the US representation activated through the X–US association (V_{X-US}) and the US representation activated through the effective X–comparator stimulus (rV_{X-i}) and comparator stimulus–US (rV_{i-US}) associative linkage. Basically, SOCR says that responding to X is not a function of the absolute value of V_{X-US}. Rather it reflects the value of V_{X-US} relative to other cues that were present when X was trained.

Similar to the first-order processes that determine responding to X, the potential of X to activate first-order comparator stimuli (rV_{X-i}) and the potential of comparator stimuli to activate the US (rV_{i-US}) are determined by comparison processes involving second-order (j) comparator stimuli, which are other stimuli that are associated with the first-order comparator stimuli and may, but not necessarily, have an association with the target cue. Specifically, the following equation was used to calculate X's potential to activate comparator stimuli:

$$rV_{X-i} = V_{X-i} - k2 \times \left(Op_{X-j-i} \times V_{X-j} \times V_{j-i} \right) \tag{4.5}$$

This equation captures the psychological intuition that the effective first-order comparator stimulus representation is determined by the representation of the first-order comparator activated directly through the association between X and the first-order comparator (V_{X-j}) compared with the representation of the first-order comparator activated through higher-order linkage (i.e., V_{X-j} and V_{j-i}). The strength of the effective, indirectly activated representation of the US (rV_{i-US}) is determined by similar, higher-order comparator processes:

$$rV_{i-US} = V_{t-US} - k2 \times \left(Op_{i-j-US} \times V_{i-j} \times V_{j-US}\right) \tag{4.6}$$

Importantly, the operator switch (Op_{X-i-US}) changes with experience in activating a representation of the US. Changes in the operator switch are modeled using the equation:

$$\Delta Op_{X-i-US} = k3 \times Salience_X \times V_{X-i} \times V_{i-US} \times \left(1 - Op_{X-i-US}\right) \tag{4.7}$$

where $k3$ ($0 < k3 < 1$) is the rate with which changes in the operator switch occur. Note that this equation applies only when $V_{X-US} = 0$. Otherwise, $\Delta Op_{X-i-US} = 1 - Op_{X-i-US}$. The starting value of Op_{X-i-US} is -1. This rule for the operator switch captures the psychological intuition that subjects must learn to discriminate between directly activated representations and indirectly activated representations.

The US-processing (USP) model

Most models of Pavlovian conditioning assume that variations in US processing drive cue interactions. However, the inadequacies of this approach prompted some researchers to consider the role of within-compound associations in retrospective revaluation (e.g., Van Hamme & Wasserman, 1994; Dickinson & Burke, 1996) and positive mediation (e.g., Rescorla, 1982; Pineno, 2007). The USP model considered in the present simulations is a hybrid of models designed to retain differences in US processing to account for cue competition and conditioned inhibition, but to use within-compound associations to explain retrospective revaluation and positive mediation. The model incorporates three important assumptions: (1) changes in associative strength function to reduce the total error across a stimulus compound and are modeled using the Rescorla–Wagner equations; (2) retrospective revaluation is driven by the retrieval of a representation of the target stimulus through within-compound associations; and (3) higher-order associative structures, including within-compound associations, support positive mediation, which varies as a function of novelty of the target cue.

The Rescorla–Wagner model was simulated as follows. First, all associative changes (ΔV) that were simulated (including both CS–US and within-compound associations) were modeled using the following equation:

$$\Delta V_{Stim1-Stim2} = \alpha_{Stim1} \times \beta_{Stim2} \times (\lambda_{Stim2} - \Sigma V_{i-Stim2}) \qquad (4.8)$$

where Stim1 and Stim2 represent two contiguous stimuli, α_{Stim1} represents the associability of Stim1 (see below for equations), β_{Stim2} represents the associability of Stim2 (see below), and ($\lambda_{Stim2} - \Sigma V_{i-Stim2}$) represents the discrepancy between the magnitude of Stim2 that occurred (λ_{Stim2}) and the magnitude of Stim2 that was expected based on all cues present ($\Sigma V_{i-Stim2}$). To reduce the number of free parameters, all λs were assumed to be fixed at 1. Notice that the parenthetical term differs from the local error-reduction system used by SOCR because it considers all cues presented on a particular trial rather than only the expectation of Stim2 based on Stim1. In the present simulations, when Stim2 was present:

$$\beta_{Stim2} = Salience_{Stim2} \qquad (4.9)$$

and when Stim2 was absent:

$$\beta_{Stim2} = k1 \times Salience_{Stim2} \qquad (4.10)$$

where $k1$ was a free parameter ($0 < k1 < 1$) that represented the diminished associability of absent stimuli. This parameter allows the model to anticipate several important phenomena, including the relative stimulus validity effect and the observation that extinction requires more trials than acquisition.

Van Hamme and Wasserman (1994) asserted that the associability of a stimulus that is absent but expected based on within-compound associations is proportional to the salience (or associability) of the stimulus when it is present, but of negative value. In their model, the strength of within-compound associations is not considered. In the present simulations, we slightly altered the Van Hamme and Wasserman model to better capture the psychological intuition that absent stimuli are retrieved through within-compound associations. Thus, in the present simulations, when Stim1 was present,

$$\alpha_{Stim1} = Salience_{Stim1} \qquad (4.11)$$

and when Stim1 was absent:

$$\alpha_{Stim1} = k2 \times Salience_{Stim1} \times \Sigma V_{i-Stim1} \qquad (4.12)$$

where $k2$ was a free parameter ($-1 < k2 < 0$) that represents the diminished (and negative) activation of a retrieved but absent stimulus. $\Sigma V_{i-Stim1}$ is the activation of the representation of the absent stimulus induced by within-compound associations. This last mechanism allows the USP model to explain several critical phenomena, such as differential retrospective revaluation as a function of within-compound associations (e.g., Witnauer & Miller, 2009). Notably, this assumption about the role of the strength of within-compound associations has precedent in the Dickinson and Burke (1996) model of retrospective revaluation.

Many researchers have asserted that within-compound associations support positive mediation in some situations (e.g., Rescorla, 1982; Pineno, 2007). We elected to add Pineno's (2007) response rule to Van Hamme and Wasserman's (1994) revision of the Rescorla–Wagner model in order to allow the USP model to explain positive mediation (and related phenomena). Pineno's model was chosen for two reasons: (1) the model is easily integrated with the Van Hamme and Wasserman model, and (2) it anticipates the transition from positive to negative mediation that is caused by increasing the number of trials in feature-negative discriminations (e.g., Stout, Escobar, & Miller, 2004). This feature is analogous to the operator switch in SOCR. According to this model, responding to X is given by:

$$R_X = V_{X-US} + \left(\Sigma N_X \times rV_{X-i} \times rV_{i-US} \right) \tag{4.13}$$

where r represents the higher-order, reiterative processes (as in SOCR) and N_X is a variable representing X's novelty. Decreases in the novelty of a stimulus are modeled by the equation:

$$\Delta N_X = \text{Salience}_X \times k3 \times (0 - N_X) \tag{4.14}$$

where $k3$ $(0 < k3 < 1)$ controls the rate of changes of novelty. N_X on Trial 1 is unity and is updated in a manner similar to associative strength (i.e., $N_X^{n+1} = \Delta N_X^n + N_X^n$). The novelty variable is an important addition in that it facilitates the model addressing the observation that second-order conditioning is observed with relatively few A+/AX− trials and conditioned inhibition is observed with relatively many of the same trials (e.g., Stout et al., 2004).

Scaling

In the present simulations, we were interested in differences between models predictions and empirical data. Consequently, we needed to scale the predictions of the models to match the scales used in psychological research. Suppression ratios were modeled in some of the present simulations. (Recall that the simulated experiments all employed fear conditioning; hence, suppression reflects the conditioned response to a fearful CS.) The suppression ratio is calculated by dividing the number of responses (lever presses in these cases) that occur during the CS (R_X) by the number of lever presses during the CS plus the number of lever presses emitted during a comparable period of time immediately before the CS ($R_{Context}$). Thus, zero represents complete suppression and 0.5 represents no suppression. To approximate the suppression ratio (SR) scale, the outputs of the models used in the present simulations response potential were scaled using the following equation:

$$SR = \left(Scaling_{SR} - R_X\right) \div \left[\left(Scaling_{SR} - R_X\right) + \left(Scaling_{SR} - R_{Context}\right)\right] \qquad (4.15)$$

where Scaling is a free parameter that was used to represent baseline levels of lever pressing (i.e., in the absence of any behaviorally relevant stimuli). Following Larrauri and Schmajuk (2008), in the present simulations that used this scaling technique, testing was conducted in a context that was not differentially excitatory, so $R_{Context}$ was assumed to be 0 in all of the suppression ratio simulations.

The critical measurement in some of the experiments simulated was the $\log_{10}$ latency to consume water for five cumulative seconds in the presence of the test CS. Following Larrauri and Schmajuk (2008), we assumed that lick suppression multiplied by a scaling factor is equal to the response potential of $X (R_X)$ as predicted by the models. In addition, we assumed that the lick suppression predicted by such proportional scaling is added to the scale's minimum (i.e., $\log_{10} 5$). Thus, in the present simulations, we approximated the lick-suppression (LS) scale using the equation:

$$LS = \log_{10} 5 + \left(Scaling_{LS} \times R_X\right) \qquad (4.16)$$

where Scaling is a free parameter used to approximate the $\log_{10}$ latency scale measured in lick-suppression situations.

Hill climbing

The statistical fit of each model was assessed by computing the sum of the squared difference between predicted (based on simulation) and observed group means (i.e., sum-of-squared-error [SSE]). The set of parameters that produced the lowest SSE was obtained using a hill-climbing algorithm. The hill-climbing algorithm searched within the set of parameter configurations immediately adjacent to the previously best-fitting (or starting) set of parameters, ultimately moving through parameter space in the direction of steepest descent on SSE. The search was terminated when it failed to find an immediately adjacent configuration of parameters that produced lower SSE. The hill-climbing algorithm was repeated four times with four widely spaced starting points in parameter space. We report the results of the simulation that produced the lowest SSE.

The hill-climbing algorithm used in the present simulations has some limitations. First, it produces a new, best-fitting set of parameters for each set of data to which it is applied. One consequence of this is that the hill-climbing algorithm is not sensitive to previously best-fitting parameters, which is consistent with each data set having been gathered with somewhat different procedural parameters such as trial spacing, cue duration, and US intensity. Another consequence is that it affords models the greatest freedom in fitting experimental data. Because we were interested (at least in part) in identifying situations in which USP and SOCR fail, we sought to test the models using a procedure that affords the greatest flexibility. This allowed us to be reasonably confident that when one or more of the models fail to fit data, it is not the result of constraining the models' parameters. Thus, a hill-climbing algorithm was used in the present simulations for the following reasons. First, we were primarily interested in comparing the performances of SOCR and the USP model. By finding the optimal set of parameters (in terms of SSE) for both models, we can conclude that differences in the fit of the models are attributable to differences between the models themselves (rather than just differences in the degree to which the parameters were optimized). Second, while Stout and Miller (2007) offered a single set of parameters that seems to hold across many SOCR simulations, no such parameters existed for the USP model. In the present simulations, parameters were allowed to take values at their boundaries (i.e., 0 and 1). This allowed for the greatest freedom in fitting experimental data. In some simulations, processes in the models were effectively disabled because their best-fitting parameters involved a value of 0 (e.g., the best-fitting extinction rate parameter in Simulation 4 was 0). We allowed this to occur because it allowed the models the greatest freedom in fitting the data. A drawback to this decision is that the models, at some points in parameter space, could be quite different from those specified by the original authors (e.g., lacking a mechanism for extinction). One might argue that the hill-climbing algorithm can be used to fit noise (rather than meaningful results); we avoided this problem by paying attention to existing significant results (rather than to potentially noise-driven tendencies). In summary, we combined two variants of the Rescorla–Wagner (1972) model in order to create a much more powerful US-processing model. We now compare it to SOCR to assess how well those two models are able to simulate experiments potentially dependent on within-compound associations. These simulations were done in a manner that optimized the performance of both models to allow for the fairest comparisons.

Simulation 1: counteraction between two blocking stimuli

One of the most challenging findings for the view that cue interactions are driven entirely by variations in US processing is the observation that multiple cue interaction treatments can counteract each other rather than summate. For example, Witnauer, Urcelay, and Miller (2008, Experiment 1) found that two independently trained blocking cues can counteract each other's potential to block a target stimulus when they are trained in compound. Half of the subjects received Phase 1 training consisting of A–US and B–US trials (i.e., experimental), whereas the other half of subjects received C–US and D–US (control) trials. Orthogonally, in Phase 2, subjects received either AX–US or ABX–US training. When X was compounded with two excitatory CSs, suppression was stronger than when X was compounded with one excitatory CS. Thus, the two potential blocking stimuli (A and B) counteracted when they were trained in compound with X. Similar counteraction effects have been observed in numerous cue competition situations (e.g., Blaisdell, Bristol, Gunther, & Miller, 1998), conditioned inhibition situations (Urcelay & Miller, 2008), and in positive mediation situations (Witnauer & Miller, in press; for a review, see Wheeler & Miller, 2008).

The USP model can explain counteraction in some situations. The account is one based on positive mediation through within-compound associations. The model asserts that, during training that involves two cue interaction treatments, the establishment of X–i and X–i–j within-compound associative structures (which serve to increase excitatory conditioned responding to X) can yield an increase in responding that outweighs the decrease in the excitatory X–US association that arises from additional cue competition. This account basically asserts that some degree of second-order conditioning occurs in counteraction situations and that within-compound associations are necessary for counteraction.

SOCR explains counteraction effects in terms of competition among comparator stimuli for the potential to reduce responding to X. Specifically, when X is conditioned in compound, the direct X–US association is down-modulated by the sum of (1) the product of Links 2 and 3 for A (i.e., the X–A and A–US associations) and (2) the product of Links 2 and 3 for B (i.e., X–B and B–US). In addition, SOCR assumes that two first-order comparator stimuli that share a within-compound association with each other can mutually down-modulate each other by serving as the other's comparator stimulus within a higher-order comparator process. For example, the X–A association can be down-modulated by the product of the X–B and B–A associations and the A–US association can be down-modulated by the A–B and B–US associations. Similar processes are assumed to operate when B's role as a first-order comparator stimulus is considered.

In Simulation 1, we applied USP and SOCR to the results of Witnauer *et al.* (2008; Experiment 2), in which the role of within-compound associations in counteractions was investigated. The design of this experiment is depicted in Table 4.1. Subjects received Phase 1 training consisting of either AB/CD pairings

Table 4.1 *Design summary of Simulation 1 (Witnauer et al., 2008, Experiment 2)*

Group	Phase 1	Phase 2	Phase 3	Test X Observed
1 Block – Ctrl	AC/BD	A+/B+	AX+	0.27
1 Block – Excite	AB/CD	A+/B+	AX+	0.21
2 Block – Ctrl	AC/BD	A+/B+	ABX+	0.17
2 Block – Excite	AB/CD	A+/B+	ABX+	0.03

Note: CSs A, B, C, D, and X were audio and visual cues. + indicates the administration of a footshock US. Slashes denote interspersed trials. Observed values are the group mean suppression ratios during testing of X (lower numbers indicate more suppression).

(Excite; which was intended to strengthen the A–B association) or AC and BD pairings (Ctrl; which controlled for exposure to A and B). In Phase 2, all subjects received A–US and B–US pairings. Orthogonal to the within-compound association manipulation, in Phase 3 subjects received training with either one blocking cue (1 Block; AX–US) or two blocking cues (2 Block; ABX–US). Witnauer *et al.* observed that responding to X was stronger when X was trained with two compounded blocking cues than with one blocking cue, and prior AB pairings increased the magnitude of this effect, yielding stronger responding relative to the absence of these prior AB pairings. These simulations were conducted with the expectation that both models would provide a reasonably good fit to the results because they both use within-compound associations to explain counteraction effects. In the present simulations only, the salience of B was assumed to equal the salience of A because, in Witnauer *et al.*'s experiments, these cues were counterbalanced (which equates salience in principle).

Results and discussion

The results of Simulation 1 are depicted in Figure 4.2. Both models provided a good fit to Witnauer *et al.*'s (2008; Experiment 2) observations in the statistical fit of the model's predictions and in anticipating the significant group differences that were observed by Witnauer *et al.* Specifically, both USP and SOCR anticipated that responding would be greater when X was trained with A and B relative to when X was trained only with A. Moreover, both models anticipated that strengthening the A–B association would increase responding to X. The average absolute difference (AAD) between SOCR's predictions and observed group means (AAD = 0.005; SSE = 0.00016) was only slightly less than the difference between USP's predictions and observed group means (AAD = 0.012; SSE = 0.00085). Both models explained much of the variance in the group means in Witnauer *et al.*'s experiment (r^2 [USP Predictions × Observed] > 0.98; r^2 [SOCR Predictions × Observed] > 0.99). Thus, both models were able to explain

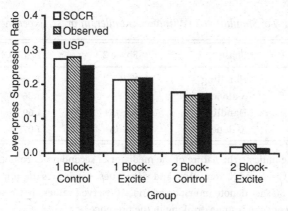

Figure 4.2 Predicted and observed conditioned lever-press suppression to X in Witnauer *et al.*'s (2008) Experiment 2. Striped bars represent observed mean suppression ratios. A score of 0 reflects complete suppression of lever pressing and a score of 0.5 reflects a complete absence of suppression. Black bars represent the best-fitting predictions of the USP model and white bars represent the best-fitting predictions of SOCR. See the text and Table 4.1 for details.

the critical differences and provided a good statistical fit to the overall pattern of data.

Simulation 2: within-compound associations in second-order conditioning

The basic observation of second-order conditioning is problematic for the original Rescorla–Wagner model. Moreover, some data suggest that a within-compound association between the target stimulus (X) and the first-order CS (A) supports second-order conditioning (Rescorla, 1982). These findings are problematic for US-processing-based accounts of second-order conditioning (e.g., Sutton, 1988). However, recent revisions of US-processing models use within-compound associations to explain positive mediation (e.g., Pineno, 2007).

Simulation 2 applied SOCR and USP to the results of Witnauer and Miller (in press), in which latent inhibition of second-order conditioning was investigated. The motivation for conducting these simulations was to determine how well SOCR and USP could account for the observation that latent inhibition of X attenuates second-order conditioning of excitation to X when A (rather than the training context) is the first-order mediating cue. Presumably, latent inhibition treatment down-modulates the X–A association as a result of a strong X–context association enhancing the indirectly activated representation of A that depends on X–context and context–A associations. The design of Witnauer and Miller's Experiment 3 is depicted in Table 4.2. Half of the subjects received

Table 4.2 *Design summary of Simulation 2 (Witnauer & Miller, in press, Experiment 3)*

Group	Phase 1	Phase 2	Test X Observed
No CS Pre – Context	Handling	X–/+	1.32
CS Pre – Context	X-alone	X–/+	1.36
No CS Pre – Punctate	Handling	AX–/A+	1.69
CS Pre – Punctate	X-alone	AX–/A+	1.07

Note: Context and Punctate indicate the nature of the mediator of second-order conditioning. Pre denotes preexposure. CSs A and X were audio and visual cues. + indicates the administration of a footshock US. Slashes denote interspersed trials. Observed values are the group mean $\log_{10}$ latencies in seconds to resume drinking in the presence of X.

non-reinforced presentations of X in the presence of A, which was made excitatory through interspersed A–US pairings, and the other half of subjects received non-reinforced presentations of X in the training context, which was made excitatory through interspersed, unsignalled US presentations in the context. Thus, all subjects received second-order conditioning (as demonstrated by other experiments in which unpaired controls were included), but the context served as the mediating cue for half of the subjects and A served as the mediating cue for the other half. Orthogonal to the nature of the mediating cue, Witnauer and Miller administered either preexposure to X (which could produce latent inhibition) or a handling control treatment. They observed that preexposure reduced responding to X when second-order conditioning involved XA pairings but did not affect responding when it involved presentations of X alone in the training context. Presumably, there was no beneficial effect of preexposure in the Context condition because the X–context pairings during Phase 2 second-order conditioning brought the X–context association to asymptote.

The USP model seemingly can account for the results of Witnauer and Miller (in press), because the model explains second-order conditioning by asserting that a within-compound association is necessary for second-order conditioning. Specifically, the model asserts that an X–context–US associative chain increases responding to X in contextually mediated second-order conditioning. Presumably, preexposure to X in the training context should have relatively little effect on the expression of the X–context association at the time of test because it should be asymptotic after several X–context trials in Phase 2. When second-order conditioning is mediated by a punctuate excitor (A), the X–A–US associative chain drives responding to X. Thus, preexposure to X should serve to latently inhibit expression of the X–A association (the mechanism being a reduction in X's novelty and, consequently, expression of the X–A association).

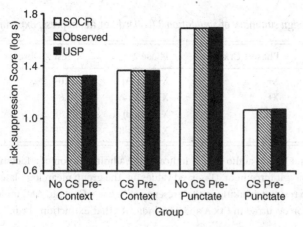

Figure 4.3 Predicted and observed conditioned lick suppression to X in Witnauer and Miller's (in press) Experiment 3. Striped bars represent observed means. Black bars represent the best-fitting predictions of the USP model and white bars represent the best-fitting predictions of SOCR. See the text and Table 4.2 for details.

Thus, USP (at least qualitatively) explains the results of Witnauer and Miller. SOCR's explanation is similar to that of the USP model's, except that SOCR explains latent inhibition by asserting that preexposure to X strengthens the X–context association, instead of explaining it in terms of a decrease in novelty. But critically, both models assert that latent inhibition results in attenuation of the expression of X–A within-compound associations.

Results and discussion

The results of Simulation 2 are illustrated in Figure 4.3. Both models were able to provide an excellent quantitative fit to Witnauer and Miller's (in press) results. They anticipated reduced responding to X when it is preexposed and second-order conditioning is mediated by A. Moreover, both models anticipated the lack of an effect of preexposure to X when second-order conditioning is mediated by the context. The USP model's predictions were slightly closer to the observed group means with respect to the AAD measurement (AAD = 0.0036) than SOCR's (AAD = 0.0038). The SSE measurement of difference between observed and predicted revealed a small advantage to SOCR's predictions (SSE = 0.000069) relative to USP's predictions (SSE = 0.000072). The USP model predicted slightly more of the variance in the group means ($r^2 = 0.9999$) than did SOCR ($r^2 = 0.9998$). Obviously, the difference between the quantitative fits of the models was small and the primary result of the analysis is that both models explained the results quite well.

Table 4.3 *Design summary of Simulation 3 (Laborda et al., in press, Experiment 3)*

Group	Phase 1 Ctx A	Phase 2	Test X Observed Ctx C
AAC–X	X+	X– (Ctx A)	1.04
AAC–XY	X+	XY– (Ctx A)	1.84
ABC–X	X+	X– (Ctx B)	1.58
ABC–XY	X+	XY– (Ctx B)	1.78

Note: CSs X and Y were audio cues. + indicates the administration of a footshock US. – denotes non-reinforcement. Observed values are the group mean $\log_{10}$ latencies in seconds to resume drinking in the presence of X. Ctx = Context. AAC indicates that Extinction occurred in Ctx A and ABC indicates that Extinction occurred in Ctx B.

Simulation 3: the role of CS–context associations in extinction

Experimental extinction in Pavlovian conditioning has recently received widespread attention in neuroscience, associative learning, and clinical application. An important phenomenon is renewal from extinction, which occurs when a context change between extinction and testing results in greater responding (i.e., less behavioral extinction) than when the extinction and test contexts are the same. AAC renewal occurs when acquisition and extinction occur in the same context (A) and testing occurs in a novel context (C). ABC renewal occurs when acquisition (Context A), extinction (Context B), and testing (Context C) all occur in different contexts. Typically, AAC renewal is weaker than ABC renewal. Laborda, Witnauer, and Miller (in press) conducted experiments that tested SOCR's account of the difference between AAC and ABC renewal. According to SOCR, when extinction occurs in Context A, the within-compound association (Link 2) between the target stimulus (X) and the context is strengthened. Strengthening of Link 2 reduces responding to X relative to when Link 2 is unaffected (or weakened) by the extinction treatment (i.e., in ABC renewal). To test this account, Laborda *et al.* (in press) conducted the design summarized in Table 4.3. In this experiment, subjects received either AAC or ABC renewal, orthogonal to which subjects received either X– or XY– extinction trials, where Y was a previously neutral stimulus. Notably, they replicated previous observations of weaker AAC than ABC renewal (i.e., responding was stronger in Group ABC–X than in Group AAC–X). Additionally, they observed that the effect of extinguishing X in the presence of Y was specific to AAC renewal. This latter finding is anticipated by SOCR because it asserts that Y overshadowed the X–Context A association (Link 2) during extinction. In Simulation 3 we simulated SOCR and USP as applied to the findings of

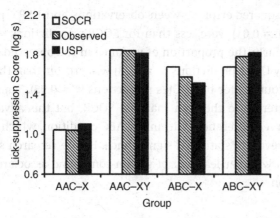

Figure 4.4 Predicted and observed conditioned lick suppression to X in Laborda *et al.*'s (in press) Experiment 3. Striped bars represent observed means. Black bars represent the best-fitting predictions of the USP model and white bars represent the best-fitting predictions of SOCR. See the text and Table 4.3 for details.

Laborda *et al.* We expected that SOCR's fit to the data would be superior to USP's because SOCR explains Laborda *et al.*'s results in terms of differences in within-compound associations, whereas USP attributes no role to within-compound associations in explaining extinction.

Results and discussion

The results of Simulation 3 are depicted in Figure 4.4. Inspection of the figure reveals that neither model explained Laborda *et al.*'s data as well as they explained the data in Simulations 1 and 2. It is also evident that both models struggled in explaining behavior within the ABC condition more than the AAC condition. SOCR asserts that the effect of Y should be completely abolished when extinction occurs in a neutral context, because Y's effect (in Context A) should be driven by overshadowing of the X–Context A association. The X–Context B association was irrelevant in the present studies because Context B could not mediate indirect activation of the US representation, because no US was administered in Context B. It is also apparent that Laborda *et al.* observed a small (nonsignificant) tendency towards greater responding in ABC–XY than in ABC–X. In contrast to SOCR, USP anticipated a larger difference between ABC–XY and ABC–X than was actually observed, and it anticipated this difference under conditions in which the difference within the AAC condition was predicted to be smaller than observed. However, both models correctly anticipated the significant differences in the AAC condition that were observed by Laborda *et al.* (in press).

Assessment of the statistical differences between the fits of SOCR and USP revealed a small advantage for USP's predictions. The average absolute difference and sum-of-squared-error between observations and USP's predictions (AAD = 0.048; SSE = 0.01) were less than for SOCR's predictions (AAD = 0.052; SSE = 0.02). Similarly, the proportion of variance in the observed group means accounted for by USP's predictions (r^2 = 0.98) was greater than the proportion of variance accounted for by SOCR's predictions (r^2 = 0.95). Thus, USP provided a slightly better fit to the data than did SOCR, but this advantage was driven by the observed differences within the ABC condition, which failed to reach conventional levels of statistical significance. Future research should seek to better establish whether learning of within-compound associations is important for extinction.

Simulation 4: the effect of CS duration on the CS's and context's response potential

Simulations 1 and 2 established that both SOCR and USP can account for data that implicate within-compound associations as necessary in positive mediation (Simulation 1) and counteraction (Simulation 2) situations. Presumably, both models' fits were improved by their use of within-compound associations to explain these phenomena. In Simulation 3, we applied the models to an experiment in extinction that suggested that within-compound associations are important for extinction, and obtained somewhat ambiguous results despite their using different mechanisms to explain the basic extinction effect. The purpose of Simulation 4 was to compare the fit of the models to an experiment in which the role of within-compound associations in cue competition was manipulated.

Urushihara and Miller (2009; Experiment 1) conducted the experiment summarized in Table 4.4 in an effort to test SOCR's assertion that the within-compound association between a target stimulus (X) and the context is directly related to competition between X and the context for behavioral control. Group X-alone was exposed only to X during training (half of the subjects received exposure to a long-duration [25.0 s] CS and half to a short-duration [2.5 s] CS). Group US-alone received exposure to the US alone. Group Short X+ received pairings of the short CS X and the US. Group Long X+ received pairings of the long CS X with the US. All subjects were tested on both X (outside of the training context) and the training context. SOCR anticipated that responding to X would be stronger when X was of relatively short duration than when it was long, because the long-duration X should establish a stronger X–context association (Link 2) than a short-duration X. This would constitute a CS-duration effect. More importantly, SOCR anticipated that the training context's response potential should also be weaker with a longer duration CS. These predictions

Table 4.4 *Design summary of Simulation 4 (Urushihara & Miller, 2009, Experiment 1)*

Group	Phase 1 Ctx A	Test Ctx A Observed	Test X (in Ctx B) Observed
X-alone	Short X/Long X	1.00	0.80
US-alone	+	2.95	1.00
Short X+	Short X+	2.55	1.90
Long X+	Long X+	2.10	1.25

Note: X was an audio cue. + indicates the administration of a footshock US. Ctx = Context. Short (Long) indicates that X was 2.5 s (25.0 s) in duration. Slashes denote interspersed trials. Observed values are the group mean $\log_{10}$ latencies in seconds to resume drinking in the presence of X and separately in the presence of Ctx A. Testing of X occurred in a neutral context (B).

were experimentally confirmed. Simulation 4 applied both SOCR and USP to these data, with the expectation that SOCR would provide a superior fit to the data because the experiment constituted a relatively direct test of the role of Link 2 in competition between a CS and context. To simulate the temporal manipulation in these experiments, we parsed simulated time into 2.5 s bins. That is, each 2.5 s bin was simulated as a single trial. Thus, long CSs consisted of ten consecutive bins (and short CSs constituted only one bin). Intertrial intervals were parsed in an identical manner.

Results and discussion

The observed group means, as well as SOCR's and USP's best-fitting predictions, are depicted in Figure 4.5. Both models anticipated most of the observed differences among the groups and both of the models' predictions fit the data reasonably well. Both models anticipated the relatively weak responding that was observed when testing on X in the control groups (i.e., X-alone–Test X and US-alone–Test X) and to the context in the X-alone–Test Ctx A condition. Moreover, both models anticipated relatively strong responding to the context when the context was reinforced with the US (i.e., in US-alone–Test Ctx A). In the experimental X+ condition, both models anticipated that when X's duration was relatively long, responding to X should be diminished relative to when X was short. SOCR anticipates this difference based on Link 2, which should be stronger with longer CSs. The USP model asserts that X's novelty should diminish during the interval preceding the US, which should reduce responding to X. This is predicted to occur because the long CS effectively constitutes 10 X presentations (whereas the short CS constitutes only 1 X presentation). Notably, with the best-fitting parameters, extinction of X during the interval between X-onset and the US should not have a strong effect on the CS-duration effect

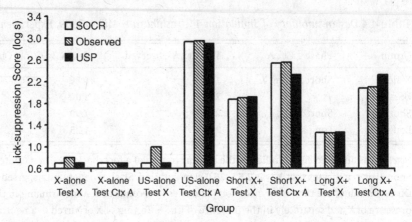

Figure 4.5 Predicted and observed conditioned lick suppression to X and the context (Ctx) in Urushihara and Miller's (2009b) Experiment 1. Striped bars represent observed means. Black bars represent the best-fitting predictions of the USP model and white bars represent the best-fitting predictions of SOCR. See the text and Table 4.4 for details.

because the best-fitting value for the weighting of absent USs was zero. With respect to the context's response potential, SOCR uniquely anticipated that an increase in X's duration should result in a decrease in the context's response potential. As with responding to X, this is anticipated because the context–X association (i.e., Link 2 for the context) should be greater with longer CSs. The USP model failed to anticipate any difference within this condition. In fact, the model's best-fitting parameters involved weighting absent USs by a factor of zero, which effectively disabled extinction during early components of the long CS. This was the best-fitting situation because extinction of X during the duration of long Xs should have resulted in increases in the context–US association (and hence increases in responding to the context) with longer CSs. That is, extinction was effectively disabled by the hill-climbing procedure so that the USP model would not erroneously anticipate greater responding to the context with a longer CS than with a shorter CS.

The sum-of-squared-error and average absolute difference between SOCR's predictions and the observed group means (AAD = 0.06; SSE = 0.10) were less than USP's (AAD = 0.12; SSE = 0.21). Similarly, SOCR explained more of the variance in the group means (r^2 = 0.99) than did USP (r^2 = 0.97). Thus, SOCR's best-fitting predictions were statistically closer to the observed group means than were the USP model's predictions. The quantitative differences between the models' fits were somewhat smaller than in other simulations (e.g., the difference in Simulation 5 was vastly greater). A greater proportion of the group means in Simulation 4 are control groups that are easily fit by both models.

For example, the difference between multiple, simple acquisition groups, and unpaired groups was simulated in Simulation 4. Thus, a huge proportion of the variability in the group means in Simulation 4 consists of differences between paired and unpaired groups, which are very easily fit by the USP (and SOCR model). USP's critical failure was dampened (in terms of r-squared) by the model fitting other points in the experiment.

Simulation 5: counteraction between latent inhibition and overshadowing

When a target stimulus (X) is presented alone prior to training, subsequent pairings of X with other stimuli (*i*) are ordinarily less effective in establishing functional X–*i* associations than when X is a novel cue at the time of the pairings. So-called latent inhibition is a well-documented phenomenon with respect to X–US associations; that is, many researchers have observed weaker excitatory responding to X as a result of latent inhibition treatment of the X stimulus. Based on the comparator hypothesis, Blaisdell *et al.* (1998) hypothesized that if overshadowing of X by A depends on the X–A association (similar to the way that excitatory responding depends on the X–US association), then latent inhibition of X should attenuate overshadowing. They further reasoned that presenting an overshadowing cue during training of X should result in reduced expression of the X–context association, which supports the latent inhibition effect according to the comparator hypothesis. These two mechanisms (latent inhibition of the X–overshadowing cue association and overshadowing of the X–context association) should effectively counteract, resulting in strong responding to X if both treatments were administered. To test this hypothesis, they conducted the experiment summarized in Table 4.5. Consistent with their hypothesis, Blaisdell *et al.* observed weak responding to X when it was either preexposed (i.e., they observed latent inhibition) or when it was trained in the presence of the overshadowing cue. When preexposure to X and overshadowing of X were administered to the same subjects, responding to X was greater than when either treatment alone was administered. SOCR anticipates these results for the aforementioned reasons. However, whether USP could account for these results was unclear. Specifically, USP can explain some counteraction effects, but Blaisdell *et al.*'s counteraction targeted the within-compound associations between X and competing cues (rather than affecting within-compound and competing cue–US associations as in other counteractions), which USP asserts are not important for cue competition. That is, Blaisdell *et al.*'s counteraction is driven entirely by presumed differences in the expression of Link 2. In Simulation 5, USP and SOCR were compared with respect to their fits to the

Table 4.5 *Design summary of Simulation 5 (Blaisdell et al., 1998, Experiment 1)*

Group	Phase 1	Phase 2	Test X Observed
No CS Pre – Elemental	Y-alone	X+	1.62
CS Pre – Elemental	X-alone	X+	1.10
No CS Pre – Compound	Y-alone	AX+	0.75
CS Pre – Compound	X-alone	AX+	1.65

Note: CSs X, Y, and A were audio and visual cues. Pre = Preexposure. + indicates the administration of a footshock US. Observed values are the group mean $\log_{10}$ latencies to resume drinking in the presence of X.

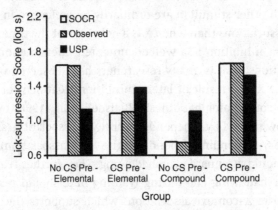

Figure 4.6 Predicted and observed conditioned lick suppression to X in Blaisdell *et al.*'s (1998) Experiment 1. Striped bars represent observed means. Black bars represent the best-fitting predictions of the USP model and white bars represent the best-fitting predictions of SOCR. See the text and Table 4.5 for details.

data of Blaisdell *et al.* with the expectation that, if within-compound associations are important for cue competition, then SOCR would provide a superior fit because of its emphasis on the role of within-compound associations in cue competition.

Results and discussion

The results of Simulation 5 are depicted in Figure 4.6. The most important finding was that SOCR's best-fitting predictions were decidedly more similar to the observed group means than were USP's best-fitting predictions. SOCR anticipated all of the critical differences between observed group means. In contrast, USP anticipated only that the overshadowing effect was stronger than the latent inhibition effect and that latent inhibition combined with overshadowing should yield more responding than either treatment alone. USP fails because it anticipates that the preexposure treatment should serve to enhance responding to X independent of whether or not X is overshadowed during conditioning. Thus, the model (under the best-fitting parameters for the present simulation) anticipates the opposite of latent inhibition, which was actually observed only in the compound condition. Note that this does not reflect a general failure of USP to anticipate either latent inhibition (because the model anticipated the latent inhibition effect in Simulation 2) or counteraction effects (because the model anticipated counteraction in Simulation 1). Instead, these results reflect a failure of the model to use within-compound associations to explain negative mediation. This failure limits USP's potential to account for counteraction between overshadowing and latent inhibition. Notably, Nakajima and Nagaishi (2005) failed to replicate Blaisdell *et al.*'s finding that latent inhibition and overshadowing counteract. Instead, they observed summation between these two treatments. It seems possible that SOCR can explain both sets of results, but more simulations (similar to the SLG simulations by Schmajuk later in this volume) are needed to illuminate the variables that SOCR predicts are critical determinants of whether summation or counteraction will occur.

The quantitative-fitting procedure revealed a strong superiority of the best-fitting predictions of SOCR, which deviated from observed group means (AAD = 0.009; SSE = 0.0005) much less than did USP's predictions (AAD = 0.317; SSE = 0.4688). The proportion of variance in the observed group means explained by SOCR's predictions ($r^2 = 0.99$) was greater than the variance explained by USP's predictions ($r^2 = 0.18$). Thus, the statistical advantage of SOCR's predictions over USP's predictions supports the view that within-compound associations contribute to cue competition.

Simulation 6: CS preexposure attenuates conditioned inhibition

The purpose of Simulation 6 was to determine whether the critical finding of Simulation 5 (SOCR's better fit to observations) would be detected if the models were applied to an experiment in which the interaction between latent inhibition treatment and Pavlovian conditioned inhibition treatment (rather than overshadowing) was examined. Specifically, Friedman, Blaisdell, Escobar, and Miller (1998) conducted the experiment summarized in Table 4.6. The design constitutes a 2 (Pavlovian [A–US/AX–] vs. Explicitly Unpaired [X/US] inhibition treatment) x 2 (CS Preexposure vs. No CS Preexposure) + 1 (Retardation Control) design. When subjects did not receive preexposure to X, strong conditioned inhibition to X was observed in both the Pavlovian and the Explicitly Unpaired conditions (relative to the Retardation Control). However,

Table 4.6 *Design summary of Simulation 6 (Friedman et al., 1998, Experiment 1)*

Group	Phase 1	Phase 2	Phase 3	Test X Observed
No CS Pre – EU	Y-alone	X–/+	X+	1.07
CS Pre – EU	X-alone	X–/+	X+	1.03
No CS Pre – Pav	Y-alone	AX–/A+	X+	1.38
CS Pre – Pav	X-alone	AX–/A+	X+	2.06
Ret Control	Y-alone	AY–/A+	X+	1.95

Note: CSs X, Y, and A were audio and visual cues. Pre = Preexposure. + indicates the administration of a footshock US. – denotes non-reinforcement. Slashes denote interspersed trials. Pav = Pavlovian conditioned inhibition treatment. EU = Explicitly Unpaired conditioned inhibition. Ret = Retardation. Observed values are the group mean $\log_{10}$ latencies to resume drinking in the presence of X.

when subjects received preexposure to X, conditioned inhibition was disrupted in the Pavlovian condition. SOCR's explanation of this is similar to its account of Blaisdell *et al.*'s (1998) experiment in which latent inhibition disrupted over-shadowing. According to SOCR, as a result of preexposure to X, the association between X and A undergoes latent inhibition (i.e., the expression of associative strength acquired in Phase 2 is slowed). Thus, X's potential to activate A should have been weaker among subjects in the CS Pre–Pav group than in the No CS Pre-Pav group, thereby resulting in less conditioned inhibition to X. Consistent with these predictions, Friedman *et al.*'s data imply that the X–A association is important for the observation of inhibition following A–US/AX– training. In Simulation 6, USP and SOCR were applied to these data.

Results and discussion

The results of Simulation 6 are illustrated in Figure 4.7. The simulations revealed that USP provided a reasonably good account of Friedman *et al.*'s (1998) results. Both SOCR and USP predicted the critical differences observed by Friedman *et al.* SOCR's account is somewhat limited by the model's prediction of a slight increase of inhibition (i.e., less responding) by CS Preexposure in the Explicitly Unpaired condition (where no difference was observed [i.e., CS Pre–EU vs. No CS Pre–EU]). SOCR explains the difference within the Pavlovian condition as being driven by a failure of X to activate an effective representation of A due to latent inhibition of X (which is driven by the X–context association). More surprisingly, USP explained the critical difference within the Pavlovian condition and it did so without predicting a difference within the Explicitly Unpaired condition. In the Pavlovian condition, the USP model anticipated stronger responding (i.e., less inhibition) with CS preexposure than in

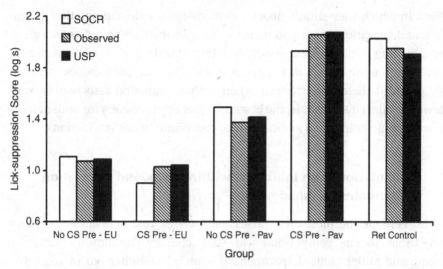

Figure 4.7 Predicted and observed conditioned lick suppression to X in Friedman *et al.*'s (1998) Experiment 1. Striped bars represent observed means. Black bars represent the best-fitting predictions of the USP model and white bars represent the best-fitting predictions of SOCR. See the text and Table 4.6 for details.

the No CS Pre–Pav group because this treatment should have strengthened the output of the X–context–US associative chain, which should drive excitatory responding to X (thereby counteracting the inhibition). The USP model anticipated a relatively small effect of the same treatment in the Explicitly Unpaired condition because the conditioned inhibition training alone in this condition should have established a near-asymptotic, X–context association. Such a strong X–context association should not have been established by Pavlovian conditioned inhibition training because Stimulus A should have overshadowed the X–context association. Thus, both models anticipate the general pattern of results observed by Friedman *et al.*, but USP provided a better explanation of the lack of an effect of CS preexposure in the Explicitly Unpaired condition.

The USP model's best-fitting predictions provided a better quantitative fit to the observed group means than did SOCR. The difference between the USP model's predictions and the observed group means (AAD = 0.03; SSE = 0.004) was less than the difference between SOCR's predictions and the observed group means (AAD = 0.10; SSE = 0.056). The USP model also explained a greater proportion of the variance ($r^2 = 0.99$) than did SOCR's predictions ($r^2 = 0.94$).

Concerning the (rather unexpected) difference between Simulations 5 and 6, USP was able to explain the results of Simulation 6 by asserting that the strength of the X–context association is directly related to excitatory responding. However, this account is incompatible with the results of Blaisdell *et al.*

(1998), in which they simultaneously demonstrated a degrading effect in the Elemental condition and a potentiating effect in the Compound condition of strengthening the X–context association. Importantly, both models were able to account for the results of Friedman *et al.* (1998) and both models presumably provided their best accounts when within-compound associations were allowed to take effect. That is, the best-fitting set of parameters for both models allowed within-compound associations to contribute to cue interactions.

Simulation 7: an inhibitory within-compound association attenuates overshadowing

Perhaps the most direct assessment of the role of within-compound associations in cue competition was conducted by Amundson, Witnauer, Pineno, and Miller (2008, Experiment 1), which is summarized in Table 4.7. They used a 2 (Phase 1: AD vs. AC) x 2 (Phase 2: X+ vs. AX+) design. In Phase 1, AD or AC presentations were interspersed with XC presentations. This resulted in an inhibitory association being formed between X and A for subjects that received XC/AC treatment (Espinet, Iraola, Bennett, & Mackintosh, 1995). The within-compound association between X and A presumably was not appreciably affected for subjects that received XC/AD presentations because there was not a common element. According to SOCR, the effective strength of Link 2 should be degraded uniquely in the Inhib condition, which should reduce the overshadowing deficit. In Simulation 7, we compared the predictions of SOCR with those of the USP model as applied to Amundson *et al.*'s data.

Results and discussion

The results of Simulation 7 are depicted in Figure 4.8. The most important aspect of these results is that USP failed to anticipate an effect of the inhibitory pretraining manipulation. In contrast, SOCR provided a reasonably good fit to Amundson *et al.*'s (2008) data. According to SOCR, the effect of the inhibitory pretraining should reduce the effective strength of Link 2 between X and A, which should function to attenuate overshadowing in the Compound condition but not in the Elemental condition. In contrast, USP predicts that such a treatment should, if anything, attenuate responding to X because within-compound associations support positive mediation in this framework. Because this prediction (more responding to X in the Inhib–Compound than in Ctrl–Compound) is contrary to the observed difference (which produces a greater SSE than would a lack of an effect), the best-fitting parameters actually called for a zero value for the salience of the common element (C). The results of the statistical comparison between the models' fits were also consistent with these conclusions.

Table 4.7 *Design summary of Simulation 7 (Amundson et al., 2008, Experiment 1)*

Group	Phase 1	Phase 2	Test X Observed
Ctrl – Elemental	XC/AD	X+	0.14
Inhib – Elemental	XC/AC	X+	0.11
Ctrl – Compound	XC/AD	AX+	0.27
Inhib – Compound	XC/AC	AX+	0.09

Note: CSs A, C, D, and X were audio and visual cues. Inhib = Inhibitory Pretraining. Ctrl = Control. + indicates the administration of a footshock US. – denotes non-reinforcement. Slashes denote interspersed trials. Observed values are the group mean suppression ratios in the presence of X.

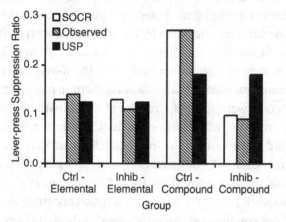

Figure 4.8 Predicted and observed conditioned lever-press suppression to X in Amundson *et al.*'s (2008) Experiment 1. A score of 0 reflects complete suppression of lever pressing and a score of 0.5 reflects a complete absence of suppression. Striped bars represent observed means. Black bars represent the best-fitting predictions of the USP model and white bars represent the best-fitting predictions of SOCR. See the text and Table 4.7 for details.

The difference between SOCR's best-fitting predictions and the observed group means (AAD = 0.01; SSE = 0.0005) was less than the difference between USP's predictions and the group means (AAD = 0.05; SSE = 0.0167). SOCR explained a greater proportion of the variance in the observed group means ($r^2 = 0.98$) than did USP ($r^2 = 0.15$). Thus, SOCR better explained the effect of within-compound associations on overshadowing than did USP.

Conclusions

The simulations and accompanying review lend strong support to the view that within-compound associations contribute to all cue interactions, including negative mediation phenomena. The strict US-processing view (e.g., Rescorla & Wagner, 1972) has been rejected by researchers in an effort to explain retrospective revaluation and positive mediation. Current US-processing models use within-compound associations to explain these phenomena, but maintain that variations in US processing support cue competition and conditioned inhibition. The present simulations compared USP with SOCR in several cue interaction situations. In Simulation 1, SOCR and USP were fit to the results of Witnauer *et al.* (2008, Experiment 2) in which the effect of increasing the strength of the within-compound association between two blocking cues was observed to increase the counteraction between these blocking cues when they were trained in compound with a target stimulus. In Simulation 2, SOCR and USP were applied to the results of an experiment in which latent inhibition attenuated second-order conditioning mediated by a punctate companion cue but not second-order conditioning mediated by the training context (Witnauer & Miller, in press, Experiment 3). In Simulation 3, SOCR and USP were applied to an extinction experiment in which overshadowing the X–acquisition context association attenuated extinction (Laborda *et al.*, 2010, Experiment 3). In Simulation 4, these models were fit to the results of Urushihara and Miller's (2009, Experiment 1) study in which increases in CS duration attenuated responding to the CS and to the context. In Simulation 5, Blaisdell *et al.*'s (1998, Experiment 1) demonstration of counteraction between latent inhibition and overshadowing was simulated. In Simulation 6, Friedman *et al.*'s (1998, Experiment 1) study in which reduced Pavlovian inhibition occurred as a result of latent inhibition of the conditioned inhibitor was simulated. In Simulation 7, USP and SOCR were fit to Amundson *et al.*'s (2008, Experiment 1) study in which establishing an inhibitory X–overshadowing cue association attenuated the overshadowing effect.

This exploration revealed that both the USP and SOCR models were able to explain data pertaining to the role of within-compound associations in counteraction (Simulation 1) and positive mediation (Simulation 2) situations, which was expected because both models assert that within-compound associations are critical to these phenomena. Second, both models failed in principled ways (although SOCR's statistical failure was slightly more pronounced) when applied to extinction data pertaining to the role of X–context associations in extinction (Simulation 3). Third, SOCR provided a much better account overall of the data pertaining to the role of within-compound associations in negative mediation (Simulations 4, 5, and 7). Thus, the clearest advantage of SOCR over USP occurred when the two models were applied to negative mediation phenomena. This advantage was not detected in Simulation 6, but USP (like SOCR) used within-compound associations to explain the critical results. Given that

Table 4.8 *Best-fitting parameters for USP*

Simulation	Sal X	Sal A (Y in Sim 3)	Sal Ctx (C in Sim 7)	Sal US	k1	k2	k3	k4	Scaling
1	0.10	0.70	NA	0.15	0.40	−1.00	0.15	0.30	0.20
2	0.35	0.55	1.00	0.45	0.25	0.00	0.05	0.60	2.05
3	1.00	0.25	1.00	0.65	0.20	−1.00	0.80	0.65	3.70
4	0.35	NA	0.90	1.00	0.00	0.00	0.30	1.00	2.20
5	0.05	0.45	0.20	1.00	1.00	0.00	0.00	1.00	2.10
6	0.25	0.30	0.05	1.00	0.40	−0.45	0.00	0.50	5.15
7	0.95	0.60	0.00	0.30	0.80	0.00	0.20	0.35	0.40

Note: Best-fitting parameters for the USP model were revealed through hill climbing on SSE. Sal = Salience. Ctx = Context. The context was not simulated when trials were widely spaced (Simulations 1 and 7; Ctx was used to simulate punctate cue C in Simulation 7). Salience of B in Simulation 1 was fixed to equal that of A because these cues were counterbalanced. k1 = absent beta dampening. k2 = absent alpha dampening. k3 = rate of changes in novelty. k4 = learning rate of CS–US associations. NA = not applicable.

SOCR's performance was better in most of the negative mediation simulations, this suggests that SOCR's account of negative mediation (which is based on within-compound associations) is superior to USP's account (which is based on variations in US processing).

Each simulation's best-fitting parameters for both models are listed in Tables 4.8 and 4.9. Notably, SOCR's predictions are based on one less parameter than are USP's predictions. More free parameters, all other things equal, should allow a model greater freedom in fitting data. Thus, SOCR's superiority is especially compelling because SOCR was at a disadvantage based on its having one less free parameter than the USP model. Also, the models were somewhat mismatched with respect to which processes were weighted by free parameters. SOCR's k2 parameter effectively dampens higher-order comparison processes, whereas USP lacked an equivalent free parameter. We elected not to implement such a free parameter in USP because it lacked a basis in previous simulations (Pineno, 2007), and adding a parameter to USP would further complicate comparison between SOCR and USP by increasing the difference in number of free parameters.

There are some limitations to the present simulations. First, one could argue that the USP model we simulated is not the most powerful US-processing model available. However, despite the existence of potentially more powerful USP algorithms (e.g., Sutton, 1988), we decided to simulate the combination of Van Hamme and Wasserman's (1994), Pineno's (2007), and Rescorla and Wagner's

Table 4.9 *Best-fitting parameters for SOCR*

Simulation	Sal X	Sal A (Y in Sim 3)	Sal Ctx (C in Sim 7)	Sal US	k1	k2	k3	Scaling
1	0.40	0.40	NA	0.85	−0.10	0.70	0.40	0.75
2	0.65	0.20	0.55	0.85	−0.10	0.75	0.05	1.70
3	0.25	0.70	0.30	0.70	0.00	0.85	0.00	2.20
4	0.30	NA	1.00	0.75	−0.30	0.55	0.30	0.75
5	0.25	0.90	0.25	0.35	−0.20	0.85	0.00	3.15
6	0.80	1.00	0.05	0.30	−0.05	1.00	0.00	3.15
7	0.30	0.40	1.00	0.75	−0.30	0.55	0.30	0.75

Note: Best-fitting parameters for SOCR were revealed through hill climbing on SSE. Sal = Salience. Ctx = Context. The context was not simulated when trials were widely spaced (Simulations 1 and 7; Ctx was used to simulate punctate cue C in Simulation 7). Salience of B in Simulation 1 was fixed to equal that of A because these cues were counterbalanced. $k1$ = extinction rate. $k2$ = comparison weighting. $k3$ = operator learning rate. NA = not applicable.

(1972) models because the combination of these is more likely to account for phenomena relevant to the present investigation (e.g., counteraction and positive mediation). Moreover, the USP model simulated here is a good match to SOCR on many dimensions, including assumptions about time (both are trial-wise rather than real-time), salience (associability), associative structure, and representation. Thus, the difference between the fits of the models is more directly attributable to the critical difference between the models (within-compound associations in negative mediation). Such a direct attribution would not be possible if we simulated other models (e.g., Schmajuk & Larrauri, 2006), because they differ from SOCR on more dimensions.

Second, our conclusions concerning the importance of within-compound associations in all cue interactions are superficially inconsistent with Melchers, Lachnit, and Shanks's (2004) observation that backward blocking is more strongly correlated with within-compound memory than is forward blocking, which was interpreted as inconsistent with SOCR. However, recent simulations in our laboratory revealed that differences in the correlation between the strength of Link 2 and the magnitude of forward and backward blocking are straightforwardly predicted by SOCR if one assumes that salience is normally distributed across a sample of subjects. In Melchers *et al.* (2004, Experiment 1), all subjects received elemental training (A+/B−) and compound training (AX+/BY+). Group Forward received elemental training (Phase 1) followed by compound training (Phase 2) and in Group Backward the order of the phases was reversed (compound training preceded elemental training). For each subject, the difference between X's rating and Y's rating was used to index the strength of the blocking effect. Also, subjects completed a recognition memory test in which they were presented with nontarget stimuli (e.g., B) and asked to indicate the target stimulus with which it had been paired (e.g., Y). This served as an index of within-compound memory. The critical finding was that the blocking effect (Y–X) was more strongly correlated with within-compound memory in Group Backward than in Group Forward. These findings were interpreted as inconsistent with the comparator hypothesis, which emphasizes within-compound associations in forward and backward blocking equally. However, because treatment of the blocking control stimulus (Y) confounded recovery from overshadowing (driven by extinction of the overshadowing cue B) with backward blocking and protection from overshadowing (driven by latent inhibition of the overshadowing cue B) with forward blocking, SOCR anticipates their results across a variety of different simulation assumptions. This is based on the model anticipating an asymmetry between latent inhibition (in forward blocking controls) and extinction (in backward blocking controls) of the blocking control cue, where the latter depends more on salience. According to SOCR, unlearning in extinction is driven by the salience of the target, $k1$, and associative strength. Latent inhibition is determined by many more factors, including the salience of the target, the salience of the context, $k2$, and the previous associative strengths. The critical difference between the two effects is that a greater proportion of the variability is attributable to salience in extinction than in latent inhibition. SOCR also predicts that the difference in correlation should disappear when more appropriate controls (involving C+ instead of B– trials) are used. Pilot data collected in our laboratory have tentatively confirmed this prediction.

The US-processing view has received widespread acceptance across multiple levels of analysis, including: neuroscience (e.g., Waelti *et al.*, 2001), extinction (Larrauri & Schmajuk, 2008), human cognition (e.g., Gluck & Bower, 1988), and animal learning (e.g., McLaren & Mackintosh, 2000; Schmajuk & Larrauri, 2006). The present results are consistent with a growing literature suggesting that this view must be qualified if not rejected (e.g., Wheeler & Miller, 2008; Witnauer & Miller, 2010). Moreover, these results suggest that a viable alternative to the US-processing view across levels of analysis might be based on within-compound associations.

Author note

This research was supported by National Institute of Mental Health Grant 33881. The authors would like to thank Mario A. Laborda, Bridget L.

McConnell, Gonzalo Miguez, and Cody Polack for their comments on an earlier version of this manuscript. Requests for information concerning this research should be addressed to Ralph R. Miller, Department of Psychology, SUNY-Binghamton, Binghamton, NY 13902–6000, USA; e-mail: rmiller@binghamton.edu.

References

Amundson, J. C., Wheeler, D. S. & Miller, R. R. (2005). Enhancement of Pavlovian conditioned inhibition achieved by posttraining inflation of the training excitor. *Learning and Motivation*, **36**, 331–352.

Amundson, J. C., Witnauer, J. E., Pineno, O. & Miller, R. R. (2008). An inhibitory within-compound association attenuates overshadowing. *Journal of Experimental Psychology: Animal Behavior Processes*, **34**, 133–143.

Blaisdell, A. P., Bristol, A. S., Gunther, L. M. & Miller, R. R. (1998). Overshadowing and latent inhibition counteract each other: Support for the comparator hypothesis. *Journal of Experimental Psychology: Animal Behavior Processes*, **24**, 335–351.

Blaisdell, A. P., Denniston, J. C. & Miller, R. R. (2001). Recovery from the overexpectation effect: contrasting performance-focused and acquisition-focused models of retrospective revaluation. *Animal Learning and Behavior*, **29**, 367–380.

Blaisdell, A. P., Gunther, L. M. & Miller, R. R. (1999). Recovery from blocking through deflation of the blocking stimulus. *Animal Learning and Behavior*, **27**, 63–76.

Brogden, W. J. (1939). Sensory pre-conditioning. *Journal of Experimental Psychology*, **25**, 323–332.

Bush, R. R. & Mosteller, F. (1955). *Stochastic Models for Learning*. New York: Wiley.

Cole, R. P., Barnet, R. C. & Miller, R. R. (1995). Effect of relative stimulus validity: learning or performance deficit? *Journal of Experimental Psychology: Animal Behavior Processes*, **21**, 293–303.

Denniston, J. C., Savastano, H. I. & Miller, R. R. (2001). The extended comparator hypothesis: learning by contiguity, responding by relative strength. In R. R. Mowrer and S. B. Klein, eds., *Handbook of Contemporary Learning Theories*. Hillsdale, NJ: Erlbaum, pp. 65–117.

Dickinson, A. & Burke, J. (1996). Within-compound associations mediate the retrospective revaluation of causality judgments. *Quarterly Journal of Experimental Psychology*, **49B**, 60–80.

Durlach, P. J. & Rescorla, R. A. (1980). Potentiation rather than overshadowing in flavor-aversion learning: an analysis in terms of within-compound associations. *Journal of Experimental Psychology: Animal Behavior Processes*, **6**, 175–187.

Espinet, A., Iraola, J. A., Bennett, C. H. & Mackintosh, N. J. (1995). Inhibitory association between neutral stimuli in flavor-aversion conditioning. *Animal Learning and Behavior*, **23**, 361–368.

Fanselow, M. S. (1998). Pavlovian conditioning, negative feedback, and blocking: mechanisms that regulate association formation. *Neuron,* **20**, 625–627.

Friedman, B. X., Blaisdell, A. P., Escobar, M. & Miller, R. R. (1998). Comparator mechanisms and conditioned inhibition: conditioned stimulus preexposure disrupts Pavlovian conditioned inhibition but not explicitly unpaired inhibition. *Journal of Experimental Psychology: Animal Behavior Processes,* **24**, 453–466.

Gluck, M. A. & Bower, G. H. (1988). From fear conditioning to category learning: an adaptive network model. *Journal of experimental Psychology: General,* **117**, 227–247.

Holland, P. C. (1999). Overshadowing and blocking as acquisition deficits: no recovery after extinction of overshadowing or blocking cues. *Quarterly Journal of Experimental Psychology,* **52B**, 307–333.

Holland, P. C. & Rescorla, R. A. (1975). Second order conditioning with food as the unconditioned stimulus. *Journal of Comparative and Physiological Psychology,* **88**, 459–467.

James, J. H. & Wagner, A. R. (1980). One trial overshadowing: evidence of distributed processing. *Journal of Experimental Psychology: Animal Behavior Processes,* **6**, 188–205.

Kamin, L. J. (1968). "Attention-like" processes in classical conditioning. In M. R. Jones, ed., *Symposium on the Prediction of Behavior: Aversive Stimulation.* Miami, FL: University of Miami Press, pp. 9–31.

Kaufman, M. A. & Bolles, R. C. (1981). A nonassociative aspect of overshadowing. *Bulletin of the Psychonomic Society,* **18**, 318–320.

Laborda, M. A., Witnauer, J. E. & Miller, R. R. (2010). Contrasting AAC and ABC renewal: the role of context associations. *Manuscript submitted for publication.*

Larrauri, J. A. & Schmajuk, N. A. (2008). Attentional, associative, and configural mechanisms in extinction. *Psychological Review,* **115**, 640–676.

Lysle, D. T. & Fowler, H. (1985). Inhibition as a "slave" process: deactivation of conditioned inhibition through extinction of conditioned excitation. *Journal of Experimental Psychology: Animal Behavior Processes,* **11**, 71–94.

McConnell, B. M., & Miller, R. R. (2010). Protection from extinction provided by a conditioned inhibitor. *Learning and Behavior,* **38**(1), 68–79.

McConnell, B. M., Wheeler, D. S., Urcelay, G. P. & Miller, R. R. (2009). Protection from latent inhibition provided by a conditioned inhibitor. *Journal of Experimental Psychology: Animal Behavior Processes,* **35**, 498–508.

McLaren, I. P. & Mackintosh, N. J. (2000). An elemental model of associative learning I: latent inhibition and perceptual learning. *Animal Learning and Behavior,* **28**, 211–246.

Melchers, K. G., Lachnit, H. & Shanks, D. R. (2004). Within-compound associations in retrospective revaluation and in direct learning: a challenge for comparator theory. *Quarterly Journal of Experimental Psychology,* **57B**, 25–53.

Miller, R. R. & Matzel, L. D. (1988). The comparator hypothesis: a response rule for the expression of associations. In G. H. Bower, ed., *The Psychology of Learning and*

Motivation (vol. 22). San Diego, CA: Academic Press, pp. 51–92.

Miller, R. R. & Schachtman, T. R. (1985). Conditioning context as an associative baseline: implications for response generation and the nature of conditioned inhibition. In R. R. Miller and N. E. Spear, eds., *Information Processing in Animals: Conditioned Inhibition*. Hillsdale, NJ: Erlbaum, pp. 51–88.

Nakajima, S. & Nagaishi, T. (2005). Summation of latent inhibition and overshadowing in a generalized bait shyness paradigm of rats. *Behavioural Processes*, **69**, 369–377.

Pavlov, I. P. (1927). *Conditioned Reflexes*. London: Oxford University Press.

Pineno, O. (2007). A response rule for positive and negative stimulus interaction in associative learning and performance. *Psychonomic Bulletin and Review*, **14**, 1115–1124.

Rashotte, M. E., Griffin, R. W. & Sisk, C. L. (1977). Second-order conditioning of the pigeon's keypeck. *Animal Learning and Behavior*, **5**, 25–38.

Rescorla, R. A. (1968). Probability of shock in the presence and absence of CS in fear conditioning. *Journal of Comparative and Physiological Psychology*, **66**(1), 1–5.

Rescorla, R. A. (1970). Reduction in the effectiveness of reinforcement after prior excitatory conditioning. *Learning and Motivation*, **1**, 372–381.

Rescorla, R. A. (1982). Simultaneous second-order conditioning produces S-S learning in conditioned suppression. *Journal of Experimental Psychology: Animal Behavior Processes*, **8**, 23–32.

Rescorla, R. A. & Wagner, A. R. (1972). A theory of Pavlovian conditioning: variations in the effectiveness of reinforcement and nonreinforcement. In A. H. Black and W. F. Prokasy, eds., *Classical Conditioning: ii. Current Theory and Research*. New York: Appleton–Century–Crofts, pp. 64–99.

Rizley, R. C. & Rescorla, R. A. (1972). Associations in second-order conditioning and sensory preconditioning. *Journal of Comparative and Physiological Psychology*, **81**, 1–11.

Rusiniak, K. W., Hankins, W. G., Garcia, J. & Brett, L. P. (1979). Flavor-illness aversions: potentiation of odor by taste in rats. *Behavioral and Neural Biology*, **25**, 1–17.

Schmajuk, N. A. & Larrauri, J. A. (2006). Experimental challenges to theories of classical conditioning: application of an attentional model of storage and retrieval. *Journal of Experimental Psychology: Animal Behavior Processes*, **32**, 1–20.

Shanks, D. R. (1985). Forward and backward blocking in human contingency judgement. *Quarterly Journal of Experimental Psychology*, **37B**, 1–21.

Stout, S. C. & Miller, R. R. (2007). Sometimes competing retrieval (SOCR): a formalization of the extended comparator hypothesis. *Psychological Review*, **114**, 759–783.

Stout, S. C., Escobar, M. & Miller, R. R. (2004). Trial number and temporal relationship as joint determinants of second-order conditioning and conditioned inhibition. *Learning and Behavior*, **32**, 230–239.

Sutton, R. S (1988). Learning to predict by the methods of temporal differences. *Machine Learning*, **3**, 9–44.

Urcelay, G. P. & Miller, R. R. (2008). Counteraction between two kinds of conditioned inhibition training. *Psychonomic Bulletin and Review*, **15**, 103–107.

Urushihara, K. & Miller, R. R. (2009). Stimulus competition between a discrete cue and a training context: cue competition does not result from the division of a limited resource. *Journal of Experimental Psychology: Animal Behavior Processes*, **35**, 197–211.

Urushihara, K., Wheeler, D. S., Pineno, O. & Miller, R. R. (2005). An extended comparator hypothesis account of superconditioning. *Journal of Experimental Psychology: Animal Behavior Processes*, **31**, 184–198.

Van Hamme, L. J. & Wasserman, E. A. (1994). Cue competition in causality judgements: the role of nonpresentation of compound stimulus elements. *Learning and Motivation*, **25**, 127–151.

Waelti, P., Dickinson, A. & Schultz, W. (2001). Dopamine responses comply with basic assumptions of formal learning theory. *Nature*, **412**, 43–48.

Wasserman, E. A. & Castro, L. (2005). Surprise and change: variations in the strength of present and absent cues in causal learning. *Learning and Behavior*, **33**, 131–146.

Wheeler, D. S. & Miller, R. R. (2008). Determinants of cue interactions. *Behavioural Processes*, **78**, 191–203.

Witnauer, J. E. & Miller, R. R. (2007). Degraded contingency revisited: posttraining extinction of a cover stimulus attenuates a target cue's behavioral control. *Journal of Experimental Psychology: Animal Behavior Processes*, **33**, 240–250.

Witnauer, J. E. & Miller, R. R. (2009). Contrasting overexpectation and extinction. *Behavioural Processes*, **81**, 322–327.

Witnauer, J. E. & Miller, R. R. (2010). The error in total error reduction. *Learning and Behavior*.

Witnauer, J. E. & Miller, R. R. (in press). Some determinants of second-order conditioning. *Learning and Behavior*.

Witnauer, J. E., Urcelay, G. P. & Miller, R. R. (2008). Reduced blocking as a result of increasing the number of blocking cues. *Psychonomic Bulletin and Review*, **15**, 651–655.

5

Associative modulation of US processing: implications for understanding of habituation

ALLAN R. WAGNER AND EDGAR H. VOGEL

Abstract

Considerable data from Pavlovian conditioning indicate that events that are associatively signaled by discrete cues are not as effectively processed as they otherwise would be. Extrapolating from early evidence of this phenomenon, especially so-called conditioned diminution of the unconditioned response (CDUR), Wagner (1976, 1979) suggested that a similar effect might be responsible for long-term habituation, as stimuli come to be "expected" in the context in which they have been exposed. In this paper we will reflect upon this reasoning in the light of more recent evidence from our laboratory and elsewhere. One major complication is that extended contexts (as well as discrete cues) can control response-potentiating, conditioned-emotional tendencies, in addition to the presumed decremental effects. Experiments that separate these effects will be exemplified, and one theoretical approach, through the models SOP and AESOP (Wagner, 1981; Wagner & Brandon, 1989) will be illustrated, with some implications for our further understanding of habituation.

In the late 1970s, Wagner (1976; 1979) presented some views about associative learning that were centered upon the notion that events that are already represented, or "primed" in active memory, are not as effectively processed as they otherwise would be. One of several forms of evidence for this supposition was the so-called conditioned diminution of the UR, a phenomenon originally reported by Kimble and Ost (1961), in the context of human eyeblink conditioning. Wagner, Thomas, and Norton (1967) had observed similar findings, while studying conditioning with electrical stimulation of the motor cortex, as the

US. They observed that after extensive CS–US pairings, dogs consistently came to show a less vigorous leg-lifting UR to the conditioning-intensity US, when it was preceded by its customary CS, than when it was occasionally presented alone. They reported this effect in dogs that never showed any detectable CRs, as well as in dogs that developed CRs, whether such CRs resembled the UR or not.

With an incautious leap, Wagner (1976, 1979) suggested that this conditioned diminution of the UR might be prototypical of what happens during long-term habituation to a stimulus. That is, when a stimulus is repeatedly presented in some context, and not otherwise, the context might serve like a CS to develop association with the habituating stimulus and cause the stimulus to be "expected," and less well processed, in that context. On this reasoning one would expect long-term habituation to be context specific, so that presenting a habituated stimulus in a context other than that of training should lead to a recovery of responding, just as the conditioned diminution of the UR is only observed when the US is preceded by a trained CS. Likewise, one would expect long-term habituation to be extinguishable as a result of exposure to the habituation context in the absence of the habituated stimulus, just as the conditioned diminution of the UR can be reversed by non-reinforced exposure to the CS alone.

Although Wagner (1979) presented experimental evidence of the extinction of habituation of the vasomotor response in the rabbit that was congruent with this notion, and pointed to other encouraging data, it is fair to say that the initial reviews of it (e.g., Mackintosh, 1987; Hall, 1991), as a useful approach to long-term habituation were less than kind. Especially challenging were the findings of Marlin and Miller (1981), who reported a series of studies of the habituation of the acoustic startle response in the rat that showed no evidence of context specificity or, indeed, of any conditioned diminution effect at all. And, both Mackintosh (1987) and Hall (1991) concluded that the only substantial evidence of the contextual control of a diminished response to a US was to be found in the work of Siegel and his students on the acquired tolerance to drugs, such as morphine (Siegel, 1975: Siegel, Hinson, & Krank, 1978). In this case, since there is also substantial evidence that the contexts come to evoke a CR that is antagonistic to the UR, one might suppose that only in such instances does it appear that something resembling habituation is context specific.

Wagner (1979) acknowledged that in some systems long-term habituation appears to result from changes intrinsic to the S–R pathway involved, and does not necessarily depend upon contextual priming. Likewise, where there is demonstrable associative influence of the context, one must, obviously, be ready to take into account the contribution of any overt CR tendencies, whether mimicking of the UR or antagonistic to it. But, the decremental effect of contextual priming, apart from CR/UR interaction, may not be as groundless a view of long-term habituation as some observed. There have now been accumulated some strong data showing such effect, with some responses, as we will mention later. And, where decisive data are lacking, there is reason to look more closely at the designs of experiments on habituation before drawing premature conclusions.

One important reason for caution in interpretation of studies of habituation is the complicating influences of emotional responses that can also be conditioned to contextual cues, and serve to potentiate the response to the habituating stimulus. A body of data collected by Brandon and others in our laboratory (Bombace, Brandon, & Wagner; 1991; Brandon & Wagner, 1991; Brandon, Bombace, Falls, & Wagner, 1991) demonstrated that the conditioned and unconditioned eyeblink responses resulting from experience with a paraorbital US were potentiated in the presence of contextual cues that had independently been paired with an aversive paraorbital or hindleg US. Thus, it is quite possible that a habituation routine involving an aversive stimulus would lead the contextual stimuli to control a conditioned diminution of the UR to that specific stimulus, but also a conditioned emotional response that would potentiate the defensive response to a variety of stimuli, including that of training. In this case changes in, or extinction of, the contextual stimuli could lead to either an increase or a decrease in the response to the target stimulus, or to some balance of the two. The supposition of both, a decremental habituation process and an incremental sensitization process as a result of iterated stimulation, is common to various theories (e.g., Groves & Thompson, 1970). But, the potential context specificity of both is a disquieting complication in relationship to the assumed tests of Wagner's interpretation of long-term habituation.

In this paper we will proceed as follows: (1) we will briefly review the kinds of data that originally encouraged the supposition that expected stimuli are not as effectively processed as they otherwise would be. This involved substantial evidence from studies using brief CSs, as well as at least one result of diminished processing that has been witnessed with extended contextual cues. The theoretical interpretation was formalized in the model SOP (Wagner, 1981); (2) we will, briefly, point to a related literature from our laboratory on the acquisition of the "conditioned emotional response" that demonstrates the potentiation of defensive URs and CRs that could obscure any conditioned diminution of the UR. The theoretical interpretation in this case was formalized in the model AESOP (Wagner & Brandon, 1989; Brandon & Wagner, 1998); (3) we will report a set of unpublished investigations by Brandon, Bell, and Wagner (unpublished manuscript) that exemplifies the kind of experimental evaluation that appears to be required to disentangle the conflicting influences. They demonstrate the way in which responding is determined by multiple associative influences, and that experiments on habituation need be designed sensitive to these influences; (4) with these data in front of us, we will attempt to show how they can be simulated via the quantitative assumptions of SOP and AESOP. The theoretical regularities involved call into question how good a basis any single response can provide for generalizing about habituation; and (5) finally, we will take the opportunity to make some additional observations about what these data and simulations might have to say about the phenomenon of long-term habituation.

The data that we will present from our laboratory will all be drawn from work with the rabbit, and the majority of it from eyeblink conditioning in which the US was a 100 msc electric shock to one or the other paraorbital regions, the UR and the CR were eyelid closures, and the CSs were either a diffusely reflected light, a vibrotactual stimulus applied to the chest, or a tone, noise, or pulsed auditory stimulus. We will ignore the specific quality of the CS in the various studies as it was always counterbalanced in within-study comparisons, and was not a differentiating variable between studies.

Diminished processing of expected USs

Our early studies demonstrated four different ways in which a US has diminished effects when it is preceded by a CS that has regularly announced it, as contrasted with being presented alone or preceded by a previously non-reinforced CS. Terry and Wagner (1975) demonstrated that a predicted US was less retained in memory over a trace interval as a discriminative stimulus than was an unpredicted US. Wagner, Rudy, and Whitlow (1973) found that a predicted US was less effective as a "distracter" in interfering with other contemporaneous Pavlovian conditioning than was an unpredicted US. A third and more familiar class of studies involved variations on the Kamin (1968) blocking effect, which showed that an expected US produces less associative learning than does an unpredicted US. This was exemplified by a study by Saavedra and Wagner (reported in Wagner, 1976), which showed that when a target CS was reinforced by a US, when in compound with another CS, the excitatory learning acquired by the target CS was diminished in proportion to the associative strength of the accompanying CS. This variation is part of what is summarized in the Rescorla–Wagner acquisition rule (Rescorla & Wagner, 1972; Wagner & Rescorla, 1972) by its stating that the reinforcement occasioned by a US is diminished by the summed associative strength of all of the cues that signal it on that trial.

The fourth demonstration of diminished processing, and the one most directly related to our concern here, was the aforementioned conditioned diminution of the UR, as seen in Donegan's (1981) dissertation studies. The

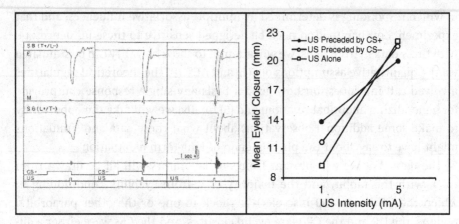

Figure 5.1 The left-hand panel depicts representative records of the three kinds of test trials from two animals in Donegan (1981, Experiment 2). The right-hand plot presents the mean amplitude of the eyeblink response to 1 and 5 mA USs when each US was preceded by CS+, CS−, or neither CS in test trials. Redrawn with permission from Donegan (1981, Experiment 2.)

experiments began with a phase of discrimination training, with CS+ reinforced and CS− non-reinforced. Then, in testing, subjects were presented with the paraorbital shock US, either in the presence of CS+ as it had previously occurred, in the presence of CS−, or alone. The left-hand panel of Figure 5.1 presents some representative records of the three kinds of test trials from two animals. As may be seen, the amplitude of the eyeblink response was attenuated when the US was preceded by CS+, in comparison with when it was preceded by CS−, or was presented alone. This occurred in spite of the fact that the conditioned response to CS+ was an anticipatory closure, which mimicked the UR, so that if no US had been given there would have been greater response on the CS+ occasions than on the CS− trials. Donegan, in fact, tested his animals with lower US intensities than the training intensity, as well as the training intensity, to see the pattern of responding reverse, as shown in the right-hand panel, from being one where CS+ facilitates eyeblink responding at the time of the US, at low US intensities, to one where CS+ diminishes eyeblink responding at the time of a more intense, conditioning-level US.

In all of these studies the US of interest was made expected by the signaling action of discrete CSs with which it had previously been paired. Rescorla and Wagner (1972), however, importantly assumed that USs administered in a context could also come to be conditioned to the extended context and, thereby, be less effective in promoting associative learning in that context. A notable study that supported the reasoning that conditioning to extended contextual cues can control a decrement in the effectiveness of a US was reported by Hinson

(1982). Hinson looked at the acquisition of eyeblink conditioned responses to a discrete tonal CS in groups of rabbits that had been pretreated over 10 sessions in which they received 20 paraorbital USs per session or had an equal number of sessions of simple confinement. Subgroups were distinguished by whether the pretreatment was in the same environment as the subsequent eyeblink conditioning or in an alternate environment, differing along multiple dimensions. The major finding was that whereas the group that received the US preexposures in the conditioning environment showed a marked reduction in acquisition of conditioned responding in comparison with the group that was simply confined in that environment, the group that received US preexposures in the alternate environment did not differ reliably from the group that was simply confined in that environment. It appeared that the decremental effects of US preexposure occurred only when the experimental context was the same in the preexposure and the conditioning phases.

In a further experiment, Hinson (1982) evaluated whether such context-specific US preexposure effects would be extinguished by exposure to the context in the absence of the US. Acquisition of eyeblink conditioned responses was observed in groups of rabbits that had received either 10 sessions of US preexposure in the conditioning environment or 10 sessions of simple confinement in that environment. Between the preexposure and the conditioning phases, subgroups received either 25 sessions of placement in the experimental environment, without the US, or rested in the home cage. The major finding was that whereas the group that had received the US preexposure and was subsequently rested in the home cage was severely retarded in eyeblink conditioning in relationship to the groups that had not received US preexposure, the group that received the US preexposure and subsequent "extinction" exposures to the experimental environment alone was reliably less retarded. As Hinson pointed out, these are just the kinds of observations that would be predicted from the assumption that US preexposure in the conditioning context causes the US to be associated with that context and to have diminished ability, in that context, to support excitatory conditioning.

Wagner's (1976, 1979) interpretation of long-term habituation was that it involves a conditioned diminution of the UR to the habituated stimulus, as seen by Donegan (1981), but controlled by contextual cues, as seen in the US preexposure effect reported by Hinson (1982).

CER potentiation of defensive responses

There are many reasons why this plausible account might be mistaken. A complication immediately presents itself in cases in which the stimulus of interest, such as the USs used by Donegan (1981) and Hinson (1982), produces not only a reflexive response such as the eyeblink, but also an appetitive or aversive reaction, itself being capable of being conditioned. A very substantial literature (e.g., Rescorla & Solomon, 1967; Davis, 1992; Brandon & Wagner, 1998) attests to the fact that conditioned emotional responses (CERs) can serve to modulate a wide range of ongoing behaviors. Of concern here is the presumption that paraorbital shock as employed as the US in the forgoing studies can be expected to support a CER being acquired by the contextual cues, which could serve to potentiate, rather than reduce, the provoked eyeblink UR as well as other defensive responses, in that context.

A series of experiments by Brandon and others in our laboratory (Bombace et al., 1991, Brandon and Wagner, 1991; Brandon et al., 1991) demonstrated this general tendency. The general design of these studies consisted of experiments in which different 30 s auditory stimuli were trained, one associated with a US placed variably 8 to 28 s into the stimulus, the other not reinforced, over a number of sessions. Subsequently, the response to different probe stimuli was evaluated, either in the presence of the previously reinforced stimulus, the previously non-reinforced stimulus, or alone. The general outcome is illustrated in Figure 5.2, which presents data drawn from the several experiments in which the training US was either a 5 mA shock to the hind leg, or an equally intense shock to the paraorbital region, and where the measured response was either the startle response to an airpuff into the auditory canal, the eyeblink UR to a paraorbital US, or an eyeblink CR to a CS that had been trained by pairing with a paraorbital US. In all cases, the measured response was potentiated in the presence of the previously reinforced stimulus, A, as compared with the previously non-reinforced stimulus, B, or when the probe was presented alone. The use of the different responses to the different stimuli, and the different locations of the aversive USs, in this research was calculated to allay any worry that the pattern of facilitation observed was attributable to some specific motor tendency that might have become conditioned to the reinforced context. The generality of the facilitation effect, instead, appears consistent with the supposition that has been mentioned, that the reinforced context came to elicit a conditioned emotional response that potentiated the defensive responses elicited by the different probes.

It may be obvious how this general potentiation effect can complicate the interpretation of studies concerning the context specificity of the conditioned diminution of the UR. However, let us illustrate by reconsidering the data from the Donegan (1981) dissertation on the conditioned diminution of the eyeblink UR using brief 1 s stimuli, shown in Figure 5.1. The essential finding was that the amplitude of the measured eyeblink following a paraorbital US was

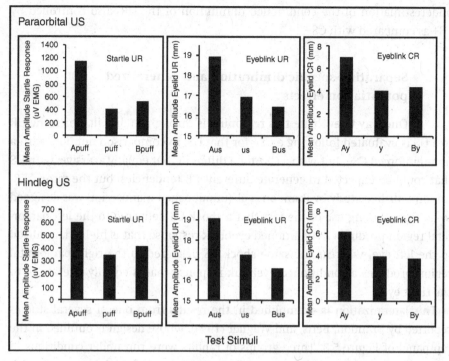

Figure 5.2 Results of six different experiments in which a 30#s contextual stimulus (A) was trained with either a para orbital shock US (top panels) or a hindleg shock US (bottom panels), while an alternative contextual stimulus (B) was nonreinforced. Responses reported are from tests in which a startle-eliciting air puff (left panels), an eyeblink-eliciting US (middle panels) or eyeblink-evoking CS, y (right panels) were presented in the context of A, B, or alone. In all instance A potentiated the response to the different test stimuli. Redrawn with permission from Bombace, *et al.* (1991), Brandon and Wagner (1991), and Brandon *et al.*, (1991).

different following a CS+ that had regularly announced the US than it was following a CS– that had regularly been non-reinforced. The striking interaction that may be seen was attributable to two tendencies controlled by the CS+. CS+ was observed to elicit an eyeblink CR alone, which was larger than the UR to a 1 mA US. This was presumed to account for the greater measured response to the 1 mA US following CS+ than following CS–. CS+ was also presumed to make the US expected, in the way that CS– would not, and thus produce a conditioned diminution of the UR. This was presumed to account for the smaller measured response to the 4 mA US following CS+ than following CS–. The complication suggested by the data of Brandon *et al.* (1991) is that the UR should also have been generally enhanced following CS+ as compared with CS– as a result of any CER tendency conditioned to the former but not to the latter. If this is so, the CER potentiation produced by CS+ as compared with CS– may have led to an underestimation of the conditioned diminution of the UR, also controlled by CS+ as compared with CS−.

Separating specific diminution and generalized potentiation effects

One way to evaluate this reasoning is through studies in which the UR to a US is evaluated following a CS+ for that US, in comparison not only with a non-reinforced CS−, but with a CS+ for a different, but equally aversive, with US that could be expected to generate different CR tendencies, but the same CER. An unpublished study by Brandon *et al.* (unpublished manuscript) was designed to do this, making use of the fact that a shock US delivered to the left paraorbital region produces a conditioned eyeblink response that is highly lateralized to the left eye, whereas the same shock US delivered to the right paraorbital region produces a conditioned eyeblink response that is equally lateralized to the right eye.

This lateralization is exemplified in the results from one of several studies reported by Brandon, Betts, and Wagner (1994), whose design is outlined in the top panel of Figure 5.3. Three groups of rabbits were run under conditions in which two CSs, CSx and CSy, were each consistently reinforced, in one case both with USs to the left eye, in another case both with USs to the right eye, and in the third case, one with a US to the left eye and the other with a US to the right eye. The bottom plot of Figure 5.3 presents the main results of this study. When the eyeblink responses were measured to each CS, it was found that the left-eye subjects learned to blink their left eye to both CSs (with few right-eye responses), the right-eye subjects learned to blink their right eye to both CSs (with few left-eye responses), and the "both eyes" animals learned to blink their left eye to one CS and their right eye to the other, with few responses with the contralateral eye.

The series of experiments conducted by Brandon *et al.* (unpublished manuscript) made use of this preparation, with a general design depicted in Figure 5.4. In each of three experiments all animals were trained over 8 sessions, each including 24 trials in which one CS, A, was paired with a 4 mA US to the left paraorbital region, another CS, B, was paired with a similar US to the right paraorbital region, and a third CS− was non-reinforced. In subsequent testing, all subjects were tested for their response to paraorbital shocks of 1 and 4 mA intensities, as in the Donegan (1981) dissertation, but now preceded, sometimes by CS+s that were the same as those with which the different probe locations of USs had been paired, or were preceded by CS+s that were different from those with which the different locations of USs had been paired, or were preceded by the CS− that was previously non-reinforeced.

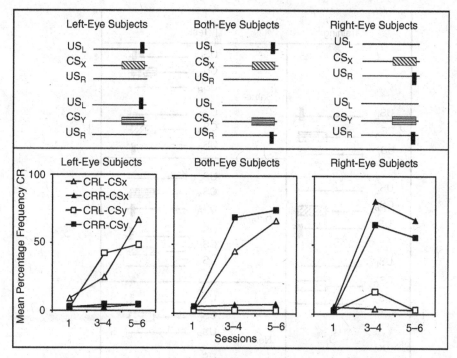

Figure 5.3 The top panel depicts the experimental arrangement of the cues during training in Experiment 1 of Brandon *et al.* (1994). In the left-eye subjects CSx and CSy were paired with a US to the left eye, in the right-eye subjects CSx and CSy were paired with a US to the right eye, and in the both-eye subjects CSx was paired with a US to the left eye and CSy was paired with a US to the right eye. All animals were tested for their conditioned responses to CSx and CSy in both eyes. The bottom plots present the mean percentage frequency of eyeblink CRs on the left (CRL) and right (CRR) eyes to the stimuli CSx and CSy across sessions for left-eye subjects (left graph), both-eyes subjects (middle graph), and right-eye subjects (right graph). Redrawn with permission from Brandon *et al.* (1994).

The left-hand panel of Figure 5.5 presents the data of Experiment 1, in which the CSs were 1 s in duration, as in the Donegan (1981) study. As may be seen, there was a replication of Donegan's findings of a conditioned diminution of the UR to the 4 mA USs when the USs were preceded by the same CSs+ as during training, as compared with the non-reinforced CS–. The important new finding is in how this difference appears to have underestimated the size of the conditioned diminution effect. Notice that the amplitude of the UR was greater on occasions when the US was preceded by a different CS+ than during training, as compared with the non-reinforced CS–. One can reasonably attribute this difference to a CER-mediated potentiation occasioned by the different CS+, and

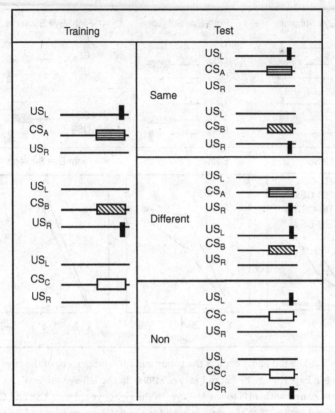

Figure 5.4 Experimental arrangement of the cues during training and testing in the three experiments conducted by Brandon *et al.* (unpublished manuscript) (2010). There was an initial phase of training in which one CS, A, was paired with a US to the left eye, another CS, B, was paired with a US to the right eye, and a third CS, C, was non-reinforced. After training, all animals were tested for their unconditioned responses when the US was preceded by the CS that was paired with the US in the same location as the probe US (same trials), by the CS that was paired with the US in the alternate location as the probe US (different trials), and by the non-reinforced CS (non-trials).

suppose that a similar, CER– mediated potentiation existed on occasions when the USs were preceded by the same CS+s as in training, but that it was then expressed in combination with the conditioned diminution peculiar to these occasions. On this reasoning, the better measure of the conditioned diminution of the UR is to be seen in the difference in the URs observed when the USs were preceded by the same CSs as compared with the different CSs, and not as compared with the non-reinforced CSs. Related reasoning is appropriate to the findings on the 1-mA tests. It can be assumed that part of the greater responding on the same and different CS tests, in comparison with the non-reinforced CS tests, is due to their common, response-potentiating CER effects, and that the better estimate of how specific CRs generated by the CSs contribute to performance at the time of the UR is to be found in the difference between the responding on the same versus different occasions.

That such separating of the more general, response-potentiating effects from the more specific conditioned diminution of the UR can be illuminating may be seen in a second experiment conducted by Brandon *et al.* (unpublished manuscript). This experiment used the same design depicted in Figure 5.4, and the same general parameters as the previous study but with CSs that were somewhat more extended and context-like, as compared with the previous study. It employed stimuli that were 10 s in duration, and, when reinforced by a US, embraced such USs variably 6, 7, or 8 s into the interval. With such stimuli, no conditioned eyeblink responses were observed to the onset of the stimuli or at sampled times within the stimuli. The data from testing can be seen in the middle plot of Figure 5.5. In this case, there was no tendency for USs preceded by CS+s that were the same as in training to be followed by a lesser UR than those preceded by the previously non-reinforced CS−. Indeed, on this comparison there was a reliable facilitation of responding following CS+. Without additional information, one would conclude that there was no conditioned diminution of the UR. However, the USs did provoke a diminished UR when they were preceded by CS+s that were the same as in training, as compared with when they were preceded by CS+s that were different than in training, in signaling the opposite USs. The reasonable conclusion is that there was a conditioned diminution of the UR when the US was signaled by its training stimulus, but that there was an even greater CER-based potentiation when the US was preceded by either of the reinforced stimuli.

A third experiment conducted by Brandon *et al.* (unpublished manuscript) was identical to the two previous studies, except that it employed yet longer context-like stimuli of 30 s, and, thus, was exactly like those employed in the aforementioned studies of modulation by Bombace *et al.* (1991), Brandon and Wagner (1991), and Brandon *et al.* (1991). In this case the reinforcement, when it occurred, was scheduled at variable intervals of 8 to 28 s into the stimulus. The results shown in the right-hand panel of Figure 5.5 were quite simple. The URs measured following the previously reinforced stimuli were reliably potentiated in relationship to those measured following the previously non-reinforced stimulus, and there was no difference in this effect between occasions in which the US was presented in the same context in which it had occurred in training, or in the context in which the alternate

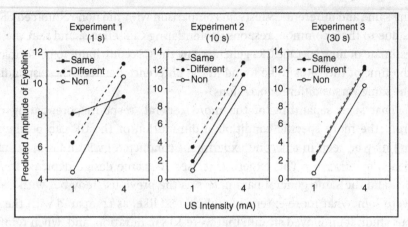

Figure 5.5 Mean amplitude of the eyeblink response to 1 and 4 mA USs when each US was preceded by the CS conditioned to the ipsilateral eye (same), the CS conditioned to the contralateral eye (different), or by the nonconditioned CS (non) in the testing phase of experiments 1 (left-hand plot), 2 (middle plot), and 3 (right-hand plot) of Brandon, *et al.* (unpublished manuscript). The duration of the CSs was 1, 10, and 30 s for experiments 1, 2, and 3, respectively.

US had occurred in training. There was clear evidence of an associative modulation of the UR, but one that might be expected from the reinforced contexts having come to control a CER, not one that might be expected from the reinforced contexts having come to control a conditioned diminution of one or the other eyeblink URs.

Brandon *et al.* (unpublished manuscript) (2010) were hesitant to accept the differential conditioned diminution effect seen with the different CS durations by such cross-experiment evidence. Thus, they conducted yet another study in which they evaluated the response to paraorbital USs when they were preceded by CS+s that either had been trained with the same US or with a US to the alternate eye. (No non-reinforced stimuli were used.) For all animals, one pair of stimuli in association with the two locations of US were 1 s in duration, as in Experiment 1, whereas another pair in association with the two locations of US were 30 s in duration, as in Experiment 3. The results depicted in Figure 5.6 were consistent with the separate prior studies. There was clear indication of a conditioned diminution of the UR when the US was signaled by the same 1-s stimulus as in training versus the different 1-s CS. There was no suggestion of a conditioned diminution of the UR when the US was signaled by the same 30-s, contextual-like stimulus as in training versus the different 30-s stimulus.

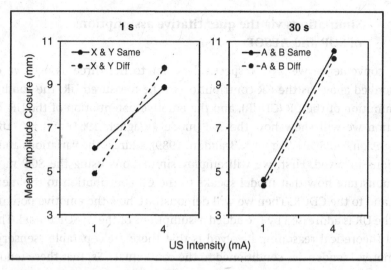

Figure 5.6 Mean amplitude of the eyeblink response to 1 and 4 mA USs when
each US was preceded by the CS conditioned to the ipsilateral eye (same) and the
CS conditioned to the contralateral eye (different) in Brandon *et al.* (unpublished
manuscript), Experiment 4. The left-hand plot presents the results for the
trials with the 1 s CSs and the right-hand plot presents the results for the trials
conducted with the 30 s CSs.

The data in this series of experiments testify to the complexity by which simple associative processes can show themselves and to the challenge to theoretical interpretation. Three different associative effects were observed. First, there
was a greater response to the same as compared with the different CS (and to
the non-conditioned CS), which was seen only under the low-US-intensity tests
with the 1 s CS. This was a replication of the effect demonstrated by Donegan
(1981) and taken to be the result of the contribution of CRs that mimicked the
tested UR – CRs that were acquired only with this CS duration and observed
in the absence of any US. Second, there was a lesser UR observed to the high-
intensity US on the occasions of the same as compared with the different CSs,
when the CSs were either 1 s or 10 s in duration. This is what is anticipated by a
conditioned diminution of the UR when there is an equating of the UR potentiating effects of any CER controlled by the comparison stimuli. Third, there was
also a potentiating effect of the reinforced CSs (same and different) versus the
non-reinforced CS that was apparent as the only tendency with the 30-s stimuli,
and as a greater response to the different CS than to the non-reinforced CS with
the 10-s and 1-s stimuli. The challenge for theoretical interpretation comes from
the complexity by which these different associative effects vary with the parameters of training and testing, most notably being the CS duration.

Simulations via the quantitative assumptions of SOP and AESOP

For convenience we will, respectively, refer to the three associative effects described above as the CR contribution to the measured UR, the conditioned diminution of the UR (CDUR), and the emotive potentiation of the UR. In this section we will show how the SOP model (Wagner, 1981) and its "affective extension," AESOP (Wagner & Brandon, 1989), address the variations and inter-actions involved. First, we will employ simulations using the SOP model to demonstrate how that model speaks to the CR contribution to the measured UR and to the CDUR. Then we will demonstrate how the emotive potentiation of the UR is addressed by the added assumptions of the AESOP model. The general theoretical reasoning involved is that there are separable "sensory" and "emotive" tendencies conditioned to the contextual CSs, that these tendencies are differentially sensitive to the duration of the CS, and that they interact with the eyeblink UR in very different ways – the sensory tendency both adding to and diminishing the measured UR (SOP), and the emotive tendency potentiating the UR (AESOP).

Figure 5.7 presents a simplified network rendition of eyeblink conditioning according to SOP. The CS (e.g., a tone) and the US (a paraorbital shock) are each assumed to activate a pair of processing units, a primary unit, $A1_i$, followed by a secondary unit, $A2_i$. The degree of activation of each unit depends on the activity of the other, and can take values between 0 (no activity) and 1 (maximal activity). At each moment of stimulation, the primary unit is activated according to the parameter $p1_i$, and subsequently drives activation of the $A2_i$ unit according to the parameter $pd1_i$. The $A2_i$ unit, in turn, recurrently inhibits the $A1_i$ unit, making it transiently less susceptible to activation by its initiating stimulus. Activity in $A2_i$ eventually decays, releasing the $A1_i$ unit according to the parameter $pd2_i$ (which is not shown in the figure). The values of p1, pd1, and pd2 are restricted to the unit interval. According to these assumptions, the momentary change in activity of the primary unit i, $\Delta A1_i$ is given by $p1_i[1-(A1_i + A2_i)] - [pd1_iA1_i]$, whereas the momentary change in activity of the secondary unit i, $\Delta A2_i$ is given by $[pd1_iA1_i] - [pd2_iA2_i]$.

Space does not allow a full quantitative description of SOP (see Wagner, 1981 for more details), but there are two parametric considerations that must be mentioned in order to facilitate the comprehension of the simulations that follow. The first is the assumption that pl is a function of relatively stable properties of the stimulus (e.g., intensity) taking a value greater than zero in the presence of the stimulus and zero in its absence. In this regard, it is generally assumed that $p1_{US} > p1_{CS}$, reflecting a difference in the saliences of the CS and the US. The second concerns the values taken on by pdl and pd2. They are

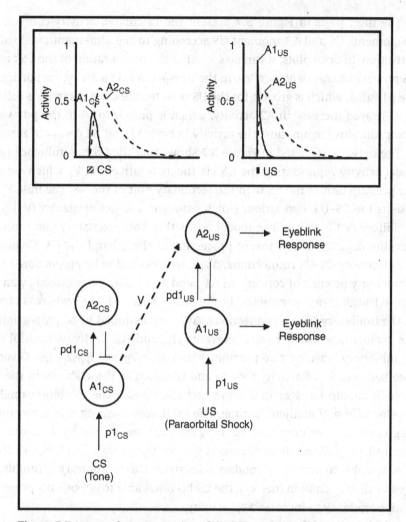

Figure 5.7 A network representation of the SOP model. Each stimulus is represented by a primary (A1$_i$) and a secondary unit (A2$_i$). The CS and the US activate their respective primary units according to their p1 values, which in turn activate the corresponding secondary units according to their pd1 values. The CS influences the activity of the US-secondary unit by means of its associative value, V. The links ending in a horizontal line represent inhibitory feedback from each secondary unit to its corresponding primary unit. The inset plots present the courses of activity for a typical CS and US.

assumed to be independent of the presence or absence of the initiating stimulus, but to be characteristics of the duration of the effective representation of the two activity states (A1 and A2). It is assumed that pd1 is greater than pd2 (which implies that A2 activity lasts longer than A1 activity), with a customary designation that pd1 = 5pd2.

The inset plots of Figure 5.7 present the calculated activity courses for a 10-moments CS and a 1-moment US according to the aforementioned rules of activation. In both plots, it can be seen that the presentation of the CS and the US provokes a transient increase in their respective A1 activity, proportional to the p1 value, which is greater for the US than for the CS. A1 activity is followed by a delayed increase in A2 activity, which is proportional to the pd1 values. Upon stimulus termination, the activity in both A1 and A2 decays to zero.

The network depicted in Figure 5.7 shows that the CS has influence on the nodal activity representing the US via the associative link V_i, which connects the primary unit of the CS with the secondary unit of the US. The link, V_i, represents the CS–US association, which expresses the net excitatory (V+) minus inhibitory (V−) learning. The model posits that both excitatory and inhibitory learning depend on concurrent processing of the CS and the US. Changes in the excitatory CS–US connections, ΔV_i+, are assumed to be proportional to the momentary product of concurrent $A1_{CS}$ and $A1_{US}$ activity multiplied by an excitatory learning rate parameter, L+ (i.e., $\Delta V_i+ = A1_{CS}A1_{US}$ L+), whereas changes in the inhibitory CS–US connections, ΔV_i-, are assumed to be proportional to the momentary product of concurrent $A1_{CS}$ and $A2_{US}$ activity, multiplied by an inhibitory learning rate parameter, L− (i.e., $\Delta V_i- = A1_{CS}A2_{US}$ L−). Given the assumed courses of activity for CSs and USs such as those shown in the inset plots, it should be clear that some excitation and some inhibition might be developed at any moment in time. The excitatory learning rate is assumed to be greater than the inhibitory learning rate, but constrained by the assumption that L+/L− = pd1/pd2. If excitation is greater than inhibition (net V+), the CS becomes able to provoke secondary US activity. On the contrary, if inhibition is greater than excitation (net V−), the CS becomes able to oppose any other associative tendency to increase $A2_{US}$ activity.

With regard to the response, SOP assumes that the presentation of the US generates a two-fold sequence in unconditioned responding, first being dependent on the activity of the US primary unit, and subsequently on added activity of the US secondary unit. As shown in Figure 5.7, the two response tendencies occasioned by a paraorbital shock US are assumed to be similar, both contributing to the eyeblink response, although they can be assumed to be antagonistic or unrelated to one another in other response systems. In contrast, the CS has its influence on behavior by activating the US secondary unit by means of its associative link. The direct effect, in this example, is an anticipatory eyeblink response that can add to the unconditioned response occasioned by a subsequent US. Notice, however, that by this action of activating the US secondary unit, the CS also has an indirect behavioral consequence by means of the recurrent inhibition from $A2_{US}$ to $A1_{US}$, of decreasing the Al activity occasioned by a

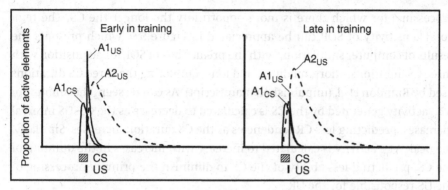

Figure 5.8 Predicted $A1_{CS}$, $A1_{US}$, and $A2_{US}$ courses of activity during training with a standard CS–US interval of 20 moments and delay conditioning according to SOP. The left-hand plot presents the predicted values in the first training trial when no learning has occurred and the right-hand plot presents the predicted values after asymptotic training. The parameters were $p1_{CS} = 0.1$, $pd1_{CS} = 0.1$, $pd2_{CS} = 0.02$, $p1_{US} = 0.85$, $pd1_{US} = 0.01$, $pd2_{US} = 0.002$, $L+ = 0.01$, and $L- = 0.002$.

subsequent US. This is the core mechanism by which this model accounts for a conditioned diminution of the UR.

According to SOP, the acquired CS–US association influences not only the probability of a conditioned response, but also the potential processing of the US. By this reasoning, if the A2 node of a US is activated by the precedence of an associated CS, the A1 node of that US will be less susceptible to activation, so as to produce a diminished UR. Figure 5.8 shows the relevant patterns of CS and US nodal activity computed to occur early and late in training for simple CS–US delay conditioning. By comparing the functions early and late in training it can be seen how the CS develops the ability to generate $A2_{US}$ activity, presumably producing the CR, and to depress $A1_{US}$ activity, presumably responsible for the conditioned diminution of the UR.

One important feature of SOP is its temporal sensitivity. The most obvious aspect of this sensitivity is that the degree of conditioning is critically dependent on the length of the CS, such that poorer learning is expected for longer-duration CSs. This effect is explained by two facts. One feature of the model is that the temporal course of A1 representation of any continuing stimulus involves a characteristic recruitment of activity followed by a decline attributable to the recurrent inhibition by the A2 activity. Thus, longer-than-optimal duration CSs will have lower $A1_{CS}$ nodal activity at the time of occurrence of the US, and thus less concurrent $A1_{CS}$ and $A1_{US}$ activity that produces excitatory learning. Furthermore, as excitatory learning does develop and the CS acquires the property of causing $A2_{US}$ activity prior to the US, this leads to the development of inhibitory CS–US associations (due to concurrent $A1_{CS}$ and $A2_{US}$

processing) for which there is more opportunity the longer the CS. The temporal sensitivity of SOP can be appreciated in Figure 5.9, which presents the results of computer simulations with the predictions of SOP for acquisition with three CS durations: short, medium, and long, emulating the three CS durations used by Brandon *et al.* (unpublished manuscript). As can be seen, the amount of $A2_{US}$ activity generated by the CS is calculated to decrease as the CS–US interval increases, predicting less CR tendencies as the CS duration increases. Similarly, the peak $A1_{US}$ activity is calculated to increase with increases in the duration of the CS, predicting less ability of the CS to diminish the primary processing of the US responsible for the UR.

The simulations depicted in Figure 5.9 employed parameters that involve a brief processing of the US (relatively large $pd1_{US}$ and $pd2_{US}$ values), which is congenial to the empirical data on eyeblink conditioning. However, Wagner and Brandon (1989) proposed that various observations concerning "response divergence" (e.g., Schneiderman, 1972), i.e., different findings among different response systems subjected to the same conditions of training, could be understood in terms of differences in the pd1 and pd2 parameters associated with the different responses. They specifically assumed in this respect that with the customary procedures of eyeblink conditioning with a paraorbital US, there is also the development of conditioned emotional responses, and that this conditioning involves US representation involving lower "decay" values and, thus, more protracted processing than the US representation implicated in the conditioning of the eyeblink response. The general idea is that a US may have separable attributes, in this case sensory attributes and emotional attributes that engage differential processing, with relatively large versus relatively small $pd1_{US}$ and $pd2_{US}$ values. They cited, as computational consequences, that this would explain how CERs could be acquired with fewer trials and over longer CS–US intervals than could the eyeblink CR, based upon the same CS–US training.

The idea that there is separable conditioning of the sensory CS–US association responsible for the CR and CDUR specific to the eyeblink, versus the CS–US association responsible for the CER, is captured by the AESOP model depicted in Figure 5.10. AESOP assumes that the presentation of the US activates two separate sets of A1/A2 units: one representing the sensory aspect of the US and the other its emotional aspects. Second, the model assumes that the association of the CS with the sensory aspect of the US controls the conditioned eyeblink response whereas the association of the CS with the emotive aspect of the US controls the CER. The model assumes that both associations follow from the rules of SOP, with any differences in acquisition reflecting only parametric differences, notable of which is that the emotive processing involves pd1 and pd2 values that are smaller (processing is more protracted) than that of the

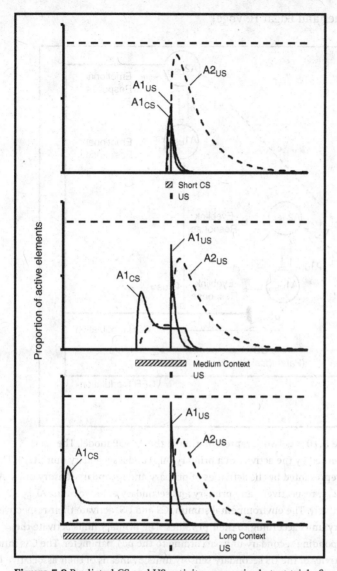

Figure 5.9 Predicted CS and US activity over a single test trial after training with three CS–US intervals according to SOP's rules of stimulus activation. The plots present simulations conducted with rapid US-processing parameters ($pd1_{US} = 0.1$, $pd2_{US} = 0.02$) that emulate data on sensory conditioning. The remaining parameters were $p1_{CS} = 0.1$, $pd1_{CS} = 0.1$, $pd2_{CS} = 0.02$, $p1_{US} = 0.85$, $L+ = 0.01$, and $L- = 0.002$. The durations for the US, short CS, medium context, and long context were 1, 10, 100, and 300 simulated moments, respectively. The US onset was at moment 220 and coterminated with the CS in the short condition, but was imbedded within the CS in the medium (US initiated at 70 percent of the CS duration) and long conditions (US initiated at 73 percent of the CS duration). The secondary activity of the CS ($A2_{CS}$) was omitted in the plots since it was assumed to have no influence in conditioning. The broken horizontal line in each plot represents the peak value of $A1_{US}$ if the US were presented alone.

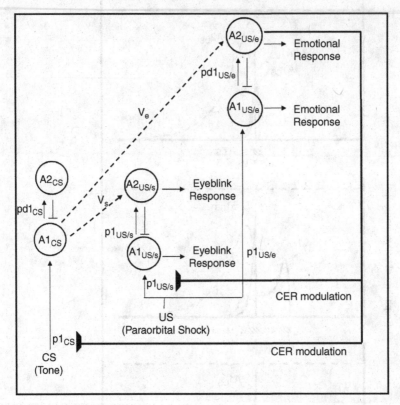

Figure 5.10 A network representation of the AESOP model. The CS is represented by the activity of a primary (Al_{CS}) and a secondary unit ($A2_{CS}$). The US is represented by the activities of primary and secondary sensory units, $Al_{US/s}$ and $A2_{US/s}$, respectively, and primary and secondary emotive units, $Al_{US/e}$, $A2_{US/e}$, respectively. The environmental stimuli, CS and US, activate their respective primary units according to their pl values. The primary units activate the corresponding secondary units according to the pd1 parameter. The CSs influence the activity of the US secondary sensory units by means of their associative links, Vs, and the activity of the US secondary emotive unit by means of their associative links, Ve. The activity of the US secondary sensory unit is responsible for the generation of a discrete CR while the activity of the US secondary emotive unit is responsible for the generation of conditioned emotional responses. The link between the emotive units and the sensory units represents the modulatory effect of the US secondary emotive unit on the activity of the CS and US sensory units. The modulatory effect is assumed to be an increment in the respective p1 values, which is proportional to $A2_{US/e}$.

sensory processing. The final critical assumption of AESOP is that the emotive $A2_{US}$ activity modulates the activation parameter, p1, of stimuli experienced in its presence. By this assumption, the processing of CSs and USs that control the eyeblink response can be expected to be potentiated by the CER.

In order to illustrate one of the core aspects of AESOP, namely the fact that the CER is predicted to be less dependent upon short CS–US durations than is the eyeblink CR, Figure 5.11 presents simulations with the same three CS durations used in the simulations in Figure 5.9, but with a US with longer processing parameters. As can be seen, there is clear evidence of conditioning at all three CS durations, apparent in the substantial anticipatory $A2_{US}$ activity, greater than that seen in the corresponding sensory eyeblink conditioning depicted in Figure 5.9. There is, in this case, also greater CDUR, evident in the diminished $A1_{US}$ at all intervals as compared with that seen with the shorter processing assumptions in Figure 5.9.

From the simulations presented in Figures 5.9 and 5.11, one can anticipate that SOP and AESOP are equipped with theoretical mechanisms for accounting for the three major effects observed by Brandon *et al.* (unpublished manuscript). Specifically, the sensory conditioned response, which depends on the $A2_{US}$ activity occasioned by the CS, is predicted to be substantial at the locus of the US so as to add to the sensory UR produced by the $A1_{US}$ activity and increment the measured response, in the case of the 1-s CS but not the longer `CSs. The same sensory tendency is also predicted to be such as to decrease the unconditioned response by diminishing $A1_{US}$ processing, in the case of the 1 and 10 s CSs, but not the 30 s CS, and the CER tendency that develops in parallel with the sensory CR is predicted to be such as to be capable of potentiating the unconditioned eyeblink response to the sensory US across the 30 s as well as shorter CS durations.

Figure 5.12 presents a summary of the three effects in accordance with the simulations depicted in Figure 5.9 (sensory effects) and Figure 5.11 (emotive potentiating effects). The left-hand panel presents the predicted eyeblink CR tendency ($A2_{US}$) as a function of the CS duration, which shows that the shorter the CS the more the contribution of the CR at the US locus. The middle panel presents the eyeblink UR tendency ($A1_{US}$) for the three CS durations and two US testing intensities. In this case, although there is generally predicted to be less conditioned diminution of the UR the longer the CS duration, the differences are not as marked as for the CR. Finally, the right panel presents the $A2_{US}$ for the conditioned emotional response that is assumed to be responsible for the sensory UR potentiation for the three CS durations. There is again a CS duration function, but one that predicts the CER to be robust at intervals for which the sensory CR and CDUR would not be.

As can be seen in Figure 5.12, although all three predicted effects exhibit some degree of dependency on the CS duration, they follow different courses that can potentially explain the data on eyeblink conditioning reported by Brandon *et al.* (unpublished manuscript). For instance, notice that the predicted

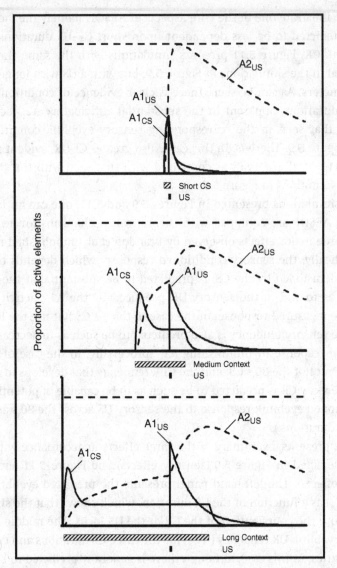

Figure 5.11 Predicted CS and US activity over a single test trial after training with three CS–US intervals according to SOP's rules of stimulus activation. The plots present simulations conducted with slow US-processing parameters ($pd1_{US}$ = 0.02, $pd2_{US}$ = 0.004), which emulate data on emotive conditioning. The remaining parameters were $p1_{CS}$ = 0.1, $pd1_{CS}$ = 0.1, $pd2_{CS}$ = 0.02, $p1_{US}$ = 0.85, L+ = 0.01, and L– = 0.002. The durations for the US, short CS, medium context, and long context were 1, 10, 100, and 300 simulated moments, respectively. The US onset was at moment 220 and coterminated with the CS in the short condition, but was imbedded within the CS in the medium (US initiated at 70 percent of the CS duration) and long conditions (US initiated at 73 percent of the CS duration). The secondary activity of the CS ($A2_{CS}$) was omitted in the plots since it was assumed to have no influence in conditioning. The broken horizontal line in each plot represents the peak value of $A1_{US}$ if the US were presented alone.

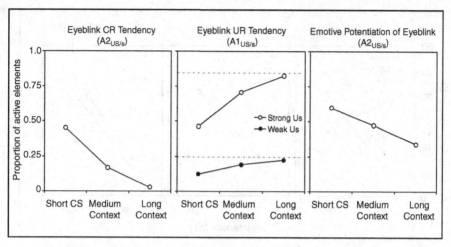

Figure 5.12 Predicted eyeblink CR tendency (left plot), eyeblink UR tendency (middle plot), and emotive potentiation of eyeblink (right plot) after asymptotic training with three CS durations. The UR tendency is plotted for test trials with a strong US ($p1_{US}$ = 0.85) and a weak US ($p1_{US}$ = 0.23). The dotted line represents the values of $A1_{US/s}$ in US-alone trials with the strong US (top line) and the weak US (bottom line). The data for the "eyeblink CR tendency" and "eyeblink UR tendency" plots were obtained from the simulations described in Figure 5.9, and the data for the emotive potentiation of eyeblink plot were obtained from the simulations described in Figure 5.11.

conditioned diminution effect for the short and medium CSs is very small when the test is conducted with the weak US (middle plot). It might be assumed that this diminution effect can be easily overcome by the substantial CR contribution (right plot) and the CER potentiation (left plot) developed by these two CS durations. On the contrary, the short and medium CSs exhibit much higher conditioned diminution of the UR with the strong US, which might not be overcome by CR addition and CER potentiation. Finally, the simulations anticipate the fact that the only noticeable effect for the longest CS is a substantial potentiation of the eyeblink response.

In order to offer an integrated account of the way in which CR, CDUR, and CER interact, we conducted computer simulations of the Brandon *et al.* (unpublished manuscript) comparisons using the same parameters used in the simulations of sensory and emotive conditioning presented in Figures 5.9 and 5.11, applying the modulation rule proposed by Brandon and Wagner (1998), and the response generation rule previously employed by Wagner (1981). The modulation rule states that $p'_{1,1} = p_{1,i}(1 + KA2_{US/e})$, where $p'_{1,i}$ is the effective p1 value for stimulus i, $p_{1,i}$ is the p1 value in the absence of modulation, and K a parameter that weights the influence of the emotive $A2_{US}$ in potentially incrementing p1.

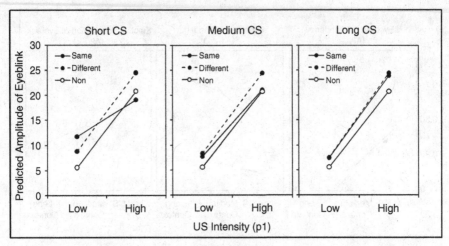

Figure 5.13 Simulation of Brandon *et al.*'s (unpublished manuscript) Experiment 1 (short CS; 10 moments), Experiment 2 (medium context; 100 moments), and Experiment 3 (long context; 300 moments) with AESOP. The US was applied at moment 220. The plots present the peak eyeblink response in a test trial. $p1_{CS} =$ 0.1, $pd1_{CS} = 0.1$, $pd2_{CS} = 0.02$; $p1_{US}$ (training) = 0.85, $pd1_{US/s} = 0.1$, $pd2_{US/s} = 0.02$, $pd1_{US/e}$ = 0.02, $pd2_{US/e} = 0.004$, k = 1. The high- and low-intensity test trials were created by setting $p1_{US}$ at 0.85 (high) and 0.23(low). The eyeblink response was computed as R = $0.245(w1A1_{US/s}+w2_{A2US/s})$. The w1 value was fixed at 100 and w2 was a linear function of $A1_{CS}$ activity (w2 = $113.92A1_{CS}+3.01$), which resulted in w2 = 54.6, = 20.3, and = 20, for the short, medium, and long CS, respectively.

For calculating the response generated by the US units, Wagner (1981) proposed that R = $f(w1A1_{US} + w2A2_{US})$, where wl and w2 are linear weighting factors, and f is a mapping function appropriate to the response measure. For the eyeblink response, in which the CR produced by $A2_{US}$ mimics the primary UR produced by $A1_{US}$, it is assumed that w1 and w2 are both positive. Finally, a dynamism factor was assumed, making w2, itself, a function of the CS trace ($A1_{CS}$ activity), which amplifies the degree to which the CR contribution from A_{US} decays over the duration of the CS, after its peak activity.

Figure 5.13 presents the major results of these computer simulations. Comparing the pattern of theoretical predictions in Figure 5.13 with the empirical data obtained by Brandon *et al.* (unpublished manuscript) shown in Figure 5.5 reveals a generally agreeable fit. The ordering of the predicted results is especially consistent with the data in the case of the high-intensity US: a strong conditioned diminution effect is predicted in the short CS condition, where the unconditioned response in the presence of CS–Same is lower than that to CS–Different and to the Non-conditioned CS; a less strong conditioned diminution effect is predicted in the 10 s CS duration condition, where it is seen only by comparing CS Same versus CS Different, but not when comparing CS Same versus CS Non; finally, the differences between CS–Same and CS–Different are predicted to be negligible in the 30-s condition, showing no detectable conditioned diminution, but both greater than CS Non, consistent with the experimental data. Likewise, the simulations of the low-intensity US tests are generally consistent with the data, predicting a greater response to CS Same than to CS Different and to CS Non in the short CS condition, a slightly diminished response to CS Same as compared with CS Different in the medium CS condition, and no diminution of CS Same as compared with CS Different, but substantial potentiation of both in comparison with CS Non in the long CS condition. There is overall a substantial fit of the model to the data.

Apart from embracing the data reported by Brandon *et al.* (unpublished manuscript) involving the rabbit eyeblink response, the assumption introduced by AESOP that different response systems may be associated with different US processing parameters, may have important implications in addressing the observed incidence of conditioned diminution of the UR in other response systems. There are, in fact, several parametric variations within the SOP/AESOP machinery that could produce different degrees of conditioned diminution of UR controlled by an extended context. As was emphasized in the preceding simulations, the most obvious parameter concerns the duration of US processing, which is instantiated in the model by the pd1 and pd2 parameters. The smaller the pd1 and pd2 values the more persistent is the processing of the US and, as a consequence of this, the higher the degree of contextual conditioning. Thus, it might be assumed that some unconditioned responses are more or less likely to be diminished by contextual conditioning depending on how slowly or rapidly the US is processed.

Another parameter of the model that influences the predicted CDUR is the weight assigned to the CR contribution to the measured UR, w2. As mentioned above, w2 is assumed to be positive for those situations in which the CR mimics the UR (as in the case of the eyeblink response), such that the CR contribution at the locus of the US adds to the measured UR, decreasing the predicted CDUR. Consequently, the more positive w2 is the less likely a CDUR would be. Alternatively, w2 is assumed to be negative in those cases in which the CR is antagonistic to the UR (as in the case of morphine as the US reported by Siegel, 1975) such that the CR contribution at the locus of the US opposes the UR, increasing the predicted CDUR. Thus, the more negative w2 is the more likely a CDUR would be.

Another potential source of variability is the potentiation parameter K, which dictates the degree to which emotive conditioning augments the measured UR. In the simulations presented in Figure 5.13, a relatively high

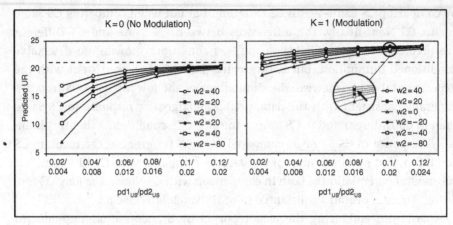

Figure 5.14 Predicted unconditioned response according to the SOP/AESOP models in a test trial in which the US is embedded within a long contextual CS that was trained to asymptote with the same US. The duration of the CS and the US were 300 and 1 moments, respectively, and the US was applied at moment 220 of the CS duration. The parameters of the model were $p1_{cs} = 0.1$, $pd1_{cs} = 0.1$, $pd2_{cs} = 0.02$, $p1_{us} = 0.85$, L+ = 0.01, L– = 0.002, and w1 = 100. The plots show the predicted UR as a function of the US decay parameters ($pd1_{us}$ and $pd2_{us}$) and the CR weighting parameter (w2). The left plot presents the predictions assuming no emotive modulation (k = 0) and the right plot presents the predictions assuming modulation by emotive conditioning developed with $pd1_{us/e} = 0.02$, $pd1_{us/e} = 0.004$. In the right plot, the bigger circle shows an enlarged view of the values for the simulation conducted with pd1 = 0.1 and pd2 = 0.02, and the arrow points to the predicted response with w2 = 20, which involves the same parameters as those used for the simulation of the study by Brandon *et al.* (unpublished manuscript) in the "same" condition with the long context and the high-intensity US depicted in Figure 5.13.

potentiation parameter of K = 1 was assumed, consistent with the fact that the conditioned emotional response is known to increase substantially the unconditioned eyeblink response in rabbits (Brandon *et al.*, 1991). It is surely the case that other responses, in other circumstances, may be more or less potentiated by conditioned emotional responses involving, thus, other values of K.

In order to provide a quantitative demonstration of the effects of the US processing ($pd1_{us}$ and $pd2_{us}$), CR contribution (w2), and emotive modulation (K) parameters in the predicted conditioned diminution of UR, we conducted a series of computer simulations of conditioning with the same 30 s contextual CS used in the previously reported simulations, but with a range of pds, w2, and K values. Figure 5.14 presents the predicted UR for six different ratios of pd1 and pd2 values, six different w2 values, and two values of K. As can be seen in the left-hand panel, in the absence of emotive modulation (i.e., K = 0) the model predicts that the UR is always diminished in the presence of the contextual CS in comparison with the UR obtained by a US imbedded in a nonconditioned context (control).

Notice, however, that the degree of conditioned diminution of the UR observed in the left-hand panel of Figure 5.14 is inversely related to the size of the pd1 and pd2 values and to the size of w2. Furthermore, there is an interaction between these factors, so that w2 has little impact when pds are large (e.g., above 0.10/0.02), but has a substantial effect when the pds are small (e.g., below 0.040/0.008). This interaction is due, on the one hand, to the fact that smaller pd1 values produce more conditioning to the context, and hence more influence of the CR on the response to the US, and on the other, to the fact that smaller pd2 values produce a more persistent $A2_{US}$ processing which causes the CR to last longer.

The right-hand panel of Figure 5.14 presents the same simulations reported in the left-hand panel, but this time assuming substantial emotive modulation, which was obtained with the same parameters used for the simulations of Brandon *et al.* (unpublished manuscript) study but for a range of pd and w2 values. Here the effects of pds and w2s are in the same direction rather than under no modulation, but potentiation rather than diminution is predicted for many of the conditions simulated. Notice that the few conditions in which a net conditioned diminution of the UR is predicted involve very small pds and negative w2 values.

Observations and conclusions

What implications should one draw from these musings? Priming theory (e.g., Wagner, 1976) was inspired by numerous observations pointing to the diminished processing of expected stimuli. Subsequent findings have continued to support the basic notion as it has been expressed within SOP (Wagner, 1981) and AESOP (Wagner & Brandon, 1989). What we have learned, however, is that there is such variation among the different indicators of associative expectation, the different measures of processing that can be influenced, and the different opportunities for these to be obscured that the implications for long-term habituation can be complicated.

One thing we have recognized is how different indicators of association between a predictive stimulus and a US can be differentially sensitive to parametric variation. In the experimental environment upon which we have focused it is known that the conditioned eyeblink as a measure of association is very dependent upon short CS–US intervals of less than two or three seconds. Thus, in the studies of Brandon *et al.* (unpublished manuscript) conditioned eyeblinks were regularly observed when the US was delivered at the end of a 1-s CS, but were never observed when the US was imbedded in either a 10 s or a 30 s stimulus. In comparison, associative blocking is not so restricted. It occurs with 1 s blocking stimuli, as in the study of Saavedra and Wagner (reported in Wagner, 1969) or with 30 s stimuli as in a study by Gewirtz, Brandon, and Wagner (1998), as well as with longer contextual stimuli as investigated by Hinson (1982). The conditioned diminution of the eyeblink UR falls someplace in between. It was observed not only under the 1 s condition, but also under the 10 s condition, although not with a 30 s stimulus.

Where to place the "sensitivity" of the conditioned diminution of the UR in this series could not be known before the fact, nor can the degree of generality of the ordering observed here in relationship to other learning situations. It may be telling that several unpublished assessments in our laboratory of the habituation of the eyeblink UR to the paraorbital shock intensities typically employed in conditioning, and used by Brandon *et al.* (unpublished manuscript), presented little evidence of any response decrement over sessions. There is a consistency in our not observing a conditioned diminution of the UR controlled by 30 s stimuli and not observing substantial habituation decrement in the UR with simple stimulus exposure.

It is similarly apparent in surveying the literature that different measures of long-term habituation can show differential sensitivity to context change. One comparison that has been investigated has been the assessments of the context specificity of habituation, as measured by the decrement in the orienting response to the habituating stimulus, versus as measured by the decreased associability of the stimulus as a CS, i.e., the so-called latent inhibition effect. Several studies (e.g., Hall & Channell, 1985; Hall & Honey, 1989) have reported that whereas stimulus exposure produces a latent inhibition effect that is context specific, it can do so without accompanying evidence that the habituation of the orienting response is similarly context specific. This might indicate different mechanisms in the two cases. However, it might also mean that latent inhibition is more sensitive in reflecting the context specificity involved, or that the studies were better designed to discriminate differences in latent inhibition versus differences in the orienting response. Recent data reported by Honey and Good (e.g., Honey, Good, & Manser, 1998; Honey & Good, 2000) attest to the conditioned diminution of the orienting response to CS-like visual stimuli. Furthermore, data reported by Jordan, Strasser, and McHale (2000) make it clear that habituation of the orienting response to similar auditory or visual stimuli is demonstrably context specific, so as to show recovery of the response when the stimulus is presented in a different, equally familiar experimental context, and to be reversed when the habituating context is extinguished in the absence of the habituated stimulus. The different outcomes in the Jordan *et al.* studies, in contrast to earlier studies comparing habituation of the orienting response and latent inhibition, is likely attributable to the greater difference in the alternative contexts employed and the greater amount of extinction given, among other differences.

A related observation is that the habituation of different URs to the same stimulus can show different degrees of context specificity. Jordan *et al.* (2000) simultaneously measured startle and lick suppression in rats produced by exposure to an intense auditory stimulus. Habituation was observed in both measures. However, whereas lick suppression showed substantial recovery with shift in context, the startle response showed no similar recovery. The lack of context control of the habituating startle response replicates the findings of Marlin and Miller (1981) with this measure, whereas the contextual control of the habituation of lick suppression supports the similar control observed in Jordan *et al.*'s aforementioned investigation of the habituation of the orienting response.

The context specificity of long-term habituation observed by Jordan *et al.* (2000) in the case of the orienting and behavioral suppression measures is supported by other studies employing habituation of a motor response. Tomsik, Pedreira, Romano, Hermitte, and Maldonado (1998) reported a context specificity and extinguishability of the habituation of the escape response of the crab to the movement of an overhead form. Rankin (2000) offered further support for the generality of such observations in her studies of habituation in the nematode *Caenorhabditis elegans*. Rankin found that the habituation of the withdrawal response to a tap of the supporting Petri plate was specific to the chemo-sensory environment during habituation and could be extinguished by exposure to the training environment between habituation and testing.

Jordan and Leaton (1982) have entertained that the habituation of the startle response, as compared with orienting and response suppression, may be governed by different mechanisms in that the two are not highly correlated and that lesions of the midbrain reticular formation severely attenuate the long-term habituation of startle without affecting the habituation of lick suppression. Jordan *et al.* (2000), however, also called attention to the different post-stimulus measurement periods in the two cases. The startle response is initiated within 10 ms of the eliciting stimulus, and its maximum amplitude is typically reached within 50 ms (although Jordan *et al.* used a 200 ms window). In contrast, the orienting response, lick suppression, and escape behavior, the habituation of which have been reported to be context dependent, have been measured over windows of seconds or tens of seconds. The theoretical simulations that we have presented might encourage the reasoning that the several responses, the habituation of which have been found to be context specific are the ones that enjoy a protracted processing, similar to that assumed to occur in the case if the CER, which should favor associative learning to the context (see Figure 5.11). In contrast, the startle response, which has not been observed to show any context dependence, may be part of a very rapid processing that affords little opportunity for learning to the context. On this reasoning the processing relevant to the eyeblink UR investigated by Brandon *et al.* (unpublished manuscript) would be argued to fall in between (see Figure 5.9), affording more opportunity for contextual control than the startle, but less than for the orienting, withdrawal, or suppression measures.

The most secure conclusion that can be drawn from the Brandon *et al.* (unpublished manuscript) studies is that the conditioned diminution of the UR can be obscured by conditioned potentiating effects, presumably reflecting the contribution of a conditioned emotional response controlled by the same CS. The conditioned diminution of the eyeblink UR, in the presence of a discrete 1-s CS with which the US had been paired, was much more apparent when measured against the amplitude of the eyeblink UR to the contralateral US in the same context than when measured against the eyeblink UR to either US in the presence of a non-reinforced CS. The conditioned diminution of the eyeblink UR, in the presence of a 10 s CS in which the US had been presented, was only detectable when measured against the eyeblink UR to the contralateral US in the same context, as the responses to both USs were potentiated in the presence of previously reinforced contexts as compared with a non-reinforced context.

There is nothing novel about the recognition that there can be incremental effects of stimulus exposure as well as decremental effects. Groves and Thompson (1970) offered an explicit "dual-process" account by which sensitization was assumed to be able to increase responding at the same time that habituation decreases responding. They also assumed different mechanisms underlying the two processes, with habituation being more specific to the exposed stimulus and sensitization reflecting more globally influential state changes. Leaton and his students (Borszcz, Cranney, & Leaton, 1989; Leaton & Cranney, 1990; Young & Leaton, 1994), studying the acoustic startle response in rats, marshaled a variety of evidence that sensitization in this circumstance is attributable to a conditioned emotional response being acquired to the contextual cues as a result of their pairing with the initially aversive startle stimulus. Such CER could be expected to potentiate the startle response and mask habituation. Its control by the experimental context should also be expected to complicate observing any tendency for habituation to be context specific. That is, a post-habituation shift in the context, or extinction of the context should be expected to produce an increment in the measured response due to a loss of habituation, but a decrement in the response due to a loss of CER-mediated sensitization.

It is noteworthy that few experiments on habituation have been designed in ways that would allow one to separate such effects. However, if long-term habituation is viewed as being relatively specific to the exposed stimulus, and long-term sensitization as being more globally influential, then even if they are both associatively mediated and context dependent, one should be able to separate the influences by tests, not only of the exposed stimulus, but of other potentially effective stimuli. That is essentially what Brandon *et al.* (unpublished manuscript) did in utilizing the lateralized eyeblink responses to paraorbital stimulation of the two eyes, and in assuming that the CS with which one US was trained would come to control a conditioned diminution of the UR specific to that US, but a CER that would equally potentiate the UR to the US of either eye.

All studies of habituation would be well served by designs that allow a separation of the response-potentiating as well as the response-diminishing effects of exposure, both of which can be context specific. Indeed, the desirability of routine use of multiple test stimuli in studies of habituation is not restricted to tests of the context specificity of the phenomena involved. As an example of the circumstances under which it would have been illuminating, consider a study that Davis and Wagner (1969) conducted on what is now called the "incremental stimulus intensity effect." They compared the acoustic startle response to 120 dB stimuli of groups of rats that had been exposed to 750 stimuli that were either a constant 120 dB, a constant 100 dB, a random order of intensities between 85 and 120 dB, or a gradually increasing order of intensities between 85 and 120 dB. As the name of the effect suggests, there was substantially less responding in test in the group that had experienced the gradually increasing intensities than in any of the other three groups. The question is whether it was due to more effective habituation under the incremental sequence or to less effective sensitization under such sequence, or, perhaps, both. Davis and Wagner could not answer that question with the simple experiment conducted. They could have commented on it if they had employed two different stimuli, perhaps one acoustic and the other vibrotactual, that have been demonstrated to have at least partially separable startle-producing features (Vogel & Wagner, 2005). Then they could have ascertained whether the exposure to one of the stimuli in the incremental versus alternative fashions produced less test responding specific to the exposed stimulus (presumably reflecting differences in habituation to that stimulus) or less test responding equally to the two stimuli (presumably reflecting differences in sensitization produced by the training). Until more studies of habituation are designed in such a way we should withhold judgment on the potential associative mechanisms involved.

Acknowledgments

We thank Susan E. Brandon, who collected and analyzed much of the unpublished data reported in this paper. We also thank Fernando P. Ponce and Jacqueline Y. Glynn for their work on the theoretical simulations and figures.

Edgar H. Vogel was supported by grants from Fondecyt (N° 1090640) and from the Program of Research on Quality of Life (Res. 387/2007, Universidad de Talca).

References

Bombace, J. C., Brandon, S. E. & Wagner, A. R. (1991). Modulation of a conditioned eyeblink response by a putative emotive stimulus conditioned with hindleg shock. *Journal of Experimental Psychology: Animal Behavior Processes*, **17**, 323–332.

Borszcz, G. S., Cranney, J. & Leaton, R. N. (1989). Influence of long-term sensitization on long-term habituation of the acoustic startle response in rats: central gray lesions, preexposure, and extinction. *Journal of Experimental Psychology: Animal Behavior Processes*, **15**, 54–64.

Brandon, S. E. & Wagner, A. R. (1991). Modulation of a discrete Pavlovian conditioning reflex by a putative emotive Pavlovian conditioned stimulus. *Journal of Experimental Psychology: Animal Behavior Processes*, **17**, 299–311.

Brandon, S. E. & Wagner, A. R. (1998). Occasion setting: influences of conditioned emotional responses and configural cues. In N. Schmajuk, ed., *Occasion Setting: Associative Learning and Cognition in Animals*. Washington, D.C.: American Psychological Association, pp. 343–382.

Brandon, S. E., Betts, S. L. & Wagner, A. R. (1994). Discriminated, lateralized eyeblink conditioning in the rabbit: an experimental context for separating specific and general associative influences. *Journal of Experimental Psychology: Animal Behavior Processes*, **20**, 292–307.

Brandon, S. E., Bombace, J. C., Falls, W. T. & Wagner, A. R. (1991). Modulation of unconditioned defensive reflexes via an emotive Pavlovian conditioned stimulus. *Journal of Experimental Psychology: Animal Behavior Processes*, **17**, 312–322.

Davis, M. (1992). The role of the amygdala in conditioned fear. In J. Aggleton, ed., *The Amygdala: Neurobiological Aspect of Emotion, Memory, and Mental Dysfunction*. New York: Wiley-Liss, pp. 255–305.

Davis, M. & Wagner, A. R. (1969). Habituation of startle response under incremental sequence of stimulus intensities. *Journal of Comparative and Physiological Psychology*, **67**(4), 486–492.

Donegan, N. H. (1981). Priming-produced facilitation or diminution of responding to a Pavlovian unconditioned stimulus. *Journal of Experimental Psychology: Animal Behavior Processes*, **7**, 295–312.

Gerwirtz, J. C., Brandon, S. E., Wagner, A. R. (1998). Modulation of the acquisition of the rabbit eye blink conditioned response by conditioned contextual stimuli. *Journal of Experimental Psychology: Animal Behavior Processes*, **24**, 106–117.

Groves, P. M. & Thompson, R. F. (1970). Habituation: a dual-process theory. *Psychological Review*, **77**, 419–450.

Hall, G. (1991). Habituation. *Perceptual and Associative Learning*, **40**, 29–68.

Hall, G. & Channell, S. (1985). Differential-effects of contextual change on latent inhibition and on habituation of an orienting response. *Journal of Experimental Psychology: Animal Behavior Processes*, **11**, 470–481.

Hall, G. & Honey, R. C. (1989). Contextual effects in conditioning, latent inhibition, and habituation: associative and retrieval functions of contextual cues. *Journal of Experimental Psychology: Animal Behavior Processes*, **15**, 232–241.

Hinson, R. E. (1982). Effects of UCS preexposure on excitatory and inhibitory rabbit eyelid conditioning: an associative effect of conditioned contextual stimuli. *Journal of Experimental Psychology: Animal Behavior Processes*, **8**, 49–61.

Honey, R. C. & Good, M. (2000). Associative modulation of the orienting response: distinct effects revealed by hippocampal lesions. *Journal of Experimental Psychology: Animal Behavior Processes*, **26**(1), 3–14.

Honey, R. C., Good, M. & Manser, K. L. (1998). Negative priming in associative learning: evidence form a serial-habituation procedure. *Journal of Experimental Psychology: Animal Behavior Processes*, **24**(1), 229–237.

Jordan, W. P. & Leaton, R. N. (1982). The effects of mesencephalic reticular formation lesions on habituation of the startle and lick suppression responses in the rat. *Journal of Comparative and Physiological Psychology*, **96**, 170–183.

Jordan, W. P., Strasser, H. C. & McHale, L. (2000). Contextual control of long-term habituation in rats. *Journal of Experimental Psychology: Animal Behavior Processes*, **26**, 323–339.

Kamin, L. J. (1968). "Attention-like" processes in classical conditioning. In M. R. Jones, ed., *Symposium on the Prediction of Behavior: Aversive Stimulation*. Miami, FL: University of Miami Press, pp. 9–31.

Kimble, G. A. & Ost, J. W. P. (1961). A conditioned inhibitory process in eyelid conditioning. *Journal of Experimental Psychology*, **61**(2), 150–156.

Leaton, R. N. & Cranney, J. (1990) Potentiation of the acoustic startle response by a conditioned stimulus paired with acoustic startle stimulus in rats. *Journal of Experimental Psychology: Animal Behavior Processes*, **16**, 169–180.

Mackintosh, N. J. (1987). Neurobiology, psychology and habituation. *Behavioral Research Theory*, **25**(2), 81–97.

Marlin, N. A. & Miller, R. R. (1981). Associations to contextual stimuli as a determinant of long-term habituation. *Journal of Experimental Psychology: Animal Behavior Processes*, **7**, 313–333.

Rankin, C. H. (2000). Context conditioning in habituation in the nematode, *C. elegans*. *Behavioral Neuroscience*, **114**, 496–505.

Rescorla, R. A. & Solomon, R. L. (1967). Two-Process learning theory: relationship between Pavlovian conditioning and instrumental learning. *Psychological Review*, **74**, 151–182.

Rescorla, R. A. & Wagner, A. R. (1972). A theory of Pavlovian conditioning: variations in the effectiveness of reinforcement and non reinforcement. In A. H. Black and W. F. Proasky, eds., *Classical Conditioning II: Current Theory and Research*. New York: Appleton–Century–Crofts, pp. 64–99.

Schneiderman, N. (1972). Response system divergencies in aversive classical conditioning. In A. H. Black and W. F. Proasky, eds., *Classical Conditioning II: Current Theory and Research*. New York: Appleton–Century–Crofts, pp. 313–376.

Siegel, S. (1975). Evidence from rats that morphine tolerance is a learned response. *Journal of Comparative and Physiological Psychology*, **89**, 498–506.

Siegel, S., Hinson, E. E. & Krank, M. D. (1979). The role of predrug signals in morphine analgesic tolerance: support for a Pavlovian conditioning model of tolerance. *Journal of Experimental Psychology: Animal Behavior Processes*, **4**, 188–196.

Terry, W. S. & Wagner, A. R. (1975). Short-term memory for "surprising" vs. "expected" unconditioned stimuli in Pavlovian conditioning. *Journal of Experimental Psychology: Animal Behavior Processes*, **1**, 122–133.

Tomsic, D., Pedreira, M. E., Romano, A., Hermitte, G. & Maldonado, H. (1998). Context- US association as a determinant of long-term habituation in the crab *Chasmagnathus*. *Animal Learning and Behavior*, **26**, 196–209.

Vogel, E. H. & Wagner, A. R. (2005). Stimulus specificity in the habituation of startle response in rat. *Physiology and Behavior*, **86**, 516–525.

Wagner, A. R. (1969). Stimulus validity and stimulus selection in associative learning. In N. J. Mackintosh and W.K. Honig, eds., *Fundamental Issues in Associative Learning*. Halifax, Canada: Dalhousie University Press, pp. 90–122.

Wagner, A. R. (1976). Priming in STM: an information-processing mechanism for self-generated or retrieval-generated depression in performance. In T. J. Tighe and R. N. Leaton, eds., *Habituation: Perspectives from Child Development, Animal Behavior and Neurophysiology*. Hillsdale, NJ: Elrbaum, pp. 95–118.

Wagner, A. R. (1979). Habituation and memory. In A. Dickinson and R. A. Boakes, eds., *Mechanisms of Learning and Motivation: A Memorial Volume for Jerzy Konorski*. Hillsdale, NJ: Erlbaum Associates, pp. 53–82.

Wagner, A. R. (1981). SOP: a model of automatic memory processing in animal behavior. In N. E. Spear and R. R. Miller, eds., *Information Processing in Animals: Memory Mechanisms*. Hillsdale, NJ: Erlbaum, pp. 5–47.

Wagner, A. R. & Brandon, S. E. (1989). Evolution of a structured connectionist model of Pavlovian conditioning (AESOP). In S.B. Klein and R.R. Mowrer, eds., *Contemporary Learning Theories: Pavlovian Conditioning and the Status of Traditional Learning Theory*. Hillsdale, NJ: Erlbaum, pp. 149–189.

Wagner, A. R. & Rescorla, R. A. (1972) Inhibition in Pavlovian conditioning: application of a theory. In M. S. Halliday and R. A. Boakes, eds., *Inhibition and Learning*. San Diego, CA: Academic Press, pp. 301–335.

Wagner, A. R., Rudy, J. W. & Whitlow, J. W. (1973). Rehearsal in animal conditioning. *Journal of Experimental Psychology*, **97**, 407–426.

Wagner, A. R., Thomas, E. & Norton, T. (1967). Conditioning with electrical stimulation of motor cortex: evidence of a possible source of motivation. *Journal of Comparative and Physiological Psychology*, **64**, 191–199.

Young, B. J. & Leaton. R. N. (1994) Fear potentiation of acoustic startle stimulus-evoked heart rate changes in rats. *Behavioral Neuroscience*, **108**, 1065–1079.

6

Attention, associations, and configurations in conditioning

N. A. SCHMAJUK, M. G. KUTLU, J. DUNSMOOR, AND J. A. LARRAURI

Abstract

This chapter describes a number of computational mechanisms (associations, attention, and configuration) that first seemed necessary to explain a small number of conditioning results and then proved able to account for a large part of the extensive body of conditioning data. We first present a neural-network theory (Schmajuk, Lam, & Gray, 1996), which includes attentional and associative mechanisms, and apply it to the description of brain activity in the amygdala, anterior cingulate cortex, dorsolateral prefrontal cortex (PFC) and insula, compound conditioning with different initial associative values, the accelerating effect of the extinction of the conditioned excitor on the conditioning of its corresponding conditioned inhibitor, super latent inhibition, recovery and absence of recovery from blocking, latent inhibition–overshadowing synergism and antagonism, summation tests in the context of extinction, and spontaneous recovery. Then we describe another neural network (Schmajuk & Di Carlo, 1992; Schmajuk, Lamoureux, & Holland, 1998) that includes configural mechanisms, and apply it to the description of response form in occasion setting. Finally, we show how the combination of attentional, associative, and configural mechanisms (Schmajuk & Kutlu, 2010) describes the effect of additivity pretraining and posttraining on blocking in causal learning.

Schmajuk, Lam, and Gray's (1996) attentional–associative model

Schmajuk *et al.* (1996) and Schmajuk and Larrauri (2006) proposed a neural-network model (SLG model) of classical conditioning. The SLG model shares properties with other associability models, including equations that portray behavior on a moment-to-moment basis (Grossberg, 1975; Wagner, 1981), the attentional control of the formation of CS–US associations (Pearce & Hall, 1980), the competition among CSs to become associated with the US (Rescorla & Wagner, 1972) or other CSs (Schmajuk & Moore, 1988), and the combination of attention and competition (Wagner, 1979). A version of the SLG program is available from the authors at www.duke.edu/~nestor.

Important properties of the SLG model include: (1) a description of the formation and *combination* of CS–CS and CS–US associations; (2) attention to the CS is controlled by the CS–US associations (as in the Pearce & Hall, 1980, model), by context-CS (CX–CS) associations (as in the Wagner, 1979, model), and by CS–CS associations (as in the Schmajuk & Moore, 1988, model, a property that explains why latent inhibition can become context independent); and (3) retrieval of CS–US and CS–CS associations is controlled by the magnitude of the attention to the CS (as in Wagner's, 1981, SOP model.)

Figure 6.1 shows a block diagram of the SLG network. The diagram includes (1) a "Short-term memory" and "Feedback" system, (2) an "Attention" system, (3) an "Association" system, and (4) a "Novelty'" system. The Attentional mechanism is regulated by the Novelty', defined as the sum of the absolute values of the difference between average expected and actual values of the US, the CSs, and the context (CX). The Attentional mechanism was designed to explain the retardation of conditioned responding following CS preexposure (latent inhibition). The Associations network is controlled by a real-time competitive rule (that describes overshadowing, blocking, and the properties of conditioned inhibition), and output from the Associative network is sent back to the input through a Feedback loop. The Feedback loop was included to describe sensory preconditioning and second-order conditioning through the combination of CS–CS and CS–US associations. The resulting model proved capable of correctly describing many experimental results for which it was not specifically designed, that is, results that are "emergent properties" of the model.

Some emergent properties of the model

Perception and imagination

As suggested by Konorski (1967), whereas environmental inputs to the short-term memory block represent a perceptual input, predictions of those inputs generated by the association system and sent to the feedback block can be regarded as imagined inputs.

Context-dependent and context-independent latent inhibition

We assume that a given CS_k can be predicted by other CSs, the CX, or itself. Therefore, either repeated presentations of that CS_k in a given context or simply repeated presentations of CS_k lead to a decrease in its novelty. Whereas

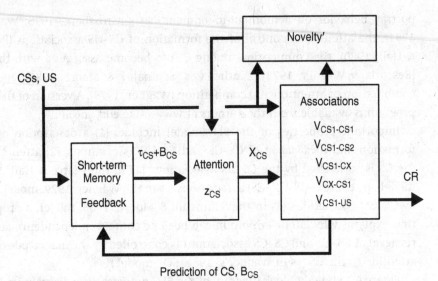

Figure 6.1 Block diagram of the Schmajuk–Lam–Gray (SLG; 1996) network. CS = conditioned stimulus; US = unconditioned stimulus; τ_{CS} = short-term memory trace of the CS; B_{CS} = prediction of the CS; z_{CS} = attentional memory; X_{CS} = internal representation of the CS; $V_{CS1-CS1}$, $V_{CS1-CS2}$, …, V_{CS1-US} = associations CS1–CS1, CS1–CS2, …, CS1–US; CR = conditioned response.

the CS_k–CS association (association of the CS_k with itself) decreases CS_k novelty in a context-independent manner, CS_j–CS_k or CX–CS_k associations decrease CS_k novelty in a context-dependent way. Because decrements in novelty are responsible for latent inhibition (LI), CS_k–CS_k associations are responsible for context-nonspecific LI, whereas CS_j–CS_k or CX–CS_k associations are responsible for context-specific latent inhibition (see Good & Honey, 1993).

Awareness

The model tends to maintain a minimum level of Novelty'. When Novelty' increases, attention to the environmental stimuli increases, associations are formed, the stimuli are predicted, and Novelty' decreases. When Novelty' decreases too much, attention decreases, existing associations are not activated, predictions decrease, and Novelty' increases again. In sum, Novelty' might decrease but rarely becomes zero.

Excitatory conditioning tends to be context independent

Excitatory $V_{CX,US}$ and excitatory $V_{CS,US}$ associations increase during the period of time when the (attentionally modulated) traces of the CX and the CS are active in the presence of (the unfiltered representation of) the US and decrease when the US is absent. Then, because the CS and the CX compete to become associated with the US, if the CS is more salient than the CX, the

CS–US association will increase more than the CX–US association. In addition, because the trace of the CX is active for a longer time (the whole duration of the "intertrial interval" [ITI]) than the trace of the CS, the excitatory $V_{CX,US}$ association will decrease more than the $V_{CS,US}$ association in the absence of the US. Therefore, because $V_{CS,US}$ increases more than $V_{CX,US}$ during the US presentation, and decreases less in its absence, $V_{CX,US}$ will be generally weaker than $V_{CS,US}$. This property is important to explain why responding at the end of conditioning tends to be CX independent and why the CX tends to become inhibitory during extinction.

Inhibitory contextual conditioning tends to be stronger than excitatory contextual conditioning

Because the SLG model assumes that B_{US} (and B_{CS}) takes on only positive values, inhibitory associations are not extinguished by CS or CX presentations. Inhibitory CX–US associations are established in extinction, during the period of time when the CS predicts the presence of the US, which is absent. These inhibitory CX–US associations do not change when the CX representation is active for the duration of the ITI, in the absence of the US. Therefore, inhibitory CX–US associations are independent of the ITI, but excitatory CX–US associations are not; a fact that has two important consequences. One is that inhibitory CX–US associations tend to be stronger than excitatory ones; a property important in extinction in which responding becomes CX dependent. Another consequence is that US presentations are more effective in decreasing the magnitude of inhibitory CX–US associations than in increasing the magnitude of excitatory CX–US associations: a property important when the effects of context reinforcement following extinction, weak conditioning (inflation), and partial reinforcement are compared. Finally, it is worth noticing that even if inhibitory CS–US and CX–US associations do not decrease with CS or CX presentations, attention to the CS or the CX might decrease with repeated presentations, thereby making the inhibitory association difficult to detect.

Limiting term for $V_{CS,US}$ associations

The SLG model incorporates a term limiting the values of all associations. This term is important in explaining the Rescorla (2000, 2001, 2002) experimental results regarding the effect of reinforced and non-reinforced presentations of an AB compound in which A and B had different initial associations with the US. Furthermore, we found that by limiting $V_{CS,US}$, the model is able to explain maximality effects on blocking (Beckers, De Houwer, Pineno, & Miller 2005), that is, the fact that blocking is present only when the prediction of the US by the blocking stimulus has not reached a maximum value and is able to predict most of the magnitude of the actual US.

Mediated acquisition and extinction

Because the representation of a $CS(B_{CS})$ is active even when that CS is absent but predicted by other CSs or the CX, all associations established by the CS can change even in its absence. This mechanism explains mediated acquisition and mediated extinction (Shevill & Hall, 2004).

Mediated changes in attention

Because a CS representation can be activated either by the CS or by its prediction by other CSs or the CX, attention to a given CS can still be modified even if that CS is absent. This is an important feature of the model that explains recovery from latent inhibition, recovery from blocking, recovery from overshadowing, backward blocking, and additivity posttraining effects on blocking.

Learning (storage) and performance (retrieval)

The representation of the CS, X_{CS}, controls both the storage (formation or read-in) of CS_1–CS_2 and CS–US associations, and the retrieval (activation or read-out) of CS_1–CS_2 and CS–US associations. Because attentional memory, z_{CS}, controls the magnitude of the internal representation X_{CS}, it indirectly controls storage and retrieval of CS_1-CS_2 and CS–US associations.

Cognitive mapping

The model can combine a series of Place–Place associations (similar to CS–CS associations) to predict whether a Place leads to a Goal (Schmajuk & Buhusi, 1997).

Attentional and associative representations in the brain

Dunsmoor, Bandettini, and Knight (2007) carried out a brain-imaging study of human fear conditioning and recorded (1) activity in the amygdala and anterior cingulate cortex (ACC), (2) activity in the dorsolateral prefrontal cortex (dlPFC) and insula, and (3) skin conductance responses. As shown in Figure 6.2 (upper panels), two distinct patterns of brain activations emerged: a linear pattern of activity that increased with the reinforcement rate was observed in the amygdala and ACC, and a greater activity to a partially reinforced CS (50% reinforcement rate) was observed in the dlPFC and insula. As shown in Figure 6.2 (lower panels), Dunsmoor and Schmajuk (2009) demonstrated that the SLG model is capable of describing those results.

The role of the amygdala in both humans and nonhuman animals has been well established as forming the association between the CS and US and producing the conditioned response (Davis & Whalen, 2001; Phelps & LeDoux, 2005). The simulations shown in Figure 6.2 (lower panels) appear to capture these functions of the amygdala: (1) predicting the US, B_{US}, based on X_{CS}–US

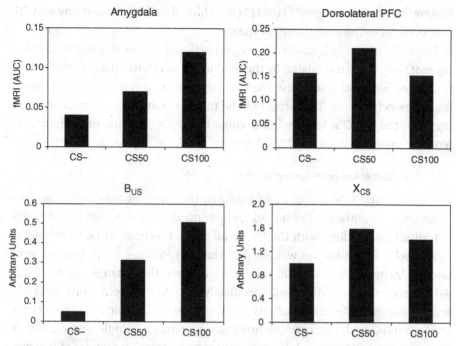

Figure 6.2 Hemodynamic response in the amygdala and the dorsolateral PFC. *Upper left panel*: area under the hemodynamic response curve (AUC) obtained with functional magnetic resonance imaging (fMRI) within the bilateral amygdala. Data from Dunsmoor *et al.* (2007). *Upper right panel*: area under the AUC within the dorsolateral PFC (dlPFC). Data from Dunsmoor *et al.* (2007). *Lower left panel*: computer simulations of the B_{US} variable for CS−, CS50, and CS100, with the SLG model. *Lower right panel*: computer simulations of the X_{CS} variable for CS−, CS50, and CS100, with the SLG model. CS−: never paired with the US, CS50: paired with the US on 50% of trials, CS100: paired with the US on 100% of trials.

associations, V_{CS-US}, and (2) using this prediction to generate the CR. However, this pattern of simulated results is not exclusive to the SLG model, as most associative learning models (e.g., Rescorla & Wagner, 1972; Mackintosh, 1975; Pearce & Hall, 1980) predict that differential reinforcement schedules affect the associative value of a CS.

Dunsmoor *et al.* (2007) characterized the pattern of responses in the dlPFC and insula as reflecting uncertainty for receiving the US, as activity was greater to the partially paired CS50 than to the CSs with more predictable outcomes (CS− and CS100). The simulations shown in Figure 6.2 (lower panels) support this suggestion. Specifically, the internal representation, X_{CS}, and attention, z_{CS}, were greatest for the CS partially paired with the US. These results are also in line with the Pearce-Hall model (1980) of associative learning, which predicts that attention is greater to CSs with more uncertain outcomes, but not in agreement with Wagner's (1981) SOP, which does not contain any variable proportional to the uncertainty of the CS.

Uniquely in the SLG model, X_{CS} is proportional to the short-term memory trace of the CS, τ_{CS}, modulated by the magnitude of attention z_{CS}. Therefore, X_{CS} is an attention-modulated, sustained activity that is closely related to a "working memory" process. This aspect of the model converges with previous findings that the dlPFC is involved in holding the representation of a stimulus in working memory (Fuster, 1973; D'Esposito, Postle, & Rypma, 2000).

Attention and error-correcting rules

Rescorla (2000, 2001, 2002) studied the effect of reinforced and non-reinforced presentations of an AB compound in which A and B had different initial associations with the US. In all cases, he reported that responding to AD (with D inhibitory) was weaker than responding to BC (with C excitatory). According to Rescorla, these results show that changes in A–US and B–US associations are different, specifically that AB+ presentations yield ΔV_B > ΔV_A, whereas AB– presentations yield $-\Delta V_A$ > $-\Delta V_B$, which contradicts the predictions of models of conditioning that rely only on a single, common-error correcting term. These models predict that the associative changes of two conditioned stimuli presented in compound are independent of the value of their initial associations.

Figure 6.3 shows responding to compounds (AD) and (BC) in which A and C are initially excitatory stimuli and B or D are initially neutral stimuli, after AB+ (Experiment 1) or AB– presentations (Experiment 2). In both cases, it was found that CR(AD) < CR(BC). Computer simulations show that the SLG model is able to explain those results as the consequence of (1) associative and attentional mechanisms acting during compound training, and (2) attentional mechanisms controlling performance during testing. Interestingly, the model's explanation of the results in terms of attentional mechanisms is supported in part by existing literature. For instance, the model suggests that, during the second phase of Rescorla's (2001, Experiment 1) blocking experiment, (1) the associative competitive mechanism leaves less room for the blocked stimulus to increase its association with the US, and (2) the attentional mechanism decreases Novelty' and attention to the blocked CS. Such decrease in attention to the blocked CS has been suggested by Mackintosh and Turner (1971), who analyzed the effect of blocking on the attention to the blocked CS.

Attention and conditioned inhibition

In a landmark experiment, Lysle and Fowler (1985) found that following conditioned inhibition, extinction of the excitatory CS decreases the retardation

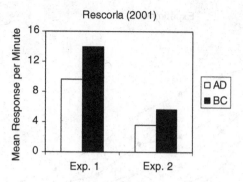

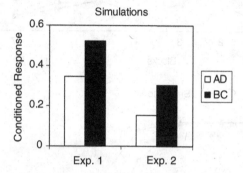

Figure 6.3 Responding to compounds (AD) and (BC). Bars represent the average responding to compounds tested in different orders. Compounds contain one previously excitatory stimulus (A or C), and one previously neutral stimulus (B or D), after AB+(Exp1) or AB–(Exp2) presentations. *Upper panel*: data from Rescorla's (2001) Experiment 1 and Experiment 2. *Lower panel*: computer simulations with the Schmajuk *et al.* (1996) attentional–associative model.

of conditioning of the inhibitory CS (Figure 6.4, upper panel). Lysle and Fowler interpreted these results in terms of a decrement in the inhibitory association of the inhibitory CS, and proposed that inhibitory associations are a "slave" process of excitatory ones. Figure 6.4 (lower panel) shows that the SLG model is able to explain these results (Kutlu & Schmajuk, in preparation). According to the model, a conditioned inhibitor shows retardation in conditioning (Group N[B]) compared with a neutral CS (groups A[C], X[C], and N[C]) because of its (1) initial inhibitory association and (2) decreased attention. Attention to both the excitor and the inhibitor decreases when they are repeatedly active together in the absence of the US. Presentation of the conditioned excitor alone (Group A[B]) increases Novelty', because the inhibitor is absent and therefore the expectation of the US is large in the absence of the US. Because the excitor, CS_A, is strongly associated with the conditioned inhibitor, the representation of the inhibitor, B_{CSB}, is active even when it is not presented, and attention to the inhibitor, CS_B,

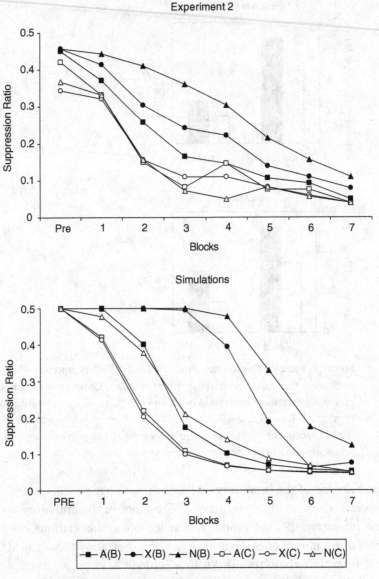

Figure 6.4 Effect of the extinction of a conditioned excitor on the retardation of conditioning of its corresponding conditioned inhibitor. *Upper panel*: mean suppression to CS$_B$ during the pretest (PRE) and retardation test. After inhibitory conditioning to either CS$_B$ or CS$_C$, the A(B) and A(C) groups received CS$_A$ extinction in the training context CX, the X(B) and X(C) groups received extinction only to CX, and the N(B) and N(C) groups received no extinction to either CS$_A$ or the CX. Data from Lysle and Fowler (1985) Experiment 2. *Lower panel*: simulations with the SLG model.

increases thereby decreasing retardation. A similar but weaker effect takes place when the context of conditioning is extinguished (Group X[B]), because the CX–CS_B association is weaker than the CS_A–CS_B association.

Most importantly, consistent with this attentional interpretation of the effect of the extinction of the conditioned excitor responsible for the establishment of conditioned inhibition, computer simulations show that the SLG model correctly describes the lack of effect of that extinction on a summation test (Rescorla & Holland, 1977, Experiment 1).

Latent inhibition

Schmajuk *et al.* (1996) showed that the SLG model describes a large number of the behavioral properties of LI. In addition, the model seems able to describe some aspects of learned irrelevance.

The SLG model seems to offer some advantages over competing theories. Although the SLG model shares with the Pearce and Hall (1980) theory the idea that attention to the CS is regulated by the mismatch between the predicted and actual values of the US, the fact that in the SLG model CS novelty also controls attention confers it with special properties. For example, only the SLG model can describe the reported LI disruption by presentation of a surprising CS (Lantz, 1973), the effect of omitting a CS preceded by other CSs on the orienting response (Wilson, Boumphrey, & Pearce, 1992), or the effect of preexposing to a compound but conditioning to a CS (Honey & Hall, 1989). In addition, because in the SLG model attention to a CS controls not only learning but also performance, the SLG but not the Pearce and Hall model describes the attenuation of LI by postconditioning exposure to the context alone, which increases Novelty' and attention to the CS (Schmajuk & Kutlu, unpublished manuscript). Finally, because the Pearce and Hall model is not a real-time model it cannot describe the effect of changing CS duration, interstimulus intervals, or intertrial intervals.

Although both the SLG model and Wagner's (1981) SOP model describe behavior in real time and the effect of postconditioning manipulation on performance (e.g., decrements in LI following contextual exposure or contextual changes), only the former is capable of describing the deleterious effect of the presentation of a surprising CS on latent inhibition (Lantz, 1973).

Also, the SLG model is the only one, at this point, that has been shown to explain super-LI. Schmajuk and Larrauri (2006) demonstrated that the model correctly replicates the De la Casa and Lubow (2002) results, using a taste-aversion preparation, for different US intensities and short and long delays between conditioning and testing (see Figure 6.5). According to the SLG model, super-LI is not due to a further decrease in attention to the target CS (flavor) in the PRE group, but to an increased attention to the stimulus representing the water (and related stimuli), which becomes a conditioned inhibitor. When the US is relatively weak, introducing a delay between conditioning and testing decreases LI because attention to the water barely changes, as a result of a relatively small increment in Novelty'. In turn, the small increase in Novelty' is the consequence of having only the unfulfilled expectation of the training context, the flavor and of a weak US, when the water is presented in their absence in the home cage. Because attention to the water does not increase during the delay, the water–US association becomes only barely inhibitory, and super-LI is absent. In addition, the increase in Novelty' causes attention to the flavor to increase and, therefore, LI decreases. Furthermore, Schmajuk and Kutlu (unpublished manuscript) showed that the SLG model also replicates Wheeler, Stout, and Miller's (2004) experiment reporting super-LI with a procedure that included sensory preconditioning.

Interactions between latent inhibition and overshadowing

Schmajuk and Larrauri (2006) showed that the SLG model describes (1) recovery from overshadowing, (2) the counteraction between latent inhibition and overshadowing, (3) the conditions under which recovery from blocking by extinction of the blocker is obtained, (4) the inability of a blocked CS to become a blocker of another CS, and (5) backward blocking and recovery from backward blocking following a retention interval. In addition, the SLG model predicts that extinction of the blocker will result in recovery from backward blocking.

Apparently the SLG model is the only one able, at this point, to give an account for the opposite results reported by Blaisdell, Gunther, and Miller (1999) and Holland (1999) for the recovery of blocking by extinction of the blocker. In addition, the SLG model is able to account for the opposite results reported for the interaction between LI and overshadowing treatments. Using a conditioned emotional response preparation, Blaisdell, Bristol, Gunther, and Miller (1998) showed that combined LI and overshadowing treatments attenuate the decrease in responding produced by each procedure alone. Interestingly, experimental results indicate that this counteraction is not obtained in taste-aversion preparations (e.g., Ishii, Haga, and Hishimura, 1999; Nakajima and Nagaishi, 2005; Nagaishi and Nakajima, 2008). Furthermore, when attenuation of latent inhibition by overshadowing was obtained, Ishii et al. (1999, Experiment 2) showed that the effect could be accounted for by the restoration of the salience of the target CS by the surprise introduction of the overshadowing stimulus, as the SLG model would predict.

The upper left panel in Figure 6.6 shows Blaisdell et al.'s (1998) reported mean time to complete five cumulative seconds of licking in the presence of the target conditioned stimulus, a measure of its level of conditioning. The results show

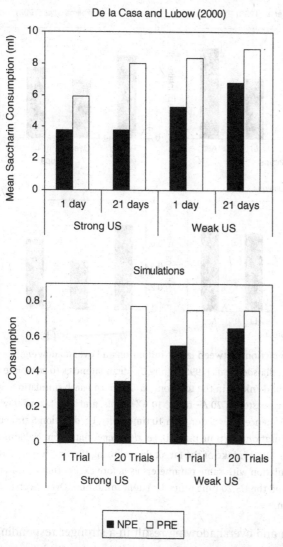

Figure 6.5 Super-latent inhibition after a post-conditioning delay with a strong US, but not with a weak US. *Upper panel*: mean Saccharin Consumption in groups that received no preexposure (NPE) or 4 preexposure days (PRE) followed by 1 day (Short Delay) or 21 days (Long Delay) in the home cage after conditioning using a Strong or a Weak US. Data from De la Casa and Lubow (2000, Experiment 2). *Lower panel*: five-trial average of simulated consumption after no preexposure (NPE) or 30 preexposure trials (Long PRE) and 1 (Short Delay) or 33 Trials (Long Delay) after conditioning using a Strong or a Weak US. The ITI was 500 t.u., the Home and Training CX salience was 0.1, the CSs were 25 t.u. in duration and of intensity 1, and the US was 5 t.u. in duration and of intensity 1.0 (strong) or 0.8 (weak).

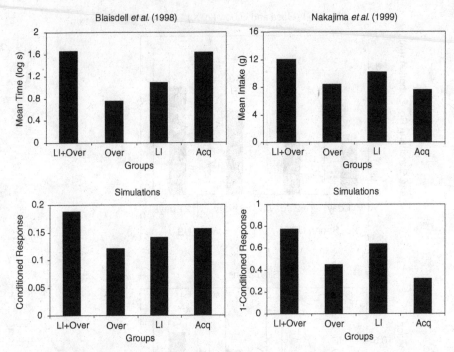

Figure 6.6 Interactions between latent inhibition and overshadowing. *Upper left panel*: data from Blaisdell *et al.* (1998, Figure 5). Mean latencies to complete the first 5 cumulative s of drinking in the test context. *Lower left panel*: simulations with the SLG model consisted of 20 A– trials, 10 AX+ trials, and 1 X– test trial with X salience = 1, A salience = 2, CS duration 10 time units, US duration 5 time units, and intertrial duration 600 time units. *Upper right panel*: data from Nakajima *et al.* (1999, Figure 1). Mean intake of the target flavor during the first testing day. *Lower right panel*: simulation with same parameters as before except that CS duration was 90 time units and the US 20 time units. LI: latent inhibition, Over: overshadowing, Acq: acquisition.

that latent inhibition and overshadowing result in a stronger responding when given together than when separated. The lower left panel of Figure 6.6 shows the simulated results. As in Blaisdell *et al.*'s (1998) experiment, preexposure and overshadowing procedures produce more responding when given together than apart. According to the model, responding in the LI + OVER group is stronger than in the LI group because the introduction of a second CS during conditioning increases Novelty' and attention to the preexposed CS, thereby accelerating conditioning. Also, responding in the LI + OVER group is stronger than in the OVER group because the value of attention to the preexposed CS in the LI + OVER group is larger than attention to the non-preexposed CS in the OVER group. Therefore, conditioning is stronger in the LI + OVER group than in the OVER group.

The upper right panel in Figure 6.6 shows Nakajima, Ka, and Imadn's (1999) reported mean intake of the solution with the target flavor, an inverse measure of the level of aversion. The results show that latent inhibition and overshadowing result in a weaker responding when given together than separated. The lower right panel of Figure 6.6 shows simulations with the same parameters as for Blaisdell *et al.* (1998) except that, because Nakajima *et al.* (1999) used a taste aversion paradigm, CS duration was 90 time units and the US duration was 20 time units. As in the experimental case, latent inhibition and overshadowing produce less response when given together than apart. According to the model, the relatively long CS results in a low level of attention at the end of preexposure. Therefore, responding in the LI + OVER group is weaker than in the LI group because the introduction of a second CS (1) increases Novelty', but this increase is not enough to increase the very depressed attention to the preexposed CS, and (2) competes with the preexposed CS to gain association with the US. Also, responding in the LI + OVER group is weaker than in the OVER group because the value of attention to the preexposed CS in the LI + OVER group is weaker than attention to the non-preexposed CS in the OVER group. Therefore, conditioning is weaker in the LI + OVER group than in the OVER group.

Extinction

Larrauri and Schmajuk (2008) showed that although associative mechanisms are sufficient to account for some of the reported results regarding extinction, additional novelty-driven attentional mechanisms, such as those included in the SLG model, are also required. Attentional processes are needed to explain extinction bursts, why contextual inhibition is not detectable in summation tests, the properties of spontaneous recovery, external disinhibition, magnitude of renewal with different procedures (ABA and ABC vs. AAB), the elimination of renewal by massive extinction, and slow reacquisition.

The upper panel of Figure 6.7 shows the model's associative values and CR, and the lower panel shows average Novelty' and the representations of CXg and the CS during conditioning and extinction, just before the time of presentation of the US on reinforced trials (the simulation corresponds to that carried out for Robbins's [1990] Experiment 1, described below). Because in this simulation CXg (which represents generalized contextual cues, common to the home cage (CX_h) and the training cage) is more salient than CX_c (which represents contextual cues specific to the training cage), Figure 6.7 shows only V_{CXg-US} and V_{CS-US}, their representations, X_{CXg} and X_{CS}, and Novelty'. In the model (see Figure 6.1), internal representations X_{CS} and X_{CXg} are proportional to attentions z_{CS} and z_{CXg} which, in turn, are modulated by Novelty'. During acquisition (trials 1 to 20), the CS–US association (V_{CS-US}) increases and the CX–US associations (V_{CXg-US}) remain close to zero. During extinction (trials 21 to 55) the association of the CS with the US decreases, but does not vanish. The CS–US association V_{CS-US} is protected by an inhibitory CXg–US association (V_{CXg-US}) that eliminates the CR. In

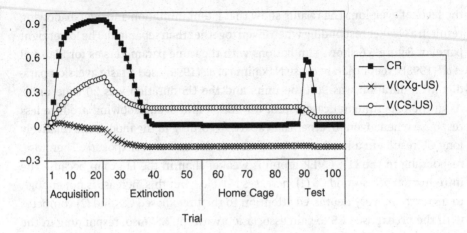

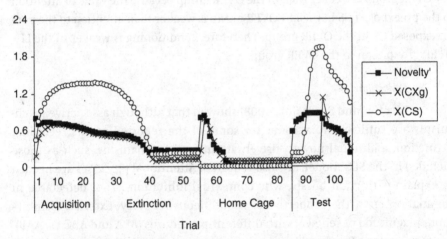

Figure 6.7 Variables of the model during acquisition, extinction, and spontaneous recovery. *upper panel*: values of the conditioned response, CR; the association between the generalized context and the unconditioned stimulus, V_{CXg-US}; and the CS–US association, V_{CS-US}; as a function of trials. *Lower panel*: values of average Novelty′; the internal representation of CXg, X_{CXg}; and the CS internal representation X_{CS}; as a function of trials. Conditioning trials 1–20, extinction trials 21–55, home-cage time periods 56–85, and test trials 86–105.

addition, during acquisition (trials 1 to 20), Novelty′ decreases, representation X_{CS} increases, and representation X_{CXg} first increases and then decreases. During extinction (trials 21 to 55), Novelty′ decreases first, followed by decrements in X_{CXg} first and, later, by decrements in X_{CS}. So, by the end of extinction, V_{CS-US} is excitatory, V_{CXg-US} is inhibitory, and representations X_{CXg} and X_{CS} are small. During the period in the home cage (trials 56 to 85) and during testing (trials 86 to 105), increments in both CXg and CS representations lag behind Novelty′. This dissociation between the orienting response (proportional to Novelty′) and attention has been reported by Hall and Schachtman (1987).

Notice that, because the CS is more salient than the CX, and the trace of the CS is present for a shorter period of time than the trace of the CX (active for the duration of the ITI), contextual associations are almost zero at the end of conditioning (see section above on "Excitatory conditioning tends to be context independent"). Therefore, the CR is context independent following acquisition. In contrast, during extinction, contextual associations are strongly inhibitory and, if attention to the context happens to increase, the CR will be context dependent following extinction. Also notice that, because CX–US associations are stronger with a short than with a long ITI, a short ITI will result in a higher Novelty' when the US is not presented during extinction. Therefore, the increased attention to the CS will facilitate extinction, a result in agreement with Cain, Blouin, and Barad's (2003) and Moody, Sunsay, and Bouton's (2006) data.

Interestingly, whereas Novelty' stays relatively high during conditioning, it decreases to a very small value during extinction. The difference is due to the fact that, during extinction, CSs and CXs can predict themselves and each other and, therefore, perfectly match predicted and actual values. In contrast, with the simulation values used in this case, the US is not perfectly predicted and Novelty' stays at a relatively high level during acquisition. Simulations with other CS and US durations and intensities show that Novelty', attention to the CS, and CR strength can decrease.

According to the SLG model, a CX–US inhibitory association formed during extinction would protect the complete elimination of the CS–US association (Chorazyna, 1962; Soltysik, 1985; Rescorla, 2003). However, Bouton and King (1983), Richards and Sargent (1983) and Bouton and Swartzentruber (1989), presented data that suggest that the context does not become inhibitory at the end of extinction. Below we show simulated results that demonstrate that even when inhibitory CX–US associations are formed, they can be difficult to detect because attention to the inhibitory CXc and CXg is small.

Summation tests following extinction

Bouton and Swartzentruber (1989, Experiment 3; see also Bouton & King, 1983, Experiment 4) evaluated whether the context of extinction becomes inhibitory or not. As shown in Figure 6.8 (left), a summation test for contextual inhibition revealed no evidence of inhibitory associations, i.e., responding in the context of extinction (Same) was not significantly different from responding in another context (Diff). The model correctly describes the statistically non significant difference in the experimental data (Figure 6.8, right).

Spontaneous recovery

Robbins (1990, Experiment 1) studied the effect of varying the interval between extinction and testing on the magnitude of spontaneous recovery. He

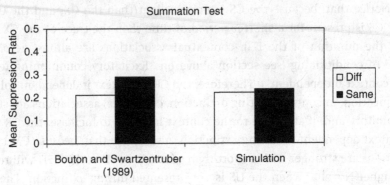

Figure 6.8 Summation test in the context of extinction. Suppression ratios to an excitatory CS when extinction to another CS had taken place in (1) another context (Diff), or (2) that context (Same). *Left*: data from Bouton and Swartzentruber (1989). *Right*: computer simulations. Conditioning sessions consisted of 20 CS1–US trials in CXA, followed by 80 CS1– trials in either CXB (Diff) or CXC (Same). After extinction, 20 CS2–US trials were simulated in CXA, followed by a summation test, which consisted of one CS2– trial in CXC. Simulations of 20 home-cage (CXh = 0.5, CXg = 0.4) time periods of duration equal to the ITI were included between the different sessions. The salience of the contexts (CXA, CXB, and CXC) was set to CXc = 0.7 and CXg = 0.4 in extinction and test sessions. The CSs had an 11 t.u. duration and salience 0.7, the US was 5 t.u. long with salience 2, and the ITI was 70 t.u.

trained pigeons in an autoshaping procedure, followed by CS extinction trials. After extinction, all the birds were tested for spontaneous recovery either 15 m, 1 day, 2 days, or 7 days after being returned to the home cage. As shown in the upper panel of Figure 6.9, he found that the recovery ratio (responding on the first three trials of recovery divided by the total level of responding on the first three trials of both extinction and recovery) increases as the interval between extinction and testing increases. As shown in the lower panel of Figure 6.9, the model correctly describes the effect of changing the extinction-test interval on spontaneous recovery.

In the framework of the model, spontaneous recovery is explained because Novelty′ increases when the CS is presented in the context of extinction after a period of absence. This increased Novelty′ increases attention to the excitatory CS first, and then to the inhibitory CX, which results in a temporary recovery of responding. Figure 6.7 also shows, in addition to acquisition and extinction, spontaneous recovery when the home-cage context is interposed between extinction and testing trials. During the time periods in the home cage (periods 56 to 85), attention to CXg initially increases due to the novelty produced by the change of the environment (CXg predicts CXc which is not present). Novelty′ later decreases as CXg and CXh (not shown) better predict each other. During

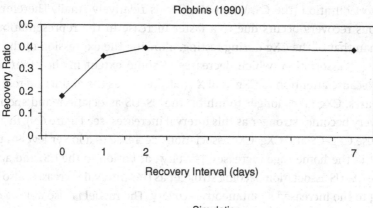

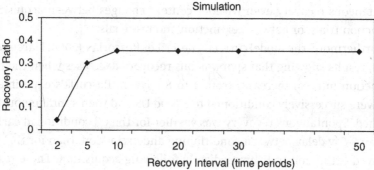

Figure 6.9 Spontaneous recovery. Recovery ratio (responding on the first 3 trials of recovery divided by the total level of responding on the first 3 trials of both extinction and recovery) as a function of the interval between extinction and testing. *Upper panel*: data from Robbins (1990). *Lower panel*: simulations. Twenty acquisition trials were simulated in the experimental chambers (CXc = 0.1 and CXg = 0.4), in which a 20 t.u. CS (salience 1) co-terminated with a 5 t.u. US (salience 2), and were followed by 35 extinction trials. The ITI was 240 t.u. To simulate the period spent by the pigeons in the housing chambers before testing, 2, 5, 10, 20, 30, and 50 time periods of duration equal to the ITI used during acquisition or extinction in that context (CXh = 0.5 and CXg = 0.4) were used. Finally, 10 test trials in the experimental context were carried out to assess the spontaneous recovery of the pecking response. Duration of each time period is equal to the intertrial interval (ITI) used during acquisition or extinction.

test trials (trials 86 to 105), CXc and the CS are present, and Novelty′ increases because CXg–CS and CXg–CXc associations had decreased in the home cage. This increase in Novelty′ triggers an increase in attention to the CS and CXg, which increases their representations, X_{CS} and X_{CXg}. However, X_{CS} increases faster than X_{CXg}, since attention to CXg had decreased more than attention to the CS during the home-cage trials. This is a basic property of the model by which attention to stimuli of long duration (the CX) will decrease more than attention to stimuli of short duration (the CS) when Novelty' is relatively small. Therefore, spontaneous recovery occurs due to a faster increase in the representation of the CS than that of the CXg during testing, allowing the expression of the remaining V_{CS-US} association (which decreases to some extent in the absence of the US). Because attention to CXg, and X_{CXg}, decreases as the extinction-test interval increases, CXg takes longer to inhibit the CS–US association, and spontaneous recovery becomes stronger as this interval increases (see Figure 6.9). In addition, because CXg–CS and CXg–CXc associations decrease to a lower level as the time spent in the home cage increases, Novelty', attention to the CS, and activation of the CS–US association become stronger as this interval increases, also contributing to the increased spontaneous recovery. The model is also able to describe spontaneous recovery even without context changes between acquisition and extinction trials, or between extinction and test trials.

Furthermore, the model correctly describes Rescorla's (2004; Maren & Chang, 2006) results showing that spontaneous recovery decreases when the training-extinction interval increases from 1 to 8 days. In Rescorla's experiment, two CSs were successively conditioned to a food US and then simultaneously extinguished. Spontaneous recovery was smaller for the CS conditioned earlier, and had an 8-day delay between conditioning and extinction, than for the one that received extinction trials immediately following acquisition. These results are well explained by the SLG model. According to the model, recovery decreases when the acquisition–extinction interval increases from 0 to 20 time periods of duration equal to the ITI used during acquisition or extinction, because increasing the interval between conditioning and extinction decreases attention to CXg. Therefore, during extinction the CS–US association will be protected only by the inhibitory CXc–US association (which is equivalent to having a weaker context), resulting in a more pronounced decrement in the CS–US association, and therefore, in a decreased spontaneous recovery.

Schmajuk and Di Carlo's (1992) associational-configural model

Schmajuk and Di Carlo (SD, 1992) introduced a real-time, single-response neural network that successfully describes many classical conditioning paradigms. In the network, a CS can establish direct, simple CS–US associations and indirect, configural H–US associations, all formed in accordance with a competitive rule. It is worth noting that CS–H associations follow a slightly different rule, which explains why even though a CS might not be able to establish strong, direct CS–US associations, it can still establish strong CS–H associations with the hidden units. Schmajuk, Lamoureux, and Holland (1998) presented an extension of the SD model, the SLH model, which includes (1) multiple response systems that establish associations with simple and configural stimuli to control different responses (e.g., headjerk to sounds and rearing to lights that precede food), (2) a system that provides both stimulus configuration and generalization to the different response systems, and (3) a system that provides inhibition to the different response systems. The SLH model offers a precise description of the different roles a CS can play in classical conditioning. A CS acts as a simple CS through its direct, simple associations with the US or as an occasion setter through indirect, configural associations with the US. As a result of their own excitatory or inhibitory associations with the output (US) units, hidden units corresponding to stimulus configurations join the action of direct excitatory and inhibitory associations of simple CSs with the US. Interestingly, hidden-unit action does not reflect a special process or function. Connections between the hidden units and the output units are not qualitatively different from direct connections between input and output units, and are both controlled by a competitive rule.

Interestingly, weak CSs can form only weak associations with both hidden and output units. However, whereas the activity of the output units is a linear function of those associations, the activity of hidden units is a highly nonlinear function that amplifies the small effect that a weak CS might have. Therefore, even though a feature CS or the CX might not be able to establish strong, direct CS–US associations, it still can control the output of the hidden units through CS–H associations, formed when those hidden units are activated by the target CS.

Occasion setting

Holland (1989) examined the acquisition of simultaneous feature-positive FP (XA+/A−) discriminations in Pavlovian conditioning, as a function of the intensity of the A target cue. The data indicated that when target A was of relatively low intensity (Group LO), feature X–US associations were formed, but if target A was of high intensity (Group HI), feature X came to modulate the action of A. These conclusions were based on observations of response form, the extent of transfer, and the effects of X extinction. For example, the upper panel of Figure 6.10 shows the incidence of responding of a form appropriate to feature X (CR_X) and to target A (CR_A) during XA compound presentations in Holland's (1989, Experiment 1) study. In Group LO, in which target A was relatively weak, responding to XA was dominated by CR_X, but in Group HI, in which target A was relatively strong, responding to XA was predominantly CR_A.

The lower panel of Figure 6.10 shows that, in agreement with experimental data, CR_A is stronger than CR_X when a relatively strong target A is used (Group

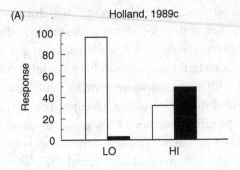

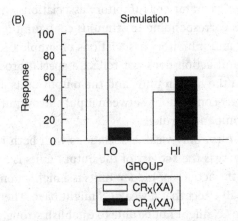

Figure 6.10 Simultaneous feature-positive discrimination. A = intensity. (A) (Data from Holland, 1989) CRA(XA) (solid bars) and CRX(XA) (open bars) responding after simultaneous feature-positive (FP) training with low- (Group Lo) or high (Group Hi)-intensity auditory A cue. (B) (Stimulation) peak CRA(XA) and CRX(XA) after 30 training trials (15 XA+ trials alternated with 15 A– trials) for Group LO (X salience 0.95, and A salience 0.3), and 250 training trials (125 XA+ trials alternated with 125 A– trials) for Group HI (X salience 0.3 and A salience 0.95).

HI), but CR_A is weaker than CR_X when a relatively weak target A is used (Group LO). In the framework of the SD/SLH model, feature X–US and target A–US associations increase with increasing intensities of target A and feature X. When feature X is more intense than target A, the feature X–US associations block target A–US associations and the FP discrimination is solved by the simple feature X–US associations. However, when feature X is less intense than A (e.g., because it temporally precedes target A and the US), the target A–US associations block feature X–US associations and the FP discrimination is solved by occasion setting. That is, target A–US associations activate CR_A, but CR_A are inhibited by the hidden units in the absence of the XA compound.

Figure 6.11 summarizes the SD/SLH model's solutions for simultaneous FP discriminations in a simplified depiction of the network where X and A

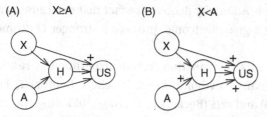

Figure 6.11 Simultaneous feature-positive discrimination. Simplified diagram of the SD/SLH network model. (A) when A is a low-intensity target, X acquires a direct excitatory association with the US. (B) When A is a high-intensity target, X acquires a direct excitatory association with the US and an inhibitory association with the hidden units (H). A acquires an excitatory association with the US and an excitatory association with the hidden units (H). The hidden units acquire an inhibitory association with the US. Associative strengths are represented by plus or minus signs placed next to the arrows connecting the nodes. Only significant associative strengths are indicated.

represent, respectively, feature and target, and H represents the hidden-unit layer. Direct associations of A and X with the US determine the response form, CR_A or CR_X. In the case of simultaneous FP discriminations with X more salient than or equally salient to A (left portion of Figure 6.11), X acts as a simple CS because it acquires strong, direct associations with the US, and A acquires weak ones. In the case of simultaneous FP discriminations with X less salient than A (right portion of Figure 6.11), X and A acquire strong, direct associations with the US. On A-alone trials, A also activates the hidden units, which then inhibit the US prediction, preventing the display of responding based on the A–US association (A acts both as an excitor and an inhibitor). But on XA trials, X weakens the inhibition normally exerted by the hidden units, enabling the performance of both CR_A and CR_X. Thus, X acts both as a simple CS because of its strong, direct excitatory association with the US, and as an occasion setter, because of its inhibitory associations with the hidden units.

Schmajuk and Kutlu (2010) attentional-configural version of the SLG model

According to associative theories (e.g., Rescorla & Wagner, 1972), blocking is the consequence of stimulus A winning the competition with X to predict the US, because the US is already predicted by A at the time of A–X–US presentations. In contrast, according to the inferential process view (see Beckers, Miller, De Houwer, and Urushihara, 2006), blocking is the consequence of an inferential process based on the assumptions of additivity and maximality. Maximality refers to the evidence that the Outcome produced by each potential cause has not reached the maximal possible value. Additivity denotes the fact that two causes, each one independently producing a given Outcome, produce a stronger Outcome when presented together.

Supporting the inferential explanation, recent experimental results have shown that both in humans (Lovibond, Been, Mitchell, Bouton, & Frohardt 2003; Beckers et al., 2005) and rats (Beckers et al., 2006), blocking was stronger if the maximal premise (the outcome of each cause does not reach the maximum possible value) and the additivity premise (the outcomes of effective causes can be added) are satisfied. In contrast, Beckers et al. (2005) showed that the Rescorla–Wagner (1972) model incorrectly predicts more blocking with an intense (maximal) than with a moderate (submaximal) outcome.

Schmajuk and Kutlu (2009) and Schmajuk and Larrauri (2008) showed that an attentional–configural version of the SLG model can describe maximality and additivity effects on blocking, and backward blocking. A simplified diagram of this attentional–configural version of the SLG model, as applied to maximality and additivity experiments in blocking, is presented in Figure 6.12. According to Figure 6.12, simultaneously active τ_A and τ_X activate configural stimulus C, and simultaneously active τ_G and τ_H activate configural stimulus C′. Attention to τ_A, τ_X, C, τ_G, τ_H, and C′ varies with Novelty′. Configural stimuli C and C′ can be associated with all other simple and configural CSs. As shown by the dashed double arrow in Figure 6.12, we assume generalization between compounds C′ (GH) and C (AX) to be strong based on Young and Wasserman's (2002) experimental data showing that generalization between simple stimuli is much smaller than generalization between compounds. In addition, the model implements generalization among elements and between elements and compounds through the presence of a common contextual stimulus that is always active.

It is important to remember that Node X (See Figure 6.12) can be activated either by τ_X or by its prediction by τ_A (or, as explained below, by $\tau_{Outcome}$). This means that z_X can still be modified by Novelty′ even if τ_X is absent. This is an important feature of the model that explains backward blocking and additivity posttraining, as described below. In our simulations, the rating of the different stimuli was given by the sigmoid Rating = Predicted Outcome^6/(Predicted Outcome^6 + β^6), where β = average of the predicted outcomes for all A, X, K, L, and Z.

Causal learning

Additivity training preceding blocking

In Beckers et al.'s (2005, Experiment 2) additivity pretraining study, one additive and one subadditive group were used. The additive group received G+/

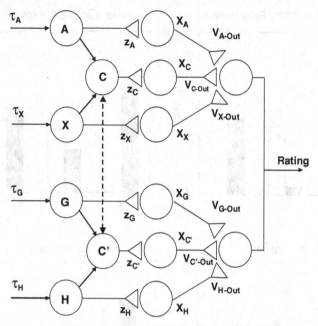

Figure 6.12 A simplified diagram of the attentional–configural form of the SLG model. τ: traces of A, X, G and H; z: attention to A, X, G, and H; X: representations of A, X, G, H, and C; Out: Outcome; V: A-Outcome, X-Outcome, C-Outcome, G-Outcome, H-Outcome or C′-Outcome associations. When simultaneously active τ_A and τ_X activate configural stimulus C, and when simultaneously active τ_G and τ_H activate configural stimulus C′. The dashed arrow connecting C and C′ represents the generalization between them. Through that generalization τ_A and τ_X can activate the $V_{C′\text{-Out}}$ association, and τ_G and τ_H can activate the $V_{C\text{-Out}}$ association. Triangles: variable connections between nodes, z and V. Arrows: fixed connections between nodes.

H+/GH++/I+/Z− alternated trials (prior training), followed by alternated A+/Z− trials (elemental training), and finally by AX+/KL+/Z− alternated trials (compound training). Whereas G, H, I, Z, A, X, K, and L denote stimuli, symbols + and ++ indicate the same outcome with different intensities. Stimuli were pictures of different foods on a computer screen, and the outcome (an allergic reaction) was represented by a red bar of different lengths on the screen. The probability, assigned by each group, of X and K (and L) to cause the outcome (ratings) were then compared. Subadditive groups received GH+ instead of GH++ presentations and I++ instead of I+ presentations. As shown in Figure 6.13 (upper left panel), although blocking was present in both groups, it was stronger in the additive than in the subadditive case.

Figure 6.13 (lower left panel), the configural version of the SLG model, correctly describes this result. Like the Rescorla–Wagner (1972) model, the

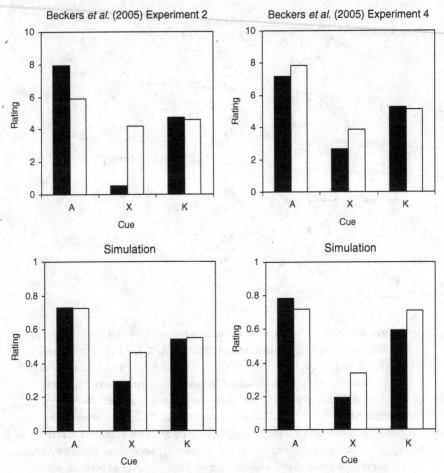

Figure 6.13 Blocking and additivity. *Upper left panel*: mean causal ratings for cues A, X, and K in a blocking experiment following additivity pre training; data from Beckers *et al.* (2005) Experiment 2. *Upper right panel*: same blocking experiment followed by additivity posttraining; data from Beckers *et al.* (2005) Experiment 4. *Lower panels*: corresponding simulations with the attentional–configural form of the SLG model. Solid Bars: Additive case, Open Bars: Sub-additive case.

SLG model explains blocking because, at the time of the presentation of X, A already predicts the Outcome (or US). As shown in Figure 6.12, compound stimulus C′, activated by τ_G and τ_H and associated with the Outcome during pretraining, is fully activated when compound stimulus C is activated by τ_A and τ_X. The $V_{C'-Out}$ association, together with the blocker stimulus A, contributes to predict the Outcome thereby increasing blocking. Because the $V_{C'-Out}$ association acquired during pre-training is stronger in the additive than in the subadditive case, blocking is stronger in the former than in the latter case (Figure 6.13, lower left panel).

Additivity training following blocking

In Beckers *et al.*'s (2005, Experiment 4) additivity posttraining study, the additive group received G+/H+/GH++/I+/Z− alternated trials, and the sub-additive group G+/H+/GH+/I+/Z− alternated trials, following blocking training. As shown in Figure 6.13 (upper right panel), although blocking was present in both groups, it was stronger in the additive than in the subadditive case.

In Figure 6.13 (lower right panel) the configural version of the SLG model correctly describes this result. In terms of the model, during the AX+ phase of blocking, Outcome–X and C–X associations are formed. During the subsequent additivity posttraining, Outcome–X and C–X associations predict X, but X is absent. In the additive case, the stronger Outcome extinguishes its Outcome–X association faster than the weaker non-additive Outcome does. During additivity posttraining, Novelty′ increases because of the presentation of the novel G and H stimuli and absence of the older A and X stimuli. Thus, because the representation of X is weaker in the additive case, attention to X increases less in the additive than in the non-additive case, because X predicts the Outcome in proportion to the product $X_X V_{X-Out}$. Therefore, the Rating is weaker (and blocking is stronger) in the additive than the non-additive case (see Figure 6.13, lower right panel).

Conclusion

The present chapter shows that the SLG model is able to describe (1) brain activity in the amygdala and anterior cingulate cortex as proportional to the prediction of the US, B_{US}, (Dunsmoor *et al.*, 2007); (2) activity in the dorsolateral prefrontal cortex (dlPFC) and insula proportional to the representation of the CS, X_{CS}, (Dunsmoor *et al.*, 2007); (3) X_{CS} as an attention-modulated, sustained activity closely related to a "working memory" process in the dlPF (Dunsmoor *et al.*, 2007); (4) the effect of reinforced and non-reinforced presentations of an AB compound in which A and B had different initial associations with the US (Rescorla, 2000, 2001, 2002); (5) the accelerating effect of the extinction of the conditioned excitor on the conditioning of its corresponding conditioned inhibitor (Lysle & Fowler, 1985); (6) super-LI as the consequence of an increased attention to a stimulus (water) that becomes a conditioned inhibitor (De la Casa & Lubow, 2002); (7) the conflicting data that result from pre-exposing a CS that is later trained in overshadowing in terms of differences in CS and US duration (Blaisdell *et al.*, 1998; Nakajima *et al.*, 1999); (8) why the context does not appear to be inhibitory at the end of extinction even when it has been reported that it is not an occasion setter (Bouton & Swartzentruber, 1989); and (9) results showing that spontaneous recovery decreases when the training–extinction interval increases (Maren & Chang, 2006). It also shows (10) how the SD/SLH model is able to describe occasion setting, and how a configural version of the

SLG model explains (11) the effect of additivity pretraining and posttraining on blocking (Beckers *et al.*, 2005).

The chapter seems to support the notion that, although apparently simple, more than one mechanism is needed to account for the reported results on classical conditioning. It is apparent that the phenomenon cannot be reduced to one simple formula, like that of the kinetic theory of gasses. Conditioning can be described by a rather complex combination of different mechanisms (see Schmajuk, 2010).

Complex models are needed

This view is supported by the fact that in the relatively short history of behavioral modeling, simple and elegant models like Rescorla–Wagner's (1972) delta rule, Pearce and Hall's (1980) attentional rule, and Miller and Schachtman's (1985) first comparator hypothesis failed to explain important aspects of conditioning. Instead, the field has moved to increasingly complex models (e.g., Le Pelley, 2004). It is clear that the complexity of these models puts them beyond the ability of our intuitive thinking and makes computer simulations irreplaceable.

Number of parameters will be large

The fact that multiple mechanisms are needed, and that those mechanisms are implemented by neural networks built by assembling "neural elements" of relatively weak computational power, implies that the number of parameters in the model will be relatively large. This number of parameters reflects the need to combine these elements in different ways in order to produce the desired functions (e.g., storage and retrieval of associations) and sub functions (e.g., maintaining a short-term memory of the CS, conveying the value of the prediction of the CS from a CS–CS memory storage to the input of the system).

Therefore, even if parsimony indicates that a small number of model parameters should be preferred, it is likely that this number will not be insignificant when a neural-network approach is used. Even a simple function such as a hyperbola, which can be mathematically defined with one parameter, needs two or three parameters to be implemented by a neural network. However, the number of parameters should not be a cause of concern given the complexity of the behavior at hand, the moment-to-moment detail with which the model describes the behavior, and the intricacy of the biological organ that regulates the behavior.

Evaluation of the models

In order to permit the comparison of experimental data and simulated results, figures in the chapter show data and simulations next to each other. In many, but not all cases, it is difficult to distinguish the experimental data from the computer-simulated results. In those cases, as suggested by Church (2001), the model has passed a Turing (1950) test by correctly "imitating" the behavior under study.

Notice that imitation refers to both the model's predictions and postdictions. We refer to "explicit correct predictions" as those cases in which the model has correctly described the experimental results before the experiment was carried out. "Implicit correct predictions" are those cases of experimental results, reported after the model was first offered, that the unmodified model correctly describes. Implicit predictions are still predictions because the model, even if capable of correctly describing the data, had not been explicitly applied to the experiment of interest. Finally, "correct postdictions" are those cases of experimental results, reported before the model was offered, that the model correctly describes. In this case, even if the data was not used to develop the model, it was already available at the time when the model was designed.

In order to quantify the quality of a model's imitation, we have used different quantitative methods. These methods include (1) correlations (e.g., Schmajuk et al., 1998), (2) χ^2 (Schmajuk, Cox, and Gray 2001), and (3) analysis of variance using the actual variance of the experimental subjects (Schmajuk & Larrauri, 2006). Of these alternative methods we prefer to use correlations because, although they disregard the importance of the variance in the data, they indicate when to reject the null hypothesis (that simulated values and experimental data are not correlated). Instead, χ^2 indicates when to accept the null hypothesis (that simulated values and experimental data are equivalent). Finally, the analysis of variance used in Schmajuk and Larrauri (2006) is rather convoluted and requires knowledge of the values of the variance of the data, which is not always reported in the experimental studies.

In addition to imitating the experimental results (e.g., Figure 6.9 for an "imitation" of spontaneous recovery), models can also explain those results, i.e., indicate how those results are reached by showing why and how they occurred. Explanations are provided by the figures illustrating the value of the variables in the model during the course of a given experiment (e.g., Figure 6.7 for an explanation of spontaneous recovery). These figures explain *why* a behavior occurs by showing its causes. For example, the cause of spontaneous recovery is the increased attention to the still excitatory CS before attention to the inhibitory context increases (see Figure 6.7). These figures also show *how* a behavior occurs by describing the series of causal processes that lead to the occurrence of that behavior. For example, spontaneous recovery is present when (1) Novelty' and attention to the CS and the CX decrease during extinction, and (2) Novelty' and attention to the CS and CX increase again when the CS is presented after being absent for a period of time (see Figure 6.7).

In sum, this chapter suggests that (1) multiple "computational" mechanisms are needed to describe classical conditioning; (2) computer simulations are needed to describe how those mechanisms work separately and together; (3) emergent properties appear when different mechanisms are integrated into one single system; (4) once behavior is captured by a model, observation of the model variables serves to identify brain structures, brain activity, and neurotransmitters that might carry out the information processing that takes place when performing a given behavior; (5) the brain-mapped models describe the effect of brain lesions, drug administration, and neural activity; (6) the models can both imitate and explain the experimental data; (7) parametric experimental studies are needed to determine the range in which the reported results can be replicated; and (8) future work should consider using model parameters appropriate for specific preparations, as well as simulation values (e.g., stimulus duration and salience, trials to criterion) that reflect the actual values used in the corresponding experiments.

References

Beckers, T., De Houwer, J., Pineno, O. & Miller, R. R. (2005). Outcome additivity and outcome maximality influence cue competition in human causal learning. *Journal of Experimental Psychology: Learning, Memory, and Cognition*, **31**, 238–249.

Beckers, T., Miller, R. R., De Houwer, J. & Urushihara, K. (2006). Reasoning rats: forward blocking in Pavlovian animal conditioning is sensitive to constraints of causal inference. *Journal of Experimental Psychology: General*, **135**, 92–102.

Blaisdell, A., Bristol, A., Gunther, L. & Miller R. (1998). Overshadowing and latent inhibition counteract each other: further support for the comparator hypothesis. *Journal of Experimental Psychology: Animal Behavior Processes*, **24**, 335–351.

Blaisdell, A. P., Gunther, L. & Miller, R. (1999). Recovery from blocking achieved by extinguishing the blocking CS. *Animal Learning and Behavior*, **27**, 63–76.

Bouton, M. E. & King, D. A. (1983). Contextual control of the extinction of conditioned fear: tests for the associative value of the context. *Journal of Experimental Psychology: Animal Behavior Processes*, **9**, 248–265.

Bouton, M. E. & Swartzentruber, D. (1989). Slow reacquisition following extinction: context, encoding, and retrieval mechanisms. *Journal of Experimental Psychology: Animal Behavior Processes*, **15**, 43–53.

Cain, C. K., Blouin, A. M. & Barad, M. (2003). Temporally massed CS presentations generate more fear extinction than spaced presentations. *Journal of Experimental Psychology: Animal Behavior Processes*, **29**, 323–333.

Chorazyna, H. (1962). Some properties of conditioned inhibition. *Acta Biologiae Experimentalis*, **22**, 5–13.

Church, R. M. (2001). A Turing test for computational and associative theories of learning. *Current Directions in Psychological Sciences*, **10**, 132–136.

Davis, M. & Whalen, P. J. (2001). The amygdala: vigilance and emotion. *Molecular Psychiatry*, **6**, 13–34.

De la Casa, L. & Lubow, R. (2000). Super-latent inhibition with delayed conditioned taste aversion testing. *Animal Learning and Behavior*, **28**, 389–399.

De la Casa, L. & Lubow, R. (2002). An empirical analysis of the super-latent inhibition effect. *Animal Learning and Behavior*, **30**, 112–120.

D'Esposito, M., Postle, B. R. & Rypma, B. (2000). Prefontal cortical contributions to working memory: evidence from event-related fMRI studies. *Experimental Brain Research*, **133**, 3–11.

Dunsmoor, J. & Schmajuk, N. (2009). Interpreting patterns of brain activation in human fear conditioning with an attentional-associative learning model. *Behavioral Neuroscience*, **123**, 851–855.

Dunsmoor, J. E., Bandettini, P. A. & Knight, D. C. (2007). Impact of continuous versus intermittent CS–UCS pairing on human brain activation during Pavlovian fear conditioning. *Behavioral Neuroscience*, **121**, 635–642.

Fuster, J. M. (1973). Unit activity in prefrontal cortex during delayed-response performance: neuronal correlates of transient memory. *Journal of Neurophysiology*, **36**, 61–78.

Good, M. & Honey, R. (1993). Selective hippocampus lesions abolish contextual specificity of latent inhibition and conditioning. *Behavioral Neuroscience*, **107**, 23–33.

Grossberg, S. (1975). A neural model of attention, reinforcement, and discrimination learning. *International Review of Neurobiology*, **18**, 263–327.

Hall, G. & Schachtman, T. R. (1987). Differential effects of a retention interval on latent inhibition and the habituation of an orienting response. *Animal Learning and Behavior*, **15**, 76–82.

Holland, P. C. (1989). Occasion setting with simultaneous compounds in rats. *Journal of Experimental Psychology: Animal Behavior Processes*, **15**, 183–193.

Holland, P. C. (1999). Overshadowing and blocking as acquisition deficits: no recovery after extinction of overshadowing or blocking cues. *The Quarterly Journal of Experimental Psychology*, **52B**, 307–333.

Honey, R. C. & Hall, G. (1989). Attenuation of latent inhibition after compound preexposure: associative and perceptual explanations. *The Quarterly Journal of Experimental Psychology B: Comparative and Physiological Psychology*, **41**, 355–368.

Ishii, K., Haga, Y. & Hishimura, Y. (1999). Distractor effect on latent inhibition of conditioned flavor aversion in rats. *Japanese Psychological Research*, **41**, 229–238.

Konorski, J. (1967). *Integrative Activity of the Brain*. Chicago, IL: University of Chicago Press.

Lantz, A. E. (1973). Effect of number of trials, interstimulus interval, and dishabituation on subsequent conditioning in a CER paradigm. *Animal Learning and Behavior*, **1**, 273–277.

Larrauri, J. A. & Schmajuk, N. A. (2008). Attentional, associative, and configural mechanisms of extinction. *Psychological Review*, **115**, 640–676.

Le Pelley, M. E. (2004). The role of associative history in models of associative learning: a selective review and a hybrid model. *The Quarterly Journal of Experimental Psychology*, **57B**, 193–243.

Lovibond, P. E., Been, S. L., Mitchell, C. J., Bouton, M. E. & Frohardt, R. (2003). Forward and backward blocking of causal judgment is enhanced by additivity of effect magnitude. *Memory and Cognition*, **31**, 133–42.

Lysle, D. T. & Fowler, F. (1985). Inhibition as a "slave" process: deactivation of conditioned inhibition through extinction of conditioned excitation. *Journal of Experimental Psychology: Animal Behavior Processes*, **11**, 71–94.

Mackintosh, N. J. (1975). A theory of attention: variations in the associability of stimuli with reinforcement. *Psychological Review*, **82**, 276–298.

Mackintosh, N. J. & Turner, C. (1971). Blocking as a function of novelty of CS and predictability of UCS. *The Quarterly Journal of Experimental Psychology*, **23**, 359–366.

Maren, S. & Chang, C. (2006). Recent fear is resistant to extinction. *Proceedings of the National Academy of Sciences of the United States of America*, **103**, 18020–18025.

Miller, R. R. & Schachtman, T. (1985). Conditioning context as an associative baseline: implications for response generation and the nature of conditioned inhibition. In R. R. Miller and N. E. Spear, eds., *Information Processing in Animals: Conditioned Inhibition*. Hillsdale, NJ: Erlbaum, pp. 51–88.

Moody, E. W., Sunsay, C. & Bouton, M. E. (2006). Priming and trial spacing in extinction: effects on extinction performance, spontaneous recovery, and reinstatement in appetitive conditioning. *The Quarterly Journal of Experimental Psychology*, **59**, 809–829.

Nagaishi, T. & Nakajima, S. (2008). Further evidence for the summation of latent inhibition and overshadowing in rats' conditioned taste aversion. *Learning and Motivation*, **39**, 221–242.

Nakajima, S. & Nagaishi, T. (2005). Summation of latent inhibition and overshadowing in a generalized bait shyness paradigm of rats. *Behavioural Processes*, **69**, 369–377.

Nakajima, S., Ka, H. & Imada, H. (1999). Summation of overshadowing and latent inhibition in rats' conditioned taste aversion: scapegoat technique works for familiar meals. *Appetite*, **33**, 299–307.

Pearce, J. & Hall, G. (1980). A model for Pavlovian conditioning: variations in the effectiveness of conditioned but not unconditioned stimuli. *Psychological Review*, **87**, 332–352.

Phelps, E. A. & LeDoux, J. E. (2005). Contributions of the amygdala to emotion processing: from animal models to human behavior. *Neuron*, **48**, 175–187.

Rescorla, R. A. (2000). Associative changes in excitors and inhibitors differ when they are conditioned in compound. *Journal of Experimental Psychology: Animal Behavior Processes*, **26**, 428–438.

Rescorla, R. A. (2001). Unequal associative changes when excitors and neural stimuli are conditioned in compound. *The Quarterly Journal of Experimental Psychology B: Comparative and Physiological Psychology*, **54B**, 53–68.

Rescorla, R. A. (2002). Effect of following an excitatory–inhibitory compound with an intermediate reinforcer. *Journal of Experimental Psychology: Animal Behavior Processes*, **28**, 163–174.

Rescorla, R. A. (2003). Protection from extinction. *Learning and Behavior*, **31**, 124–132.

Rescorla, R. A. (2004). Spontaneous recovery varies inversely with the training-extinction interval. *Learning and Behavior*, **32**, 401–408.

Rescorla, R. A. & Holland, P. C. (1977). Associations in Pavlovian conditioned inhibition. *Learning and Motivation*, **8**, 429–447.

Rescorla, R. A. & Wagner, A. (1972). A theory of Pavlovian conditioning: variations in the effectiveness of reinforcement and non-reinforcement. In A.H. Black and W.F. Prokasy, eds., *Classical Conditioning II: Current Research and Theory*. New York: Appleton–Century–Crofts, pp. 64–99.

Richards, R. W. & Sargent, D. M. (1983). The order of presentation of conditioned stimuli during extinction. *Animal Learning and Behavior*, **11**, 229–236.

Robbins, S. J. (1990). Mechanisms underlying spontaneous recovery in autoshaping. *Journal of Experimental Psychology: Animal Behavior Processes*, **16**, 235–249.

Schmajuk, N. A. (2010). *Mechanisms in Classical Conditioning: A Computational Approach.* Cambridge, UK: Cambridge University Press.

Schmajuk, N. A. & Buhusi, C. V. (1997). Spatial and temporal cognitive mapping: a neural network approach. *Trends in Cognitive Sciences*, **1**, 109–114.

Schmajuk, N. A. & Di Carlo, J. J. (1992). Stimulus configuration, classical conditioning, and the hippocampus. *Psychological Review*, **99**, 268–305.

Schmajuk, N. A. & Kutlu, M. G. (2009). The computational nature of associative learning. *Behavioral Brain Science*, **32**, 223–224.

Schmajuk, N. A. & Kutlu, M. G. (2010). A computational model that provides an associative interpretation of outcome additivity and maximality effects on blocking. In E. Alonso and E. Mondragon, eds., *Computational Neuroscience for Advancing Artificial Intelligence: Models, Methods and Applications*. Hershey, PA: IGI Global.

Schmajuk, N. A. & Larrauri, J. A. (2006). Experimental challenges to theories of classical conditioning: application of an attentional model of storage and retrieval. *Journal of Experimental Psychology: Animal Behavior Processes*, **32**, 1–20.

Schmajuk, N. A. & Larrauri, J. A. (2008). Associative models describe both causal learning and conditioning. *Behavioral Processes*, **77**, 443–445.

Schmajuk, N. A. & Moore, J. (1988). The hippocampus and the classically conditioned nictitating membrane response: a real-time attentional-associative model. *Psychobiology*, **16**, 20–35.

Schmajuk, N. A., Cox, L. & Gray, J. A. (2001). Nucleus accumbens, entorhinal cortex and latent inhibition: a neural network model. *Behavioral Brain Research*, **118**, 123–141.

Schmajuk, N. A., Lam, Y. & Gray, J. A. (1996). Latent inhibition: a neural network approach. *Journal of Experimental Psychology: Animal Behavior Processes*, **22**, 321–349.

Schmajuk, N. A., Lamoureux, J. A. & Holland, P. C. (1998). Occasion setting: a neural network approach. *Psychological Review*, **105**(1), 3–32.

Shevill, I. & Hall, G. (2004). Retrospective revaluation effects in the conditioned suppression procedure. *The Quarterly Journal of Experimental Psychology B: Comparative and Physiological Psychology*, **57B**, 331–347.

Soltysik, S. (1985). Protection from extinction: new data and a hypothesis of several varieties of conditioned inhibition. In R.R. Miller and N.E. Spear, eds., *Information Processing in Animals: Conditioned Inhibition*. Hillsdale, NJ: Lawrence Erlbaum.

Turing, A. M. (1950). Computing machinery and intelligence. *Mind*, **59**, 433–460.

Wagner, A. R. (1979). Habituation and memory. In A. Dickinson and R. A. Boakes, eds., *Mechanisms of Learning and Motivation*. Hillsdale, NJ: Lawrence Erlbaum.

Wagner, A. R. (1981). SOP: a model of automatic memory processing in animal behavior. In N. E. Spear and R. R. Miller, eds., *Information Processing in Animals: Memory Mechanisms*. Hillsdale, NJ: Erlbaum, pp. 5–47.

Wheeler, D. S., Stout, S. C. & Miller, R. R. (2004). Interaction of retention interval with CS-preexposure and extinction treatment: symmetry with respect to primacy. *Learning and Behavior*, **32**, 335–347.

Wilson, P. N., Boumphrey, P. & Pearce, J. M. (1992). Restoration of the orienting response to a light by a change in its predictive accuracy. *The Quarterly Journal of Experimental Psychology*, **44B**, 17–36.

Young, M. E. & Wasserman, E. A. (2002). Limited attention and cue order consistency affect predictive learning: a test of similarity measures. *Journal of Experimental Psychology: Learning, Memory, and Cognition*, **28**, 484–496.

7

Computer simulation of the cerebellum

MICHAEL D. MAUK

Abstract

The connection between eyelid conditioning and the cerebellum arose from the search for the site of plasticity that mediates eyelid conditioning, but the cerebellum is far more than the site of plasticity for eyelid conditioning and eyelid conditioning is far more than a cerebellum-dependent behavior. The specific relationships between the stimuli used in eyelid conditioning and cerebellar inputs, as well as between cerebellar output and behaviour, make eyelid conditioning a powerful tool for empirical and computational analysis of cerebellar learning and information processing. This relationship makes the well-established behavioral properties of eyelid conditioning a first approximation of the rules for input–output transformations in the cerebellum – that is, for what the cerebellum computes. The practical experimental advantages of eyelid conditioning greatly facilitate analysis of how the neurons and synapses of the cerebellum accomplish this computation. Finally, the close correspondence between eyelid conditioning and the cerebellum provides a rare opportunity to implement biologically relevant and quite stringent tests on the successes and failures of computer simulations of the cerebellum. From these advantages is emerging an increasingly clear and specific story of what the cerebellum computes and how its neurons and synapses produce this computation. One way that this is revealed is in the many ways that current large-scale computer simulations of the cerebellum qualitatively and sometimes quantitatively mimic the many intricate behavioral properties of eyelid conditioning. I will briefly outline previous work laying the foundation for simulation of the cerebellum and identifying the essential basics of learning in the cerebellum. I will then describe a number of new computational findings that are moving toward a relatively precise picture of the essential computational unit of cerebellum and how it functions against the backdrop of noisy inputs.

There is a long history of using eyelid conditioning as a way to study the behavioral properties and neural mechanisms of learning. Early studies in humans, monkeys, and rabbits were aimed at identifying the rules governing associative learning (Gormezano, Kehoe, & Marshall, 1983; Lavond, McCormick, & Thompson, 1984; Kehoe & Macrae 1998, 2002). Mechanistic studies beginning in the 1970s initially emphasized localization, which for delay eyelid conditioning revealed the cerebellum as the site of plasticity that is necessary and sufficient to explain the acquisition and expression of conditioned responses (McCormick *et al.*, 1982; McCormick & Thompson, 1984a, 1984b; Thompson, 1986). There remain spirited debates over the number of plasticity sites and their relative contributions to learning. Computer simulations of the cerebellum may play an important role in helping bring these debates to a satisfying conclusion.

Our work has been guided by the belief that these studies produced something far beyond localization. The deeper revelation was that eyelid conditioning represented an especially powerful means to study the cerebellum in terms of what it computes and how its neurons and synapses accomplish this computation. This utility of eyelid conditioning stems from the relatively direct ways in which the training stimuli activate cerebellar inputs and from the way cerebellar output relatively directly drives the motor neurons responsible for expression of the conditioned responses. This close relationship between the cerebellum and delay eyelid conditioning has important conceptual and practical advantages. Conceptually, this relationship makes the behavioral properties of eyelid conditioning a first approximation of the input to output transformations of the cerebellum – that is, of *what* it computes (Ohyama, Nores, Murphy, & Mauk, 2003). The ability to use eyelid conditioning experiments to control cerebellar inputs and to have a relatively easy measure of cerebellar output is a practical advantage that greatly facilitates analysis of how the cerebellum computes, including its mechanisms of learning.

The close relationship between delay eyelid conditioning and the cerebellum has an additional and extremely important advantage when it comes to the use of computer simulations (Mauk & Donegan, 1997; Medina & Mauk, 2000). The ability to build a computer simulation of the cerebellum is currently not the limiting factor; the speed of current computers and the wealth of data available regarding the synaptic organization and physiology of the cerebellum ensure that this is so. The limiting factor is the ability to test in a biologically meaningful way the quality of the simulation – the extent to which it behaves like the real cerebellum. Eyelid conditioning greatly obviates this limitation for analysis of cerebellum using computer simulations. Since data are available for (1) how the stimuli used in eyelid conditioning activate cerebellar inputs, (2) how cerebellar output translates into the observed behavioral responses, and (3) the expected behavioral consequences for a wide range of variations in the training protocol, eyelid conditioning provides stringent ways to test the performance of a computer simulation of the cerebellum. Inputs to the simulation can be arranged to mimic inputs to the real cerebellum during a given training protocol, and published results of the behavioral consequences of such training indicate the proper output.

With such advantages then, computer simulations of the cerebellum represent an approach to the general topic of associative learning mechanisms that can provide quite concrete tests of various ideas, including relatively abstract theories of association and stimulus processing. I will briefly describe the relationship between eyelid conditioning and the cerebellum, our approach to simulations of the cerebellum, and ways that it has contributed to our understanding of cerebellar mechanisms of learning and information processing, and then outline various new ideas that stem from ongoing simulation work. One hope is that various debates about the nature of associative learning and its mechanisms may find focus or small insights from the relatively concrete ideas that emerge from this highly bottom-up, computational approach to learning.

Eyelid conditioning and the cerebellum

The procedures of eyelid conditioning are relatively straightforward. Animals are trained by presenting training trials in which a relatively neutral conditioned stimulus (CS) such as a tone is paired with an unconditioned stimulus (US) that is mildly threatening to the eye. In years past the US was usually a puff of air directed at the cornea. We now favor mild electrical stimulation through sub dermal electrodes implanted on both sides of the eye. This stimulation US is not aversive and indeed appears to be far less bothersome to the animals than the air-puff US. Initially the US elicits a reflex response, the eyelids close, whereas there is no response to the CS. With training the CS acquires the ability to elicit increasingly large eyelid responses, until in the well-trained animal the rate of responding is near 100% and each response is a full closure of the eyelids (~ 6 mm). An example is shown in Figure 7.1.

The behavioral properties of eyelid conditioning are quite well characterized. Briefly, eyelid conditioning shows robust acquisition that, depending on conditions, requires 2–4 sessions to reach peak responding. There is rapid extinction of responding with either CS-alone trials or unpaired presentations of the CS and US on separate trials. Robust savings are generally seen where the rate of relearning after extinction is much greater than the rate of initial learning. One of the key behavioral properties is the dependence of eyelid conditioning on the interstimulus interval (ISI) – that is, the time between the onset of the CS and the onset of the US. This interval determines whether or not the animal learns and, as seen in Figure 7.1, the timing of the responses when learning occurs. Learning requires the use of an ISI of at least 150 ms and less than approximately 2000 ms. Robust learning requires an ISI between 250 and 750 ms (Figure 7.2). These temporal properties of eyelid conditioning will represent an important part of the ideas that follow.

The relationship between eyelid conditioning and the cerebellum has been revealed using a combination of lesion, stimulation, and recording studies. The reader is referred to the numerous reviews for a comprehensive treatment of these studies (Thompson, 1986; Thompson & Krupa, 1994; Ohyama, Medina, Nores, & Mauk, 2002). Briefly, the essence of this vast literature reveals that (1) output of the cerebellum via the anterior interpositus nucleus drives the expression of conditioned responses, (2) presentation of the CS is conveyed to the cerebellum via activation of certain mossy fiber afferents, and (3) presentation of the US is conveyed to the cerebellum via excitation of certain climbing fiber afferents (Figure 7.3). Lesions of the anterior interpositus nucleus either before or after training prevent the expression of conditioned responses (Garcia & Mauk, 1998). Lesions of mossy fiber inputs produce effects on learning equivalent to omitting the CS in training (Steinmetz et al., 1987). Lesions of climbing fiber inputs have been reported either to produce extinction of responses (as if the US was omitted) or to abolish responses (McCormick, Steinmetz, & Thompson, 1985). The interpretation of these lesion data is complex and will be discussed further later on. Electrical stimulation of mossy fibers can be used as a substitute for the tone CS, and stimulation of the correct region of the dorsal accessory olive (a source of climbing fibers afferents) can substitute for the US (Mauk, Steinmetz, & Thompson, 1986). Indeed, Steinmetz and others showed that stimulation of mossy fibers as the CS and climbing fibers as the US can support normal conditioning in the same animal (Steinmetz, Lavond, & Thompson, 1989). Finally, recording studies have shown that neurons in the anterior interpositus nucleus respond vigorously just prior to the expression of conditioned responses, that CS presentation activates mossy fibers, and that US presentation activates climbing fibers. Thus, bursts of activity in the appropriate anterior interpositus nucleus neurons are necessary and sufficient for the expression of conditioned responses, assuming that the downstream pathways are intact. Likewise, activation of mossy fiber inputs is a necessary and sufficient CS input to the cerebellum, and climbing fiber activation is a necessary and sufficient US input.

SESSION 1   SESSION 2

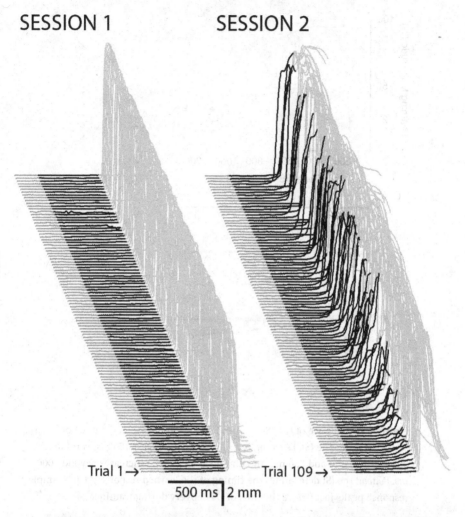

Trial 1 →   Trial 109 →

500 ms | 2 mm

Figure 7.1 Example raw data from two sessions of eyelid conditioning. Each horizontal sweep represents a single trial with the time of CS presentation indicated in black. Eyelid closure is seen as an upward deflection of the trace. In the first session (left) the reflex responses to the US are seen in the gray upward deflections. Conditioned responses with increasing amplitude are seen in the second session. Note also the precise timing of the conditioned responses in the second session. The onset of the responses is delayed so that the response peak occurs near the time of US presentation.

These data reveal that eyelid conditioning is not only a cerebellum-dependent task, but that eyelid conditioning can be used as a powerful tool to study the cerebellum. Eyelid conditioning permits a fair degree of control over the inputs to the cerebellum and allows for a simple behavioral readout of cerebellar output. As discussed in the introduction, eyelid conditioning therefore

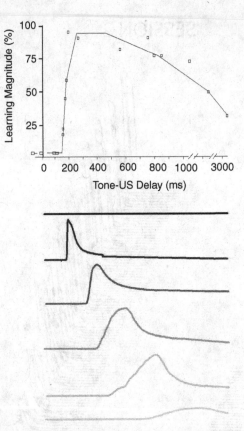

Figure 7.2 Influence of the ISI on eyelid conditioning. *Top*: magnitude of learning as a function of the ISI. Learning requires an ISI of at least 150 ms, is robust for ISIs between 250 and 750 ms, and diminishes as the ISI increases beyond 1000 ms. *Bottom*: the ISI determines the timing of the learned responses. Each sample response peaks just before the time of US delivery during training.

provides the ability to study the cerebellum in terms of its input to output transformation, and to test the performance of computer simulations of the cerebellum.

What the cerebellum computes

Given these relationships between the cerebellum and eyelid conditioning, the behavioral properties of eyelid conditioning can be used to construct a relatively simple view of what the cerebellum computes. Although all of the behavioral properties of eyelid conditioning ultimately reveal something about cerebellar computation, a simple view of cerebellar learning requires attention to only three key aspects of eyelid conditioning: that it is associative, the influence of the ISI on acquisition, and on response timing (Ohyama *et al.* 2003).

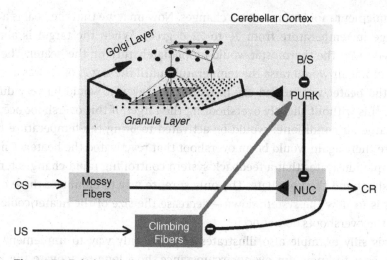

Figure 7.3 Relationship between eyelid conditioning and the cerebellum. The two training stimuli activate cerebellar afferents. The CS activates mossy fibers and the US activates climbing fibers. Cerebellar output via the anterior interpositus nucleus (NUC) drives the expression of conditioned responses. Plasticity necessary for the expression of conditioned responses occurs at two synapse types (shown as triangles): the granule–Purkinje (PURK) synapses in the cerebellar cortex and the synapses between mossy fiber synapses in the interpositus nucleus. B/S: basket and stellate cells

For clarity of explanation it may be better to begin with the key assertion about what the cerebellum computes and then to use properties of eyelid conditioning to defend this assertion. The assertion is that the essential job of the cerebellum is to make rapid feed-forward predictions and that the properties of cerebellar learning revealed by eyelid conditioning are properly suited for this task.

In principle, there are two ways in which information (sensory input) can be used to make decisions for subsequent action: through feedback and feed-forward prediction. The need for feed-forward predictions can be illustrated by evaluating the limitations of feedback as a means of control. Everyone is familiar with feedback control, as we all make use of it with the thermostats that control room temperature. A thermostat measures room temperature and compares it with the target temperature. If the measured temperature differs from target, the heater or air conditioner is activated to bring the temperature back to target. This feedback process is simple and effective, but it has the limitation of being inherently slow. This can be illustrated with an odd but simple thought experiment. Imagine that the task is to use a thermostat to make rapid changes in room temperature on demand. To accomplish this would require a very large heating/cooling system that can inject large amounts of air to implement rapid temperature changes. Now imagine that the goal is a rapid change in temperature from 70 to 72 degrees. When the target is abruptly shifted to 72, the thermostat would immediately turn on the heater. The large rush of hot air would raise the temperature until the target of 72 was achieved and the heater was turned off. In reality, however, it would be very difficult to do this without slightly overshooting the target. If this overshoot occurred, the large air conditioner would be activated to bring the temperature down, where there again would be an overshoot that reactivated the heater. This silly example illustrates that a feedback system controlling rapid changes tends to overshoot and then oscillate. The only surefire way to eliminate these oscillations is to slow the system down – decrease the size of the heater/cooler – so that the overshoots do not occur.

This silly example also illustrates that the only way to implement rapid changes is to know, for every circumstance, how long to activate the heater to achieve the target. This is the idea of feed-forward control; to use previous experience to predict the proper response for the present circumstance. In our silly example, a hypothetical feed-forward thermostat would react to the sudden change in target from 70 to 72 to predicting how long to activate the heater so that the room temperature moves to 72 exactly. In simple situations these predictions can be calculated ahead of time and preprogrammed, but in complex situations this is not possible and the only recourse is to learn predictions based on previous experience.

The key assertions can now be restated more specifically. The cerebellum's contributions to movement are to make rapid feed-forward predictions to help control the accuracy of movements. If the further assertion is that these predictions are learned from previous experience, what would the properties of this learning be? The learning should be error-driven, that is to say, changes are only required when the response is incorrect. So we might expect that our smart feed-forward thermostat would have an input that signals incorrect responses. How should it react to an error signal? First, we can presume that this signal should be bidirectional to handle situations where the heater was activated for too short a time when it was activated for too long. This learning should be associative, which means that an error signal should only modify the response to the previous input, not to all other inputs. To implement this specificity, the thermostat would require many sensors to provide input regarding relevant factors such as temperature, size of the temperature change, humidity, number of people in the room, number of windows open, how much wind might be blowing in through the windows, etc. Associative learning would mean that an error signal would only alter the subsequent responses for inputs similar to those that contributed to the output that drove the error signal in the first place. Finally, we would expect that as this system operates over time it would be able to solve a certain type of temporal credit-assignment problem, which we will examine shortly.

As a first step it should be clear that the properties of cerebellar learning revealed by eyelid conditioning match with these expectations. The learning is associative, is relatively specific to the training input (the CS), and is error-driven (the US). The way that eyelid conditioning depends on the ISI (Figure 7.2) reveals insights about timing and this temporal credit-assignment problem. To produce learning the CS (mossy fiber input) must precede the US (climbing fiber) by at least 150 ms and by not more than about 2000 ms. Within this range, training promotes the acquisition of conditioned responses that are timed to peak just before the US. To connect this to the feed-forward learning idea, we must look closely at the implications of these properties for how the cerebellum responds to an error input (to activation of a climbing fiber).

Consider a feed-forward device that has just used the inputs from its various sensors to make a prediction, that this prediction was wrong, and that because of this the device has received an error input (indicating, for example, that the prediction was too small). Since the point is to make adjustments to the connections that produced the bad prediction in the first place, the wrong thing to do would be for that error signal to adjust the weights of currently active inputs. Instead, the weights of recently active inputs should be adjusted. The time frame of "recently active" would depend on the delays between making the prediction and the eventual arrival of the error signal. This idea is represented schematically in Figure 7.4. The arrival of a climbing fiber error signal should alter processing that contributed to the previous output (dotted line to the black box) that turned out to be incorrect (Raymond & Lisberger, 1998).

Figure 7.4B expands this notion to consider the sensor signals; in the case of the cerebellum these are conveyed by mossy fiber inputs. Here I make a presumption: I presume that it would be a very limited feed-forward system that could only make use of sensor signals immediately preceding the time of prediction. Instead, it seems a far more adaptable system could make use of sensory signals that occur over a span of time preceding the prediction. In the case of our smart thermostat, this would be useful should the impact of various events that could be signaled by the sensors have different delays. Opening a window, for example, might have a more immediate impact on subsequent decisions than would the entry of two more people into the room. I also presume that there are limits to this time span. The likelihood that a signal might be useful in making a decision should decrease the further back in time that it occurred relative to the decision. Opening a window yesterday, for example, would provide no new information beyond that conveyed by the current temperature

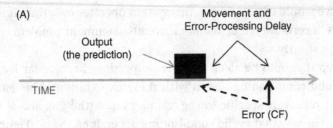

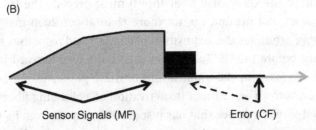

Figure 7.4 The temporal credit-assignment problem for feed-forward learning. Errors conveyed by climbing fibers (CFs) must modify synapses responsible for prior output (black box). The mossy fiber (MF) inputs that may contribute to this input are shown in the gray shaded region. Learning must display temporal flexibility so that mossy fiber inputs occurring over this can alter output at the same time, here indicated by the black box. (Refer to text.)

in the room. The gray shaded area in Figure 7.4B conveys this notion, that the utility of signals declines the further back in time they occurred. This gray region defines the likelihood that a sensory signal was useful to the decision. It increases as the time to the decision approaches, is highest just before the time of decision, and then abruptly falls to zero as the decision is made. With this capability there would also be the additional computational demand of solving a temporal credit-assignment problem. The consequence of any learning driven by an error signal must still affect the output at the same fixed time point shown by the black box in Figure 7.4B.

These two constraints define the type of learning the feed-forward system needs. The error signal should be able to modify the weights of inputs occurring of the time range indicated by the shaded gray region. The height of the region at each point in time should define how strong the learning would be for a signal (mossy fiber input) arriving at that time. The learning must then show temporal flexibility. Since the error signal should only fix the errant output produced by the prediction (black box), the system must have the capacity for flexibility in the temporal relationship between the sensory input (mossy fiber) and the error input (climbing fiber). When a mossy fiber input consistently precedes the arrival of an error input some time later, learning should modify the predictions made in the time just before the arrival of the error (black box). Mossy fiber inputs that precede climbing fiber inputs by short intervals should produce a change in output to that mossy fiber input with a short latency, so that the altered output occurs before the error. Mossy fiber inputs that precede climbing fiber inputs by longer intervals should produce changes in output that are delayed with respect to the mossy fiber input so that again, the change in output is properly timed – it is time-locked prior to the error.

In sum, the specific assertion is this: the properties of learning just described are identical to the properties of cerebellar learning revealed by eyelid conditioning (shown in Figure 7.2). Learning is associative, error-driven, and stimulus specific. Moreover, the shape of the interstimulus-interval function is as predicted: mossy fiber inputs must precede climbing fiber inputs by at least ~ 150 ms to support learning, and learning fades as that ISI increases beyond 750 ms. Finally, the timing of the conditioned eyelid responses shows the predicted temporal flexibility. Since the responses must be time-locked to occur just before the time of US delivery, the latencies vary depending on the ISI – that is, on the time interval between the arrival of the mossy fiber and climbing fiber inputs.

I propose that these properties of cerebellar learning, as revealed by eyelid conditioning, suggest the purpose of learning in the cerebellum. This learning is in the service of a system whose purpose is to make feed-forward predictions to improve the accuracy of movements that can be rapid. These feed-forward predictions are improved and informed by the type of associate cerebellar learning revealed by the eyelid conditioning (Ohyama *et al.* 2003).

A brief summary of previous findings

Most work in this field has dealt with the other side of the coin: how the circuitry, cells, and synapses within the cerebellum accomplish the above computation. This work began with lesions of the cerebellum and the corresponding debates about the relative roles of the cerebellar cortex and the cerebellar deep nuclei. There are numerous reviews regarding this debate, and it is true that there does not yet exist a consensus on this topic. If we limit consideration to rabbit eyelid conditioning, however, I believe the following interpretation enjoys by far the best support from the experiments with the strongest controls. Almost everyone agrees that lesions in, or reversible inactivation of, the cerebellar anterior interpositus nucleus prevents the expression of conditioned responses (Garcia & Mauk, 1998). This is not terribly informative, however, about the relative contributions of cerebellar deep nucleus versus cerebellar cortex, since the sole output of the cerebellar cortex is via the deep nuclei. So the real issue, and the source of the most controversy, has been lesions of the cerebellar cortex (Yeo, 1991). The range of observations extends from complete abolition of conditioned responses to no effect whatsoever (McCormick & Thompson, 1984a, 1984b; Yeo, Hardiman, & Glickstein, 1985; Lavond & Steinmetz, 1989). We have observed that with careful attention to the placement of the lesions that the effect on already trained responses is a disruption of response timing. The normally well-timed responses, delayed to peak near the time of US presentation, are replaced by responses with relatively fixed and short latencies to onset (Perrett, Ruiz, & Mauk, 1993; Perrett & Mauk, 1995; Garcia & Mauk, 1998; Medina, Garcia, Nores, Taylor, & Mauk, 2000). For convenience I will refer to these responses as "short-latency responses" or SLRs. An example produced by an infusion of a GABA antagonist into the interpositus nucleus is shown in Figure 7.5.

We interpret the SLR effect as evidence for two sites of plasticity in the cerebellum, one in the cerebellar deep nuclei revealed by the SLRs, and one in the cerebellar cortex revealed by the abolition of learned timing of the conditioned responses. We have recently demonstrated directly that the SLRs seen after inactivation of the cerebellar cortex are mediated by learning-dependent and associative plasticity in the cerebellar deep nucleus (Ohyama, Nores, Medina, Riusech, & Mauk, 2006).

These data speak to the effects of cerebellar cortex lesions on response expression, but the real controversy has been whether or not the cerebellar cortex is necessary for acquisition and extinction of responses. We have demonstrated that lesions of the cerebellar cortex prevent acquisition of responses and prevent extinction of existing (short-latency) responses (Perrett & Mauk, 1995; Garcia, Steele, & Mauk, 1999). From this, we have proposed the following sequence of events to mediate the acquisition of conditioned eyelid responses. Paired presentation of CS + US initially induces plasticity in the cerebellar cortex that teaches the Purkinje cells to decrease or even pause their ongoing activity during the CS. These pauses, in turn, serve as a signal for the induction of plasticity in the anterior interpositus nucleus. Once this latter plasticity is induced, full and robust expression of conditioned responses is possible. This hypothesis accounts for the necessity of the cerebellar cortex for acquisition and extinction, because the Purkinje cells both undergo plasticity and control the induction of plasticity in the cerebellar deep nuclei.

Computer simulation of cerebellar learning

The cerebellum is particularly amenable to the use of bottom-up computer simulations to study mechanisms of information processing and learning. The synaptic organization and synaptic physiology of the cerebellum are particularly well known, and as described above, the relationship between the cerebellum

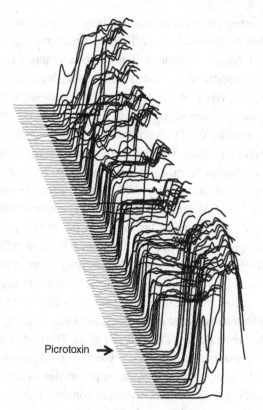

Picrotoxin →

Figure 7.5 The effects of a temporary blockade of the cerebellar cortex output
via picrotoxin infusion in the deep nucleus. Responses at the front are before
the infusion and show proper timing; they peak just before the US. Post-infusion
responses have a short-fixed latency to onset. CS presentation is indicated by the
black portion of each trace.

and eyelid conditioning provides a variety of stringent tests on the performance
of simulations. Our work in this area was initially motivated by attempts to understand the learned timing of conditioned eyelid responses and the underlying temporal coding in the cerebellum (Buonomano & Mauk, 1994; Medina *et al.*, 2000).
The essential idea was that interactions between the granule cells and Golgi cells
converted mossy fiber inputs into patterns of granule-cell activation that encoded
not only the presence of a stimulus (such as the CS), but also produced a temporal
code with different subsets of granule cells being active at different times during
the tone. Because the synaptic organization connecting these neurons was well
known, and the synaptic physiology was (at the time) somewhat known, we built
a large-scale computer simulation to test this idea.

The details of these simulations have been presented elsewhere, so the
description here will be brief (Medina & Mauk, 2000; Medina *et al.*, 2000; Medina,
Nores, & Mauk, 2002; Mauk & Ohyama, 2004). Neurons are represented with a

single-compartment, leaky, integrate-and-fire model. There is sometimes confusion about the nature of this representation. Difference equations are used to solve for membrane potential based on the leak conductance, synaptic conductances, and any other relevant conductance that is not voltage-dependent, such as calcium-activated potassium. Synaptic conductances are modeled with step increases upon synapse activation followed by exponential decay as constrained by the literature. The main contrivance of this representation is the lack of explicit representation of active conductances, which are extremely computationally intensive to calculate. In its simplest form, an integrate-and-fire representation simply assigns the occurrence of an action potential when membrane potential crosses an assigned threshold. This captures the essential synaptic-integration process that drives action-potential activity, but omits many of the processes that are mediated by the properties of active conductances, such as refractory periods (absolute and relative), and spike threshold accommodation. It is, however, fairly easy to implement such processes in the integrate-and-fire representation by using a dynamic rather than static threshold. As a simple example, absolute and relative refractory periods are easily obtained by increasing spikes to increases in threshold that then decay in the proper ways. The end result is a computationally efficient representation that can serve as a good phenomenological model of the synaptic integration and spiking properties of any target neuron. The first step in building a simulation is then to construct an integrate-and-fire representation of each neuron type that is properly constrained by what is known about the physiology of that neuron type.

Building a simulation that properly represents the real synaptic organization (wiring diagram) is a particular challenge for the cerebellum, in part because of the enormous number of granule cells that are present. It was not possible at the time (early 1990s) to build simulations that fully matched the numeric, divergence, and convergence ratios of cerebellar circuitry (it still is not practical); compromises were necessary. The early simulations were comprised of 600 mossy fibers, 10 000 granule cells, 900 Golgi cells, 200 stellate/basket cells, one Purkinje cell, and one climbing fiber. By comparison, our current "standard simulation" has 600 mossy fibers, 12 000 granule cells, 900 Golgi cells, 200 stellate cells, 128 basket cells, 24 Purkinje cells, 8 deep nucleus cells, and 4 climbing fibers. Since there are approximately 200 000 synapses in simulations of this magnitude it would not be practical to program each connection by hand. Instead, we devised algorithms to construct the connectivity based on constraints of the real circuitry. Forming the Golgi cell synapses for one granule cell can serve as an example of the essentials of this process. Each neuron is assigned a position in the 2-dimensional representation of the cortex. Given the granule cell's location, the geometry of its t-shaped axon extending in opposite directions along the folium, and the cylindrical geometry of the Golgi cells, a long and narrow rectangle can be defined on the 2-dimensional cortex. The Golgi cells within this rectangle represent those that could physically receive a connection given the location and geometry of each cell. The next step is to determine the actual connections within this rectangle, which is constrained by the divergence ratio of granule-to-Golgi connections: how many Golgi cells does each granule cell contact? The algorithm randomly selects this number of Golgi cells from within the rectangle as candidate synaptic targets, pending evaluation of a final constraint. For each candidate Golgi cell, the convergence ratio is used as a final constraint. In essence, this constraint asks: would this synapse exceed the proper number of granule cell synapses onto the candidate Golgi cell? If not, the connection is stored. If it would exceed the convergence limit, the algorithm selects a new candidate from the rectangle, and this process is repeated until all required connections are formed.

Once the cellular representations are established, the connectivity is determined, and rules for plasticity are implemented (as described below), running the simulation requires only a means to create proper mossy fiber activity as the input. In our simulations each mossy fiber is assigned an average background firing rate and is assigned, if appropriate, an identity as a neuron activated by the CS. CS-activated neurons can then be further identified as either responding to this CS with tonic activity or with a phasic burst at CS onset, as dictated by published responses of mossy fibers to auditory stimuli. These properties are used to determine the likelihood of synaptic inputs to the mossy fibers, either during background or during the CS, which creates activity that is noisy but that produces, with averaging, the proper peri-stimulus histograms.

Sites and rules for synaptic plasticity

The question of sites and rules for plasticity in the cerebellum is related to the relative contributions of cerebellar cortex and deep nuclei, and is equally contentious. Rather than present an exhaustive review of both sides I will present the view that we favor (Mauk, 1997; Nores, Medina, Steele, & Mauk, 2000), in part because recent evidence from slice work provides strong new support. In the simulation we represent plasticity at the granule–Purkinje cell synapses that is controlled by the climbing fiber input to the Purkinje cell. Based on strong empirical support, these synapses are decreased in strength when active in the presence of a climbing fiber input and are increased when active in the absence of a climbing fiber input. There exist debates about the overall existence of cerebellar learning and there are certainly unresolved issues regarding other potential sites of plasticity within the cerebellar cortex, but there appears to be general agreement that climbing fibers control plasticity of this sort at the granule–Purkinje cell synapses. We also implement plasticity at the mossy fiber synapse onto the deep nucleus cells that is controlled by Purkinje cell inputs. In this regard we have been the minority view for many years. We originally proposed this based on analytic analysis of the cerebellum using linear models, with later support from simulation work. We built three simulations that differed only in the rule for plasticity induction in the deep cerebellar nucleus: Hebbian, controlled by climbing fiber collaterals and by Purkinje cell inputs (Medina & Mauk, 1999). We found that although all three simulations learned, two of the three were unstable in that they displayed persistent induction of plasticity that, over time, led to the saturation of synaptic weights in the cortex and deep nuclei. These processes degrade the expression of previously learned responses and eventually lead to the inability of the system to learn. The simulation where deep nucleus plasticity was controlled by the Purkinje cells was the only one of the three that did not have this flaw. The idea that Purkinje cells control induction of long-term potentiation (LTP) and long-term depression (LTD) at the mossy fiber synapse in the cerebellar deep nucleus is directly supported by recent slice work (Pugh & Raman, 2006, 2008).

Successes and failures

As mentioned above, our initial simulation work involved testing ideas regarding temporal coding in the granule–Golgi system of the cerebellum. These early simulations show some success in supporting this general idea regarding temporal coding, and example peri-stimulus histograms showing temporal coding in granule cells are shown in Figure 7.6. These simulations were in all other ways a surprisingly terrible failure. Our belief at the time was that the general process for learning in the cerebellum was sketched in, whereas timing and temporal coding were open issues. What we discovered instead is that the simulation was wholly unable to learn. In fact, without implementation of gratuitous contrivances to keep weights from drifting, learning could not even be tested in the simulations. Even short simulation runs produced strong drift and saturation of weights, indicating a severe lack in our understanding of the basic mechanisms of learning.

The solution revealed by further simulation analysis was surprisingly simple. Bidirectional control of plasticity requires not only a bidirectional signal, such as the presence or absence of a climbing fiber input, but proper regulation of that signal to prevent long-term drift of synaptic weights to saturation. For the cerebellum the solution appears to be inhibitory control of climbing fiber activity by output from the cerebellar deep nuclei (Medina et al., 2002).

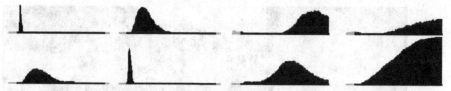

Figure 7.6 Peri-stimulus histograms of simulated granule cells from a simulation presented where mossy fiber inputs mimic a tone CS. Note the variety of latencies ranging from just after CS onset to delayed activity peaking near the end of the CS. The black region indicates the presence of the CS for each trace.

This inhibitory projection has been known for some time, but simulations help reveal its fundamental importance. The solution also provides insight into a long-time dilemma about the cerebellum: why do climbing fibers show spontaneous activity of about 1 Hz and how can this activity be reconciled with the putative role for climbing fibers in controlling the induction of plasticity in the cerebellar cortex? Would spontaneous activity not lead to saturation of synaptic weights, and how can a climbing fiber spike acting as an error signal provide information against the multitude of spontaneous spikes? To appreciate the need for spontaneous climbing fiber activity that is controlled by cerebellar output, consider the consequences of its absence on an already learned response. Previous learning would have made those granules–Purkinje synapses that are activated by the CS relatively weak. Any subsequent activity of these synapses would increase their strength. Over time, synapses would continue to increase until the memory was erased. This is the inverse of what many people speculated would occur because of spontaneous climbing fiber activity. Each active synapse would be weakened until eventual saturation was reached, also erasing any memory of previous learning.

This perpetual drift and eventual saturation of synaptic weights, all at either the maximum or minimum value, was precisely the misbehavior displayed by our early simulations. What is needed to prevent this drift is the right amount of spontaneous activity, precisely calibrated so that the chances of increases and decreases in synaptic weights are equal and opposite. The only reasonable way to achieve this level precisely enough is to have the output of the cerebellum control the ongoing activity in a negative-feedback mode. When we expanded our early simulations to include deep nucleus neurons and their inhibitory projection to the climbing fibers, the simulations exhibited a natural equilibrium in which granule–Purkinje synaptic weights would drift until the proper level of climbing fiber activity was achieved. This equilibrium is shown in the raster plots of Figure 7.7. This simulation was initiated with overly weak synapses between granule and Purkinje cells. The resulting low level of Purkinje activity

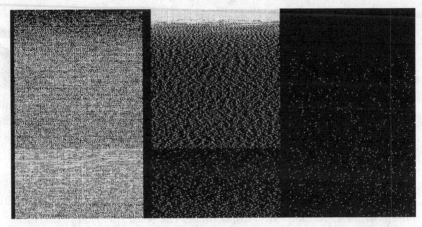

Figure 7.7 Raster plots for three cells in a simulation of the cerebellum: Purkinje cell on the left, deep nucleus cell in the center, and climbing fiber on the right. Each row is a two-second snippet of activity taken every two minutes, and each row shows the same time for the three cells. The simulation began with a weak synapse onto, and thus sparse activity in, the Purkinje cell. This produced robust activity in the nucleus cell and sparse activity in the climbing fiber. The sparse climbing fiber activity led to net increases in strength of the synapses onto the Purkinje cell, and thus a drift toward an equilibrium level of activity for each cell. Toward the bottom, the synapses on the Purkinje cell were artificially increased in strength to show the drift back to equilibrium from the other direction. At equilibrium there is no net drift in synaptic weights.

(left) resulted in high activity of nucleus cells (center) and thus a paucity of activity in the climbing fiber (right). Each row is separated by a few simulated minutes and thus the progression toward equilibrium can be seen top to bottom. The low level of climbing fiber activity induced net increases in the weights of synapses onto the Purkinje cells. As their activity increased the activity of the nucleus cells and the climbing fiber decreased and increased, respectively. Midway down, the granule–Purkinje synapses were artificially increased to show how the inverse move toward equilibrium also occurs.

This simulation work showed that spontaneous climbing fiber activity is not a problem for learning-based ideas of cerebellar function. Instead, they suggest that activity of this sort is necessary for an input that controls the induction of bidirectional plasticity. With cerebellar output coupled to control of climbing fibers, the system will always adjust itself to the right levels of activity to prevent spontaneous net drift of synaptic weights.

Rescorla–Wagner in the cerebellum

Not only does this control of spontaneous climbing fiber activity prevent the drift of synaptic weights, it provides the mechanism for the bidirectional signals needed for both acquisition and extinction, it improves response timing, and it endows this system with many of the advantageous properties explained by the Rescorla–Wagner model of associative learning (Rescorla & Wagner, 1972). Since the spontaneous climbing fiber activity prevents net changes in synaptic weights, learning and extinction of responses must now be understood against the backdrop of this activity. The three raster plots in Figure 7.8 parallel those of Figure 7.7: the Purkinje cell activity is on the left, deep nucleus cell activity is in the center, and climbing fiber activity is on the right. Presentation of the CS is indicated by the gray boxes and, in addition, CS-onset is indicated by the arrows at the bottom. The top rows begin with CS-alone trials in an untrained state. Note that the climbing fiber activity is moderate, at the equilibrium level that produces no net changes in synaptic weights. The row in which training trials commence is apparent in the climbing fiber raster plot, where the US initially produces near certainty of a climbing fiber response, which appears as a straight vertical line. Over many training trials high likelihood of climbing fiber activity induces net decreases in the strengths of CS-activated synapses onto the Purkinje cells. This is reflected in the decrease in Purkinje activity during the CS that intensifies as training proceeds. The temporal specificity of this decrease is the result of the temporal coding in granule cells, as shown in Figure 7.6. Only those granule cells that are active toward the end of the CS are affected, and thus the decrease in Purkinje cell activity is specific to this time.

The expression of conditioning in the simulation can be seen in the deep nucleus activity depicted in the center raster plot. The well-timed bursts of activity in this cell toward the end of the CS represent expression of a well-timed conditioned response.

The other consequence of this activity is seen in the climbing fiber raster plot on the right. The burst of deep nucleus activity inhibits the climbing fiber activity to a level well below its normal equilibrium value. When the US is omitted in the last few trials at the bottom, there is an abject absence of climbing fiber activity during the CS, which results in net increases in the strengths of the CS-activated granule to Purkinje synapses, restoration of the strong Purkinje cell activity during the CS, which suppresses deep nucleus activity during the CS, and thus promotes the extinction of the conditioned responses.

A clear prediction from these simulations is that transiently blocking the inhibitory connection between the deep nucleus cells and the climbing fibers should prevent the extinction of conditioned responses. Prolonged blockade of this inhibition should promote upward drift of the strength of granule to Purkinje synapses to the point of saturation and abolition of any previous learning. With a transient blockade of these synapses, there would be no decrease in

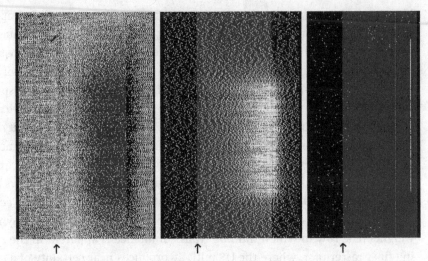

Figure 7.8 Acquisition and extinction in a simulation of the cerebellum. Raster-plot format and cells are the same as for Figure 7.7. The time of CS presentation for each cell is shown by the gray rectangle, with CS onset also indicated by arrows at the bottom. The first few rows represent CS-alone presentations to the untrained simulation. The US-driven climbing fiber responses aligned toward the end of the CS can be seen on the right. Their presence indicates the onset of paired training of the simulation. The training gradually results in decreases in Purkinje cell activity during the CS, which contributes to the increases in nucleus activity (center) that are the conditioned responses of the simulation. These increases also inhibit the climbing fiber, which suppress the ability of the US to activate the climbing fiber, contribute to response timing, and are the signal for extinction when the US is omitted. (Refer to text.)

climbing fiber activity during unreinforced presentation of the CS to a trained simulation (as in the lower-right corner), and thus no ability for extinction. We have confirmed this prediction empirically; it thus appears that inhibition of the climbing fibers is a signal controlling extinction learning in the cerebellum (Medina *et al.*, 2002).

We expect that this inhibition also endows this system with the many associative learning features addressed by the Rescorla–Wagner model of learning. Because expression of conditioned responses suppresses the effectiveness of the US – a key feature of this model – learning phenomena such as negatively accelerating acquisition, blocking, and conditioned inhibition may occur in this system in ways that nicely parallel the explanations of the phenomena by Rescorla–Wagner. One such parallel in cerebellar learning has already been tested. Blocking inhibition of the climbing fibers precludes the phenomenon of blocking in eyelid conditioning (Kim & Thompson, 1998).

Back to conditioned response timing

These mechanisms of learning superimposed on regulation of climbing fibers also turn out to affect response timing. The basic implication is that at ISIs long enough to promote responses where latency to onset is delayed beyond the minimum, each training trial can engage both mechanisms of acquisition and mechanisms of extinction. This process can be seen in a somewhat exaggerated form in the climbing fiber raster on the right of Figure 7.8. Note that once learning begins to change Purkinje cell and deep nucleus cell activity, there is also inhibition of the climbing fibers early in the CS. These changes implement a two-phase opposing process in which granule-cell synapses active early in the CS are increased in strength (suppression responding) and those activated late in the CS are decreased in strength (encouraging response expression). This process naturally sharpens the timing of the conditioned responses by suppressing responding early in the tone. We found empirical support for this mechanistic prediction using small lesions of the cerebellar cortex in already-trained rabbits (Medina *et al.*, 2000). These lesions presumably damage some, but not all, of the relevant Purkinje cells. The result was the unmasking of short-latency responses similar to but smaller than those in Figure 7.5. Like the simulation following partial removal of the Purkinje cells, further training with these rabbits resulted in partial to complete restoration of normal timing, presumably because the spared Purkinje cells underwent additional learning to suppress responding early in the CS.

In summary, computer simulations of the cerebellum have been useful in revealing the fundamentally important role of spontaneous climbing fiber activity and its regulation by inhibition by the deep nuclei in cerebellar learning. This Rescorla–Wagner-like regulation of the US pathway acts to enforce equilibrium levels of activity that preclude net drift of synaptic weights. All learning, acquisition, extinction, and that related to response timing, must then be understood against the backdrop of this equilibrium activity. For example, these processes provide a simple means of bidirectional signaling for extinction as well as acquisition. Increases in probability of climbing fiber activity above equilibrium during the CS, as occurs with the pairing of the US in an untrained animal, result in acquisition. Decreases in climbing fiber probability below equilibrium during the CS, as occur during unreinforced presentation of the CS to trained animals, result in extinction. Finally, the coupling of conditioned response expression with inhibition of the US pathway implements a form of US processing envisioned by the Rescorla–Wagner model, with the associated potential for all of the learning phenomena addressed by this model, including blocking, conditioned inhibition, and negatively accelerating learning curves.

Open questions and future directions

In many ways computational analysis of learning mechanisms in the cerebellum is moving full circle toward Marr's original approach. In his classic theory of the cerebellar cortex (Marr, 1969), Marr attempted to specify the contributions of each cerebellar neuron type, as well as the sites and rules for induction of plasticity, to the computation and learning of the cerebellum. Ongoing simulation studies are similarly focused. Preliminary data suggest the need for certain types of homeostatic plasticity in the cerebellar cortex to prevent long-term drift of synaptic weights. While the climbing fiber equilibrium mechanisms outlined above can keep the average activity of Purkinje cells, nucleus cells, and climbing fibers in order, over long periods of time the individual cells in these categories can diverge from the average, increasing the variance of their average activities but not changing the average. This work reveals the need for a better appreciation of the essential computational unit of the cerebellar cortex and how the individuals within the unit are regulated to act in harmony. Preliminary results suggest strong contributions in this regard from a better appreciation of the role played by the interconnections between Purkinje cells and basket cells, as well as a new appreciation for the computational relevance of electrotonic coupling between olivary neurons – the cell bodies of the climbing fiber afferents.

However these results play out, computer simulation of cerebellar learning will continue to illustrate how a proper combination of empirical studies with computational models can lead to more specific ideas about the mechanisms of associative learning. Such computationally oriented and specific hypotheses can lead to better experiments and have the great advantage of being specific enough in their expression to permit rejection by such experiments. I believe many of the long-time debates about mechanisms of associative learning will one day be made clearer by such studies.

References

Buonomano, D. V. & Mauk, M. D. (1994). Neural network model of the cerebellum: temporal discrimination and the timing of motor responses. *Neural Computation*, **6**(1), 38–55.

Garcia, K. S. & Mauk, M. D. (1998). Pharmacological analysis of cerebellar contributions to the timing and expression of conditioned eyelid responses. *Neuropharmacology*, **37**, 471–480.

Garcia, K. S., Steele, P. M. & Mauk, M. D. (1999). Cerebellar cortex lesions prevent acquisition of conditioned eyelid responses. *Journal of Neuroscience*, **19**, 10940–10947.

Gormezano, I., Kehoe, E. J. & Marshall, B. S. (1983). Twenty years of classical conditioning research with the rabbit. *Progress in Psychobiology and Physiological Psychology,* **10**, 197–275.

Kehoe, E. J. & Macrae, M. (1998). Classical conditioning. In W. O'Donogue, ed., *Learning and Behavior Therapy.* Needham Heights, MA: Allyn & Bacon, pp. 36–58.

Kehoe, E.J. & Macrae, M. (2002). Fundamental behavioral methods and findings in classical conditioning. In J. W. Moore, ed., *Classical Conditioning: a Guidebook for Neuroscientists.* New York: Springer, pp. 171–231.

Kim J. J. & Thompson, R. F. (1998). Inhibitory cerebello-olivary projections and the blocking effect in classical conditioning. *Science,* **279**, 570–573.

Lavond, D. G. & Steinmetz, J. E. (1989). Acquisition of classical conditioning without cerebellar cortex. *Behavioral Brain Research,* **33**, 113–164.

Lavond, D. G., McCormick, D. A. & Thompson, R. F. (1984). A nonrecoverable learning deficit. *Physiological Psychology,* **12**, 103–110.

Marr, D. A. (1969). A theory of cerebellar cortex. *Journal of Physiology,* **202**, 437–470.

Mauk, M. D. (1997). Relative contributions of cerebellar cortex and nuclei in motor learning: contradictions or clues? *Neuron,* **18**(3), 343–349.

Mauk, M. D. & Donegan, N. H. (1997). A model of Pavlovian eyelid conditioning based on the synaptic organization of the cerebellum. *Learning and Memory,* **4**(1), 130–158.

Mauk, M. D. & Ohyama, T. (2004). Extinction as new learning versus unlearning: considerations from a computer simulation of the cerebellum. *Learning and Memory,* **11**, 566–571.

Mauk, M. D., Steinmetz, J. E. & Thompson, R. F. (1986). Classical conditioning using stimulation of the inferior olive as the unconditioned stimulus. *Proceedings of the National Academy of Science USA,* **83**, 5349–5353.

McCormick, D. A. & Thompson, R. F. (1984a). Cerebellum: essential involvement in the classically conditioned eyelid response. *Science,* **223**, 296–299.

McCormick, D. A. & Thompson, R. F. (1984b). Neuronal responses of the rabbit cerebellum during acquisition and performance of a classically conditioned nictitating membrane-eyelid response. *Journal of Neuroscience,* **4**, 2811–2822.

McCormick, D. A., *et al.* (1982). Initial localization of the memory trace for a basic form of learning. *Proceedings of the National Academy of Sciences,* **79**, 2731–2735.

McCormick, D. A., Steinmetz, J. E. & Thompson, R. F. (1985). Lesions of the inferior olivary complex cause extinction of the classically conditioned eyeblink response. *Brain Research,* **359**, 120–130.

Medina, J. F. & Mauk, M. D. (1999). Simulations of cerebellar motor learning: computational analysis of plasticity at the mossy fiber to deep nucleus synapses. *Journal of Neuroscience,* **19**, 7140–7151.

Medina, J. F. & Mauk, M. D. (2000). Computer simulation of cerebellar information processing. *Nature Neuroscience,* **3**, 1205–1211.

Medina, J. F., Garcia, K. S., Nores, W. L., Taylor, N. M. & Mauk, M. D. (2000). Timing mechanisms in the cerebellum: testing predictions of a large scale computer simulation. *Journal of Neuroscience*, **20**, 5516–5525.

Medina, J. F., Nores, W. L. & Mauk, M. D. (2002). Inhibition of climbing fibres is a signal for the extinction of conditioned eyelid responses. *Nature*, **416**, 330–333.

Nores, W. L, Medina, J. F., Steele, P. M. & Mauk, M. D. (2000). Relative contributions of cerebellar cortex and cerebellar nucleus to eyelid conditioning. In D. S. Woodruff-Pak and J. E. Steinmetz, eds., *Eyeblink Classical Conditioning: Volume II Animal Models*. Boston: Kluwer, pp. 205–228.

Ohyama, T., Medina, J. F., Nores, W. L. & Mauk, M. D. (2002). Trying to understand the cerebellum well enough to build one. *Annals of the New York Academy of Sciences*, **978**, 1–15.

Ohyama, T., Nores, W. L., Murphy, M. & Mauk, M. D. (2003). What the cerebellum computes. *Trends in Neuroscience*, **26**(4), 222–227.

Ohyama, T., Nores, W. L., Medina, J. F., Riusech, F. A. & Mauk, M. D. (2006). Learning-dependent plasticity in cerebellar nucleus. *Journal of Neuroscience*, **26**(49), 12656–12663.

Perrett, S. P. & Mauk, M. D. (1995). Extinction of conditioned eyelid responses requires the anterior lobe of cerebellar cortex. *Journal of Neuroscience*, **15**(3), 2074–2080.

Perrett, S. P., Ruiz, B. P. & Mauk, M. D. (1993). Cerebellar cortex lesions disrupt the learning-dependent timing of conditioned eyelid responses. *Journal of Neuroscience*, **13**(4), 1708–1718.

Pugh J. R. & Raman I. M. (2006). Potentiation of mossy fiber EPSCs in the cerebellar nuclei by NMDA receptor activation followed by postinhibitory rebound current. *Neuron*, **51**(1), 113–123.

Pugh J. R. & Raman I. M. (2008). Mechanisms of potentiation of mossy fiber EPSCs in the cerebellar nuclei by coincident synaptic excitation and inhibition. *Journal of Neuroscience*, **28**(42), 10549–10560.

Raymond, J. L. & Lisberger, S. G. (1998). Neural learning rules for the vestibulo-ocular reflex. *Jornal of Neuroscience*, **18**, 9112–9129.

Rescorla, R. A. & Wagner, A. R. (1972). A theory of Pavlovian conditioning: variations in the effectiveness of reinforcement and nonreinforcement. In A. H. Black and W. F. Prokasy, eds., *Classical Conditioning ii: Current Theory and Research*. New York: Appleton-Century-Crofts.

Steinmetz, J. E., *et al.* (1987). Initial localization of the acoustic conditioned stimulus projection system to the cerebellum essential for classical eyelid conditioning. *Proceedings of the National Academy of Science USA*, **84**, 3531–3535.

Steinmetz, J. E., Lavond, D. G. & Thompson, R. F. (1989). Classical conditioning in rabbits using pontine nucleus stimulation as a conditioned stimulus and inferior olive stimulation as an unconditioned stimulus. *Synapse*, **3**, 225–233.

Thompson, R. F. (1986). The neurobiology of learning and memory. *Science*, **233**, 941–947.

Thompson, R. F. & Krupa, D. J. (1994). Organization of memory traces in the mammalian brain. *Annual Review of Neuroscience*, **17**, 519–549.

Yeo, C. H. (1991). Cerebellum and classical conditioning of motor responses. *Annals of the New York Academy of Sciences*, **627**, 292–304.

Yeo, C. H., Hardiman, M. J. & Glickstein, M. (1985). Classical conditioning of the nictitating membrane response of the rabbit. II. Lesions of the cerebellar cortex. *Experimental Brain Research*, **60**, 99–113.

8

The operant/respondent distinction: a computational neural-network analysis

JOSÉ E. BURGOS

This chapter presents an analysis of the distinction between operant (instrumental) and respondent (Pavlovian, classical) conditioning, in terms of a computational, neural-network model. The importance of this distinction cannot be overemphasized, judging by the extensive literature on it (e.g., Asratyan, 1974; Bindra, 1972; Davis & Hurwitz, 1977; Dykman, 1976; Gormezano & Tait, 1976; Gray, 1975; Guthrie, 1935; Hearst, 1975; Henton & Iversen, 1978; Hineline, 1986; Hull, 1943; Kimmel, 1976; Konorski & Miller, 1937a, 1937b; Logan, 1960; Mackintosh & Dickinson, 1979; Miller & Konorski, 1928; Mowrer, 1960; Pear & Eldrige, 1984; Ray & Brown, 1976; Rehfeldt & Hayes, 1998; Rescorla & Solomon, 1967; Schlosberg, 1937; Schoenfeld, 1966; Sheffield, 1965; Skinner, 1935, 1937; Spence, 1956; Trapold & Overmier, 1972). Obviously, this abundance of analyses is too long to summarize in a way that does them justice. Instead, I will begin with how the distinction has been treated in the field of computational modeling of conditioning.

A glance at the field reveals that most models are of respondent conditioning (e.g., Gibbon & Balsam, 1981; Klopf, 1988; Mackintosh, 1975; Pearce & Hall, 1980; Rescorla & Wagner, 1972; Schmajuk & Moore, 1986; Stout & Miller, 2007; Sutton & Barto, 1981; Wagner & Brandon 1989), or operant conditioning (e.g., Dragoi & Staddon, 1999; Killeen, 1994; Machado, 1997), with little if any communication between the two types of models. The field is thus deeply divided. If there is any validity to the motto "United we stand, divided we fall," the field has fallen long ago.

More unification efforts are needed, and this chapter presents one such effort. I do not mean to dismiss dividing efforts, because they are steps towards a scientific understanding of conditioning. I am only saying that science is not *only* about division, but *also* unification. Divide and conquer has been a tried-and-true strategy in science, but not the only one. Unification too has been tried and true. Given the great complexity of conditioning, it seems unwise to restrict research efforts to one strategy. The more strategies we try, the better our chances to build adequate theories.

A few computational neural-network models consider both types of conditioning explicitly (e.g., Grossberg, 1987; Schmajuk, 1994), and this allows them to achieve some degree of unification. However, like most other models, they are strongly top-down and thus use cognitive categories that hinder computational unification. A list of such categories makes my point: associative strength, attention, drive, emotion, expectancy, habit, incentive, information, internal representation, learning, memory (short-term, medium-term, long-term), motivation, processing, storage, and retrieval. With this morass of categories, computational unification becomes exceedingly difficult. Besides, they are too nontechnical (defined in too many different, often ambiguous, ways), which makes unification even harder. Perhaps they are a reason why there are so few unification efforts in the field. In order to facilitate my analysis, then, I will abandon such categories and hence the differences they engender.

I will attempt this through a more strongly bottom-up model that appeals to computational neural-network interpretations of neural categories, guided by empirical evidence about certain neural correlates of both types of conditioning. Some of the categories allow for a relatively high degree of computational unification, perhaps higher than other models. Other categories honor *behavioral* differences that in my view should not and cannot be eliminated by any unification effort, as they involve *basic categories of analysis* of conditioning. Against Dickinson's (1979) adage, then, which belittles the theoretical status of behavior as "but a spade to disinter thought" (p. 553), behavioral categories will be integral to my analysis. However, neural categories will be *equally* integral, not to displace, eliminate, or replace, but to *complement* behavioral categories and thus achieve a more *holistic* treatment of the distinction.

The rest of the chapter will elaborate the above overview. The first and second sections will give the behavioral and computational neural frameworks of my analysis, respectively. The third section lays out the analysis itself, in terms of both frameworks and with the aid of computer simulations. The chapter ends with concluding remarks about limitations and future directions.

The behavioral framework

The behavioral framework consists of what seem to me to be the most basic behavioral categories that are typically used to make the operant/respondent distinction in the literature. I will not propose anything fundamentally new here. The categories are standard in conditioning theory, although I will organize them somewhat differently. They are very general and thus exclude many specific categories that are also used to make the distinction. I shall focus on the operant/respondent distinction in its simplest form.

I derive the categories from the following more basic ones: R, S^*, R^*, and S. I will use this notation instead of a more standard one because the latter promotes the sort of conceptual division I am trying to avoid. The notation promotes unification. For instance, S^* includes US (unconditioned stimulus) and S^R (operant primary reinforcer), and S includes CS (conditioned stimulus) and S^D (discriminative stimulus). Also, R^* includes UR (unconditioned response) and CR (conditioned response). My intention with the general categories is not to eliminate but only to *bypass* the differences between US and S^R, CS and S^D, or CR and UR as obstacles to a unified computational treatment of the operant/respondent distinction. The more general categories preserve such differences in ways that I will show later on.

I will characterize the general categories very simply and intuitively, via typical examples and without trying to be exhaustive. Thus, my characterization will involve no necessary or sufficient conditions, or strictly common properties. Nor do I intend to separate the categories sharply. Their differences and those they engender strike me as fuzzy rather than crisp. Also, my characterization will focus on how they are typically used in conditioning laboratory research, appealing to standard apparatuses, observations, and manipulations. Their occurrence in natural settings is a far more complex affair that goes well beyond this analysis.

The basic categories comprise four classes of events typically studied in conditioning research. One is the class S^* of biologically relevant stimuli, which concern an organism's survival more or less directly, like food, water, shock, a loud noise, a puff of air to an eye, drugs that induce various sorts of physiological states (e.g., the nausea-inducing LiCl), and so on. The other stimulus class is S, which comprises exteroceptive sensory stimuli such as lights, tones, smells, tastes, and quiet noises. Class R refers to response topographies that are typically observed in experimental environments where organisms are relatively unrestrained, like Skinner boxes (e.g., bar-pressing, key-pecking, chain-pulling, locomotion, wing-flapping, nose-poking, head-turning, etc.). The last basic category, R^*, includes response topographies the observation of which typically requires more restrictive environments, like Plexiglas restrainers and harnesses of various sorts (e.g., salivation, eye blink, swallowing, heartbeat, galvanic skin response, stomach and intestinal movements, gill-retraction, etc.).

Table 8.1 summarizes the framework as consisting of nine categories organized into two rows (operant and respondent) and three columns that show a

Table 8.1 *Basic behavioral categories of the operant/respondent distinction. The categories are based on the following ones: R (e.g., bar-pressing, key-pecking, etc.), S* (e.g., food, water, shock, etc.), R* (e.g., salivation, eye blink, swallowing, etc.), and S (lights, tones, noises, smells, etc.). The dashed line represents the fuzzy character of the distinction, meaning that operant and respondent conditioning may share some of the more basic categories.*

	BEFORE REINFORCEMENT	REINFORCEMENT	AFTER REINFORCEMENT
OPERANT	*Emission:* Low R frequency does not depend on any stimulus.	*R-dependent (unsignaled):* S* depends only on R. *R-dependent/S-dependent (signaled):* S* depends on R and S. (Elicitation is possible).	*Free operant:* High R frequency. *Discriminated operant:* R depends on S. (R* can become dependent on S).
RESPONDENT	*Elicitation:* R* depends on S*. *Neutrality:* R* does not depend on S.	*S-dependent/response-independent:* S* depends only on S. (Emission is possible).	*Conditioned response (CR):* R* depends on S. (R can become dependent on S).

temporal sequence of different types of experimental scenarios or situations, namely: before, during, and after reinforcement.

Such organization suggests that, behaviorally, the operant/respondent distinction has different meanings in different scenarios. The whole behavioral distinction is the combination of these categories. The fuzzy character of the distinction is visually represented by the dashed line dividing the two rows of the table. This line means that the distinction may share some of the more basic behavioral categories I characterized above.

In the first column, before any reinforcement operation, the operant/respondent distinction typically refers to three basic types of stimulus–response relations, namely: emission in the case of operant conditioning, and elicitation and neutrality in the case of respondent conditioning. Emission is a low frequency of occurrence of R independently of any apparent evoking stimulus, particularly S*. Elicitation is the dependence of R* on S*, which captures the notion of an unconditioned reflex as consisting of US closely and reliably followed by UR. Neutrality is the independence of R* on S, which captures the notion of the CS as initially neutral with respect to the UR.

In the reinforcement column, the operant–respondent distinction typically refers to three basic types of explicit reinforcement operations, where S*

is programmed to depend on certain events (I thus exclude adventitious or accidental reinforcement, so I will not be concerned with superstitious conditioning, important as it is). In operant reinforcement, S^* depends *at least* on R. Operant reinforcement, then, is R-dependent.

Operant reinforcement can be purely R-dependent, where S^* depends *only* on R, which defines unsignaled operant reinforcement. S^* can also depend on R and S, which defines signaled operant reinforcement. In respondent reinforcement, S^* depends only on S, which captures the standard notion of CS–US pairing. Hence, in respondent reinforcement, S^* does not depend on *any* response. That is to say, respondent reinforcement is S-dependent *and* response-independent. These operations do not prevent two possibilities that I have included (in parentheses), namely: elicitation can occur during operant reinforcement, and emission can occur during respondent reinforcement. Both have received empirical support and are directly relevant to the operant–respondent distinction.

In the third column, the operant–respondent distinction usually refers to different types of typical maintenance effects of each type of reinforcement operation. The typical effect of unsignaled operant reinforcement is a high R frequency. The typical effect of signaled operant reinforcement is known as discriminated operant responding, where R depends on S. The typical effect of respondent reinforcement is a dependence of R^* on S. This effect captures the notion of a conditioned reflex as consisting of CS reliably followed by CR.

These effects do not preclude two more that I have enclosed in parentheses and are directly relevant to the operant–respondent distinction, namely: R^* can become dependent on S as an effect of signaled operant reinforcement, and R dependent on S as an effect of respondent reinforcement. An example of the latter possibility is autoshaping. Since its discovery (Brown & Jenkins, 1968), it has been much discussed in relation to the distinction (e.g., Hearst & Jenkins, 1974; Schwartz & Gamzu, 1977). The reason is well known: the phenomenon implies that a dependence of R^* on S is not the only possible effect of respondent reinforcement. Respondent reinforcement can also result in a dependence of R on S. This implication will be the means by which the neural-network model I describe in the next section approximates operant conditioning.

The implication does not mean that "the operant/respondent distinction lost most of its utility" (Staddon, 2001, p. 67). As I have characterized them, all the differences depicted in Table 8.1 remain valid, useful descriptions of basic manipulations and observations in conditioning research. In particular, autoshaping neither invalidates nor makes useless the differences between R and R^*, response-dependent versus stimulus-dependent/response-independent reinforcement, and their typical effects. Such differences are basic behavioral categories of analysis of conditioning, and hence, not only valid and useful, but also inevitable.

Table 8.1 does not include the context: the constellation of static or tonic cues of the situation where the other categories occur. I excluded it because it has not been a typical subject matter in discussions about the operant–respondent distinction. Nowadays, however, this exclusion seems implausible, and it can be remedied by including the category C of contextual cues in Table 8.1. For instance, contextualized elicitation can be characterized as a dependence of R^* on S in C, and so on (C and S differ only in complexity and spatiotemporal relation; S is simpler than and occurs within the spatiotemporal span of C). The model I summarize next will contemplate C, although in a simplified manner that focuses on its tonic character.

The computational neural framework

The neural framework is provided by a neural-network model whose neuroscientific and behavioral rationale have been discussed elsewhere (e.g., Donahoe, Burgos, & Palmer, 1993; Donahoe & Palmer, 1994; Donahoe, Palmer, & Burgos, 1997a, 1997b). Here, I will only summarize its bare essentials, to permit the points that I seek to make here, namely: the stronger bottom-up character of the model, and its identification of two levels of theoretical analysis (computational and network).

To motivate the model, Table 8.2 provides a list of the respondent-conditioning phenomena that it has simulated thus far. This initial focus on respondent conditioning has been motivated by practical reasons. On the one hand, neural-network models of conditioning have focused on respondent conditioning. On the other hand, respondent conditioning is simpler. As can be seen, the model can simulate a fair number of phenomena, although delay conditioning and autoshaping are the most directly relevant ones to the operant–respondent distinction as I characterized it in the previous section and will interpret in the next section.

Admittedly, the list excludes many phenomena. However, this does not necessarily mean that the model cannot simulate them, but rather that they await investigation with the model.

The model consists of two submodels, namely: neurocomputational and network. They are related in that a network consists of connected units, the functioning of which is described by the neurocomputational model. Moreover, some of the neural categories of one submodel appear in the other, so summarizing any of the submodels first will force me to anticipate categories that I will describe later. Despite these relations, each submodel constitutes a level of

Table 8.2 *Respondent conditioning phenomena simulated by the model thus far*

Delay conditioning[a]
Extinction[a]
Faster reacquisition[a]
Blocking[a,l]
Discrimination[a]
Dependence on US magnitude[a]
ISI function[b,c,d]
Overshadowing[e,l]
Reinforcement reevaluation[f]
CS-preexposure effects[g]
Effects of the C/T ratio[h]
Simultaneous conditioning[i]
Context specificity and renewal[j]
Autoshaping and automaintenance[k]
Second-order conditioning[m]
Conditioned inhibition[n]

[a] Donahoe, Burgos, & Palmer (1993).
[b] Burgos (1997).
[c] Burgos & Donahoe (2000).
[d] Donahoe & Burgos (1999).
[e] Donahoe, Palmer, & Burgos (1997a).
[f] Donahoe & Burgos (2000).
[g] Burgos (2003).
[h] Burgos (2005).
[i] Burgos, Flores, García, Díaz, & Cruz (2007).
[j] Burgos & Murillo-Rodríguez (2007).
[k] Burgos (2007).
[l] Burns, Burgos, & Donahoe (unpublished manuscript).
[m] Sánchez, Galeazzi, & Burgos (2010).
[n] Burgos & Ponce (unpublished manuscript).

theoretical analysis with distinct categories. For convenience, I will summarize the neurocomputational submodel first.

Neurocomputational submodel

Like most neural-network models, the neurocomputational submodel consists of an activation rule and a weight-change rule. These rules describe the functioning of the units and connections that constitute a neural network. Figure 8.1 shows a generic unit, labeled as *j*. The unit is an abstraction of a

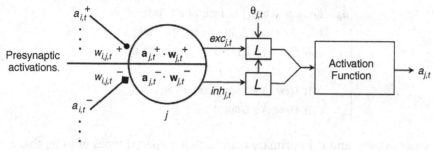

Figure 8.1 A generic neural computation unit, labeled as j. Unit j receives connections from presynaptic units that can be excitatory (+) or inhibitory (−), and influence j separately at t. $a_{i,t}$+: excitatory presynaptic activation at t. $a_{i,t}$−: inhibitory presynaptic activation at t. $w_{i,j,t}$+: weight of a connection from an excitatory presynaptic unit to j at t. $w_{i,j,t}$−: weight of a connection from an inhibitory presynaptic unit to j at t. **a**: presynaptic activation vector. **w**: weight vector. **a·w**: inner product of activation and weight vectors. $exc_{j,t}$: amount of excitation on j at t. $inh_{j,t}$: amount of inhibition on j at t. L: logistic function. $\Theta_{j,t}$: Gaussian threshold on $L(exc_{j,t})$ ($L(inh_{j,t})$ is another threshold). $a_{j,t}$: activation of j at t. All activations and weights are real numbers between 0 and 1.

relatively small cluster of neurons (circle) that can be influenced by other units via connections symbolizing bundles of synapses (lines). The connections' efficacies or strengths are indicated by weights that change according to the weight-change rule (see below). This submodel thus corresponds roughly to the cellular and synaptic levels of organization of nervous systems.

Unit j can receive connections from excitatory and/or inhibitory units. If both, they influence j separately, in a manner similar to Fukushima's (1975) cognitron. However, as a simplification, the present analysis focuses on excitatory units, because they suffice for my present purposes (inhibition, as important as it might be, does not seem directly relevant to a neural-network analysis of the operant–respondent distinction in its simplest form). I will only say that the distinction between excitation and inhibition in this model does not take the usual form of a distinction between positive and negative values. All activations and weights in this model are real numbers between 0 and 1, which allows for neurobiological interpretations in terms of proportions. An activation can thus be interpreted as a proportion of members of a neuron cluster that fire at t. A weight can be interpreted as a proportion of postsynaptic receptors that are influenced by a presynaptic process.

The activation rule is a conditional function that determines the activation of unit j at t ($a_{j,t}$). It has two general possible states: primary and secondary. Secondary activation has three possible states: reactivation, decay, and deactivation. Each state obtains as follows:

$$
a_{j,t} = \begin{cases}
a_{s^*,t} \text{ if } a_{s^*,t} > 0 \text{ and } j \text{ is a } vta \text{ or } r^* \text{ unit; otherwise,} \\
L(exc_{j,t}) + \tau L(exc_{j,t-1})[1 - L(exc_{j,t})] - L(inh_{j,t}) \\
\quad \text{if } L(exc_{j,t}) > L(inh_{j,t}) \text{ and } L(exc_{j,t}) \geq \theta_t \\
a_{j,t-1} - \kappa a_{j,t-1}(1 - a_{j,t-1}) - L(inh_{j,t}) \\
\quad \text{if } L(exc_{j,t}) > L(inh_{j,t}) \text{ and } L(exc_{j,t}) < \theta_t \\
0 \quad \text{if } L(exc_{j,t}) \leq L(inh_{j,t})
\end{cases}
\tag{8.1}
$$

where s^*, vta, and r^* in primary activation are special types of units that I will describe in the network submodel. Suffice it to say that primary activation simulates some of the effects of S^* on a nervous system.

In secondary activation,

$$
L(x) = \frac{1}{1 + e^{\frac{-(x-\mu)}{\sigma}}}
\tag{8.2}
$$

is the logistic function with constant mean $\mu = 0.5$, variable standard deviation σ (a free parameter that determines an above-zero activation with an argument of zero; in most simulations, $\sigma = 0.1$, which gives an activation of approximately 0.007 with an argument of zero). The argument (x) is the dot or inner product between presynaptic activation and connection-weight vectors, widely used in neural-network modeling and defined algebraically as:

$$
x = \sum_{i=1}^{n} a_{i,t} w_{i,j,t}
\tag{8.3}
$$

where n is the total number of units connected to j. This argument is computed separately for excitatory presynaptic units and inhibitory units. In the first case, $x = exc_{j,t}$; in the second, $x = inh_{j,t}$. The rule has two other free parameters: temporal summation (τ) and decay (κ), where typically $\tau = 0.1$ (used in all simulations with the model) and $\kappa = 0.1$ (in some simulations, $\kappa = 0.15$). The Gaussian threshold θ_t has a constant mean of 0.2 and standard deviation of 0.15 (used in all simulations with the model). The free parameters of the rule, as well as those of the weight-change rule, are values between 0 and 1.

The weight-change rule describes how connection weights change in time. It has two possible states, weight gain and weight loss, related as follows:

$$
\Delta w_{i,j,t+1} = \begin{cases}
\alpha(a_{j,t}, d_t, p_{i,t}, r_{j,t}) \text{ if } d_t \geq 0.001 \\
-\beta(w_{i,j,t}, a_{i,t}, a_{j,t}), \text{ otherwise}
\end{cases}
\tag{8.4}
$$

where α (rate of weight increment) and β (the rate of weight decrement) denote the two free parameters of the rule (typically, $\alpha = 0.5$ and $\beta = 0.1$; in some simulations, like those described later on, $\beta = 0.05$). The other terms of the rule are:

$a_{i,t}$: activation level of i (presynaptic unit);

$a_{j,t}$: activation level of j (postsynaptic unit), computed by the activation rule;

$d_t = d_{ca1,t} = |a_{j,t} - a_{j,t-1}| + d_{vta,t}(1 - d_{ca1,t-1})$ if j is a $ca1$ unit; $d_t = d_{vta,t} = a_{j,t} - a_{j,t-1}$ if j is a vta unit (see network submodel for the distinction between $ca1$ and vta units; if a network consists of several $ca1$ and/or vta units, d_t is the average discrepancy across the corresponding units);

$$p_{i,t} = \frac{a_{i,t}w_{i,j,t}}{N}, \text{ where } N = exc_{j,t} \text{ if } i \text{ is excitatory, or } N = inh_{j,t} \text{ if } i \text{ is inhibitory};$$

$$r_{j,t} = 1 - \sum_{i=1}^{s} w_{i,j,t}$$

(8.5)

The key factor is d_t. Its inclusion in the model was guided by evidence on the roles of hippocampal ($ca1$) and dopaminergic (vta) systems in conditioning, evidence that has received further confirmation in recent years (e.g., Nutan & Meti, 2000; Pan, Schmidt, Wickens, & Hyland, 2005; Sharf, Lee, & Ranaldi, 2005; Tronson, Schrick, Guzman, Huh, Srivastava, Penzes *et al.*, 2009; Yun, Wakabayashi, Fields, & Nicola, 2004). This evidence suggests that *when present*, such systems play a role in *both* types of conditioning, *regardless of whether or not they are necessary*. They thus seem like good candidates for a common mechanism.

The value of d_t is computed as a difference in the activations of certain types of units ($ca1$ and vta; see network submodel) in moments $t - 1$ and t. In this sense, d_t is a "discrepancy" factor. It also is a "diffuse" factor, in that it affects *all* weight changes at t. In early simulations, the threshold for d_t was zero. Since Burgos (2003), the value has been increased to an arbitrary value slightly above zero (0.001) to simulate the CS-preexposure effect as a decrease in certain initial weights (see Burgos, 2003). The simulations I describe later on use the new threshold.

The rule also has a Hebbian import in that weight increments and decrements depend (partly) on the pre- and postsynaptic activations. Hence, stronger pre- and/or postsynaptic activations promote larger weight changes than weaker ones, everything else being equal. Also, $p_{i,t}$ makes weight gain competitive in that two or more connections on the same postsynaptic unit compete for a maximum weight (1.0), and strong connections with a strong presynaptic activation gain more weight, following a rich-get-richer-poor-get-poorer competition scheme (excitatory and inhibitory units do not compete with each other; competition obtains only within each type of unit). The amount of weight that is gained in such competition, however, is limited by the total amount of weight

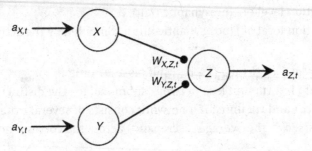

Figure 8.2 Part of a neural network to exemplify how the weight-change rule works. Units are depicted as circles, labeled as X, Y, and Z. Connections are depicted as lines. X and Y are connected to Z (i.e., X and Y are presynaptic and Z is postsynaptic). X and Y are excitatory. $a_{X,t}$: activation of X at t. $a_{Y,t}$: activation of Y at t. $w_{X,Z,t}$: weight of connection from X to Z. $w_{Y,Z,t}$: weight of connection from Y to Z. $a_{Z,t}$: activation of Z at t.

available on j at t, which is determined by $r_{j,t}$. As connections gain weight, there will be less available weight to be gained by any connection unit at t.

In a typical simulation, all initial connection weights are set to a low value. In early simulations, the value was 0.01 for all connections. In later simulations, some initial weights have been set to 0.15, to simulate latent inhibition as a loss of initial connection weights (see Burgos, 2003). The present account follows this latter strategy.

To show how the rule works, consider a simple numerical example. The example will show that a connection can gain considerably more weight than another if the former's presynaptic unit is activated more strongly, everything else being equal.

Let X, Y, and Z denote three units such that X and Y are connected to Z (i.e., X and Y are presynaptic, and Z is a postsynaptic unit), as in Figure 8.2 (assume that X and Y are excitatory). Each unit can be activated at t at levels equal to $a_{X,t}$, $a_{Y,t}$, and $a_{Z,t}$, respectively. There are two connections, one from X to Z and one from Y to Z, indicated by thin lines with a button-like cap on one end (which indicates a one-directional connection). Their weights are denoted by $w_{X,Z,t}$ and $w_{Y,Z,t}$, respectively.

The figure exemplifies only part of a neural network in this model. Exactly which part depends on the types of units that I describe in the network sub-model. I will thus treat the units in the diagram as generic ones, for the sake of the example. The task is to compute $\Delta w_{X,Z,t+1}$ and $\Delta w_{Y,Z,t+1}$. For this, let $a_{X,t} = 0.8$, $w_{X,Z,t} = 0.01$, $a_{Y,t} = 0.2$, $w_{Y,Z,t} = 0.01$, and $a_{Z,t} = 0.01$ (computed according to the activation rule, assuming that $L[exc_{Z,t}] > \theta_t$). That is to say, X is more strongly activated than Y, both connections have the same near-zero weight (0.01), and Z is weakly activated.

Also, let $d_t = 0.9$, a near-maximal value (the maximum possible is 1) that results from a large temporal difference in the activations of certain types of units (see network submodel below). Again, this value depends on the activations of certain types of units (*ca1* and *vta*), which I examine later in the network submodel. Here, it will suffice to say that a large d_t indicates a low activation of those units (say 0.05) at $t - 1$, and a high activation (say 0.95) at t (hence, $d_t = 0.95 - 0.05 = 0.90$). The high activation can be either primary (via activation of s^*) or secondary (via activation of other units).

Clearly, d_t far exceeds the 0.001 threshold, so both connections will gain weight, proportionally to α, $a_{z,t}$, d_t, $p_{i,t}$ ($p_{X,t}$ for the X–Z connection, $p_{Y,t}$ for the Y–Z connection), and $r_{z,t}$, where

$$p_{X,t} = \frac{(0.8)(0.01)}{(0.8)(0.01) + (0.2)(0.01)} = 0.8 \tag{8.6}$$

$$p_{Y,t} = \frac{(0.2)(0.01)}{(0.8)(0.01) + (0.2)(0.01)} = 0.2 \tag{8.7}$$

$$r_{z,t} = 1 - (0.01 + 0.01) = 0.98 \tag{8.8}$$

Assuming that $\alpha = 0.5$, the following obtains:

$$\Delta w_{X,Z,t+1} = (0.5)(0.01)(0.9)(0.8)(0.98) \approx 0.0035 \tag{8.8}$$

$$\Delta w_{Y,Z,t+1} = (0.5)(0.01)(0.9)(0.2)(0.98) \approx 0.0009 \tag{8.9}$$

As a result, $w_{X,Z,t+1}$ will be larger than $w_{Y,Z,t+1}$. If at $t + 1$, the discrepancy units are activated as strongly as in t (0.95), d_{t+1} will be zero (if activated less strongly, d_{t+1} will be negative, if the unit is a *vta*) and hence below 0.001, which will cause the connections to lose weight. Such weight loss, however, will be much less considerable than the weight gain, if β (the weight-loss free parameter) is much smaller than α (the weight-gain free parameter), which is the typical case. The rule thus allows connections to progressively accumulate weight, to a point where presynaptic units can activate postsynaptic units strongly. For one of the discrepancy units (*vta*), this means that secondary activation can cause a sufficiently high d_t to prevent significant weight losses in the absence of primary activation. This mechanism allows for the simulation of maintenance under intermittent primary reinforcement, second-order conditioning, and conditioned reinforcement.

Many other examples are possible, but I trust the above one will give a sense of how the rule works. The key consideration is that the rule is the *only* one used in the model to change connection weights. Hence, it is the *same* one for all variable connections. It does not distinguish between *fundamentally different* types of variable connections, at least not in any way that corresponds to the two types of reinforcement operations shown in Table 8.1.

The relevance for conditioning is that most if not all neural-network modelers agree that a change in connection weights simulates what the neuroscientific evidence strongly suggests as a crucial neural substrate of numerous behavioral phenomena, including both types of conditioning, namely: changes in synaptic efficacies. In fact, this sort of rule is more often referred to in the neural-network literature as a "learning" rule. However, I have not used this term here because learning is one of the categories I seek to avoid as a hindrance to a unified treatment of the operant–respondent distinction.

Network submodel

The network submodel is a classification of the types of units that can constitute a neural network in this model, and a few suggestions on how to connect them, guided by considerations on "gross neuroanatomy." This submodel thus corresponds very roughly to the structural or architectural level of organization of nervous systems. Some of the unit types (s^*, $ca1$, vta, and r^*) appeared in the neurocomputational submodel, and will reappear here.

Figure 8.3 shows an example of a complete neural network in this model (it is the same network used in the computer simulations described in the next section). It is a system of units (circles) related by connections (lines). The network is the simplest one thus far used in research with this model, so it has not been tested with most of the phenomena depicted in Table 8.2 (although it was tested for delay conditioning and autoshaping, as will become apparent in the next section). Also, it consists only of excitatory units. Despite its simplicity, it will suffice for my present purposes.

Like networks in other models, the present network has a "feed-forward architecture," where units can be classified into input, hidden, and output layers. However, I prefer a more neurobiological classification into two types of units that constitute two subnetworks: "sensory" and "motor." The sensory subnetwork consists of s' (for "primary sensory"), s'' (for "secondary sensory"), and $ca1$ (for "Cornu Ammonis 1," the hippocampal area) units. The s' units are subdivided into s, c, and s^*, their activations being the network's "inputs." Motor units are classified into m' (for "primary motor"), vta (for "ventral-tegmental area," the dopaminergic nucleus), and m'' (for "secondary motor"). The m' units are subdivided into r and r^*, their activations being the network's "outputs."

One difference between sensory and motor units is that some of the former, the s' units, are not activated according to the activation rule, but rather a *training protocol* that simulates aspects of the reinforcement operations depicted in Table 8.1. Activations of s, c, and s^* thus correspond roughly to the intensities of members of S, C, and S^*, respectively. The model does not give a more concrete interpretation of such activations, particularly regarding sensory modality. An

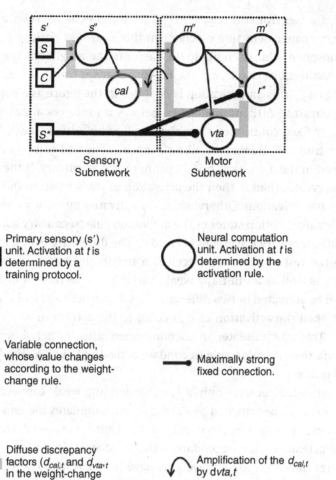

Primary sensory (s′)
unit. Activation at *t* is
determined by a
training protocol.

Neural computation
unit. Activation at *t* is
determined by the
activation rule.

Variable connection,
whose value changes
according to the weight-
change rule.

Maximally strong
fixed connection.

Diffuse discrepancy
factors ($d_{cal,t}$ and $d_{vta,t}$
in the weight-change
rule).

Amplification of the $d_{cal,t}$
by $d_{vta,t}$

Figure 8.3 Example of a complete neural network. The network consists of a
sensory subnetwork and a motor subnetwork. The sensory subnetwork consists
of the s′ (for "primary sensory") or "input," s″ (for "secondary sensory"), and *cal*
(for "Cornu Ammonis 1") units and their connections. The motor subnetwork
consists of the connection from s″ to m″ (for "secondary motor"), and the m″,
vta (for "ventral tegmental area"), and m′ (for "primary motor") units and their
connections. The m′ ("output") layer consists of r (which receives only a variable
connection from m″) and r* (which receives a variable, initially weak connection
from m″ and a fixed, maximally strong connection from s*). All units are excitatory.

s activation, then, could simulate a light, a tone, or some other sensory exteroceptive stimulus, and an s* activation, food, water, or even shock.

Another difference between sensory and motor units is the source of d_t,
depicted in the figure as shaded areas. For the sensory connections (s′–s″,

s''–$ca1$), d_t arises from $ca1$ (i.e., $d_t = d_{ca1,t}$; see weight-change rule), and simulates a sensory change-detection mechanism that is always positive (hence the use of the absolute value to compute this factor in the weight-change rule). For the motor connections (s''–m'', m''–vta, m''–m'), d_t arises from vta (i.e., $d_t = d_{vta,t}$) and amplifies $d_{ca1,t}$ (this amplification is depicted in the figure as a curved arrow).

In contrast to $ca1$, and like r^* (see below), vta receives a maximally strong, excitatory fixed connection from s^*, as well as an initially weak, variable connection from m''. Hence, vta, like r^*, can be activated in two different ways, described in the activation rule as primary and secondary. If the activation of s^* at t is greater than 0, then the activation of vta is equal to the activation of s^* (primary activation). Otherwise, vta is activated by m'' via one of the three conditional-activation states of the activation rule (secondary activation).

Finally, there are the m' units, r and r^*. The difference is that r^*, like vta and unlike the rest of the units, receives a maximally strong, fixed connection from s^*, as well as an initially weak, variable connection from m''. Hence, r^* also can be activated in two different ways. If the activation of s^* at t is greater than 0, then the activation of r^* is equal to the activation of s^* (primary activation). This way simulates an unconditioned reflex. Otherwise, r^* is activated by m'' via the activation rule (secondary activation), which simulates a conditioned reflex.

In contrast, r receives only a variable initially weak connection from m'. Hence, r cannot be activated by s^*. This feature simulates the non-elicited character of emission, as described in Table 8.1. Unit r can be activated only by m'' via the activation rule (secondary activation). Such activation will be strong only after the corresponding weights have increased enough for s' to activate s'', s'' to activate m'', and m'' to activate r. The necessary weight increases will result from exposing the network to a training protocol that simulates the reinforcement operations depicted in Table 8.1.

Taking stock

As is apparent in the above summary, the model is more strongly bottom-up than others, in the sense that all of its categories were inferred directly from neural correlates of conditioning. This strategy contrasts to the top-down one followed by other models, where cognitive categories are first inferred from behavioral categories, and then made to correspond to neural correlates. The present model omits the inference of cognitive categories and starts directly with neural correlates. This strategy allows the model to dispense with the usual cognitive categories of other models and this promotes a more unified treatment of the operant–respondent distinction.

The strategy also allows for the identification of two levels of theoretical analysis, namely: neurocomputational and network. Albeit they are intimately related, each comprises a distinct set of neural categories. The categories of the neurocomputational level constitute the activation and weight-change rules (unit, activation, connection, weight, etc.). The categories of the network level are the types of units that can constitute a neural network (s', s'', $ca1$, etc.).

The analysis

In the previous sections, I laid out the behavioral and computational neural frameworks for my analysis. In this section, I proceed with the analysis itself, in two parts. One is an analysis at the neurocomputational level. The other is an analysis at the network level. The previous sections have anticipated the basics of both parts, but I elaborate them here.

The key consideration regarding the first part is the use of a single activation rule for all units and a single weight-change rule for all connections. At this level, the model makes *virtually* no distinction between operant and respondent underlying mechanisms, particularly regarding weight changes under the two types of reinforcement operations depicted in Table 8.1. The feature of the neurocomputational submodel that is closest to the distinction is the difference between primary and secondary activation in the activation rule. This difference relies on separating r^* units from the rest, including r, which entails a distinction between r and r^* units. As will become clear shortly, this separation corresponds to one aspect of the operant–respondent distinction (i.e., the difference between emission and elicitation).

The neurocomputational submodel, then, does not eliminate all the differences that comprise the distinction. Therefore, the submodel only achieves a partial computational unification. However, it is reasonably high, perhaps higher than other neural-network models. The difference between primary and secondary activation is as far as the neurocomputational submodel goes into a distinction between operant and respondent underlying processes, which is not very far.

The neurocomputational submodel allows for a higher degree of unification also because it dispenses with the usual cognitive categories of other models. None of the submodel's categories corresponds to any cognitive category. Hence, the submodel need not distinguish between types of associations, associated internal representations, memory systems, learning processes, attentional processes, cognitive mappings, storage and retrieval systems, and so on. Nor does it need to distinguish between drive, incentive, motivation, and reinforcement, because it appeals only to reinforcement and conceives it in a purely behavioral, operational manner, without any cognitive import.

The analysis at the network level is far more differential, as it preserves all the behavioral differences of the operant–respondent distinction, as depicted in Table 8.1. This preservation takes the form of a correspondence between the neural categories of the network submodel and the distinction's basic behavioral categories. At this level, then, the model achieves no unification. However, this is deliberate, under the conviction that the behavioral categories are fundamental to any analysis of conditioning.

The correspondence in question requires a way to simulate responses, and this can be done in the model on the basis of m' (r and r^*) activations. These activations are continuous, whereas responses typically are binary. Hence, m' activations do not simulate responses. Responses can be simulated through a "response rule" that transforms m' activations into binary events. The model does not determine a unique rule, so indefinitely many are possible. A simple one used in previous simulations defines a response as an m' activation of 0.5 or more, and I shall use it here. Henceforth, I shall refer to above-criterion m' activations as "responses."

At the network level, then, the before-reinforcement categories in Table 8.1 can be interpreted as follows: r responses do not depend on s^* activations (non-elicitation aspect of emission; see below), r^* responses depend on s^* activations (elicitation), and r^* responses do not depend on s activations (neutrality). To simulate this interpretation, two copies of the architecture depicted in Figure 8.3 (N1 and N2) were used (the simulator can be obtained as freeware, upon request to the author). N1 received a training protocol consisting of 300 1-moment s^* activations of 1.0 (corresponding roughly to a maximally intense US), separated by a fixed interval of 30 moments. N2 received 300 5-moments s activations of 1.0 (corresponding roughly to a maximally salient CS), separated by a fixed interval of 25 moments.

For both networks, c had a constant activation of 0.2 throughout the entire simulation, to simulate the presence of a mildly salient context. Initial s'–s'' and s''–$ca1$ weights were set to 0.15, to be consistent with a previous simulation study (e.g., Burgos, 2003). The initial weights for the rest of the connections were set to 0.01. The values of the free parameters were $\sigma = 0.1$, $\tau = 0.1$, $\kappa = 0.1$, $\alpha = 0.5$, and $\beta = 0.05$. The update procedure was asynchronous-random, where activations and weights were updated in random order at each moment. Weights for each individual unit were also updated in random order at each moment.

The results are shown in Figure 8.4, which depicts the mean r and r^* activations in the presence of s^* (N1) or s (N2) activations. The output activations were recorded in blocks of five consecutive moments. For N1, each block consisted

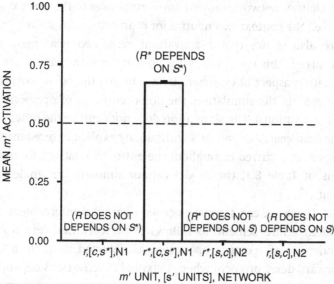

Figure 8.4 Mean m' (r and r^*) activations in a simulation of the non-elicited aspect of emission, and elicitation and neutrality (see Table 8.1, first column), with two copies N1 and N2 of the architecture depicted in Figure 8.3. The graph shows the mean m' (r and r^*) activations in the presence of s' (s, c, and s^*) activations across 1500 moments, grouped into 300 blocks of five consecutive moments each. For N1, a block consisted of five consecutive moments where c and s^* were activated at the first moment, and c was activated in the following four moments ($a_c = 0.2$, $a_s^* = 1.0$). For N2, s and c were activated in the five moments ($a_s = 1.0$). The dashed line shows the activation criterion used as a response rule (0.5). The square brackets enclose simultaneous s' activations. The simulated behavioral relations are shown in parentheses. Error bars represent standard errors.

of the activations of c and s^* at the first moment, and the activation of c in the next four moments. For N2, each block consisted of the activations of s and c throughout the five moments. The simulation consisted of 300 blocks, for a total of 1500 moments. The means shown in Figure 8.4 were computed across these 1500 moments.

As the figure shows, all r activations were near zero, whereas r^* activations were well above 0.5 (about 0.7) in the presence of s^* activations, but near-zero in the presence of s activations. These results simulate the three behavioral relations shown in the before-reinforcement column of Table 8.1, as follows. N1 simulated the non-elicitation aspect of emission as the non-occurrence of r responses in the presence of s^* activations. N1 simulated elicitation as a frequent occurrence of r^* responses in the presence of s^* activations (elicitation). N2 simulated neutrality as the nonoccurrence of r^* responses in the presence of

s activations. Neither network showed any r^* responses to the context (c activations) alone (i.e., the context was neutral for r^* activations as well).

The figure also shows that r activations remained near zero, so no r responses occurred. This result raises a problem: the simulation captures only the non-elicitation aspect of emission, that is to say, the *non-occurrence* of R in the presence of S^* (in the simulation, the non-occurrence of r responses in the presence of s^* activations). The simulation does not capture the other aspect of emission, the *occasional occurrence* of R without any explicit antecedent stimulus (i.e., no r responses occurred throughout the entire simulation). Consequently, and in terms of Table 8.1, the model cannot simulate unsignaled operant reinforcement.

The model, however, can simulate *signaled* operant reinforcement but only after respondent reinforcement, as follows. A network first receives a simulated respondent-reinforcement operation, as depicted in Table 8.1, in the form of a forward-delay protocol where maximal s^* activations depend on (are "paired" with) maximal s activations. At the outset of training, maximal s^* activations cause near-maximal vta discrepancies, which in turn amplify the $ca1$ discrepancies. These discrepancies, combined with the maximal s activations, promote the increase of s–s'' weights. Thanks to this increase, s activations eventually become capable of activating s'' strongly. This activation, combined with a high vta discrepancy, promotes an increase in the s''–m'' weights, which allows s'' to activate m'' strongly. This activation, combined with a high vta discrepancy, promotes an increase in the m''–r weights. The overall result of this feed-forward chain of weight and activation increases is that, after a number of s–s^* pairings, s also becomes capable of activating r (via s'' and m''), enough for r activations to satisfy the response rule and hence allow for an operant-reinforcement protocol.

To simulate this, a second experiment was run with a third copy of the same architecture (N3), using the same initial weights and free parameters as the first simulation. In a first phase, N3 received a simulated respondent-reinforcement protocol consisting of 470 s–s^* pairings, where s had an activation of 1.0 for five moments and s^* an activation of 1.0 at the last s moment (for an interstimulus interval of four moments), *regardless of the m′ activations* (this simulates the response-independent character of the arrangement). Successive s activations were separated by a fixed interval of 25 moments between the offset of an s activation and the onset of the next (which simulates the intertrial interval). The presence of a mildly salient context was simulated as before. This protocol simulates a standard forward-delay respondent procedure, which satisfies the basic respondent reinforcement operation depicted in Table 8.1 (the dependence of S^* on S).

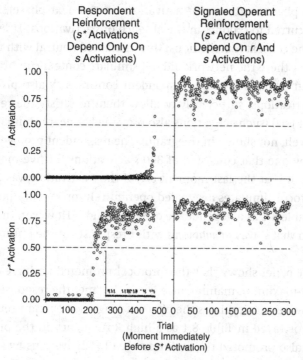

Figure 8.5 Mean m' (r and r^*) activations in a simulation of two types of reinforcement operations (respondent and signaled operant) and their basic effects (see Table 8.1, second and third columns, respectively). *Upper left panel*: r activations during respondent reinforcement, defined as 470 s–s^* pairings (a_s = 1.0 for five moments, a_s^* = 1.0 at the last s moment, regardless of the m' activations). *Lower left panel*: r^* activations during respondent reinforcement. *Upper right panel*: r activations during signaled operant reinforcement, where s^* was activated at the last s moment only if the r activation met the response criterion (0.5, indicated by the dashed line). *Lower right panel*: r^* activations during signaled operant reinforcement. Both m' activations were recorded at the moment immediately before the s^* activation.

The results are shown in the left panels of Figure 8.5, which depict the activations of r (upper left panel) and r^* (lower left panel) at the second-to-last moment of each successive s activation. As the lower left panel shows, after about 200 s–s^* pairings, the protocol promoted an increase in the activation of r^* by s to maintenance levels that met the response criterion in all the remaining trials. The results simulate the basic effect of a respondent reinforcement operation, namely, a dependence of R^* on S.

The inset of the lower left panel shows that, in this phase, r^* activations during the five moments immediately before s activations remained near zero, well below the response criterion (comparable results were obtained with r

activations in this phase, and r and r^* activations in the next phase). Hence, no r^* responses occurred to c alone, in the absence of s activations, at least for those moments. The context (c activations) thus remained neutral with respect to r^*, indicating that there the network did not simulate context conditioning.

As the upper left panel shows, the respondent contingency also promoted an increase in r activations, sufficiently to allow them to satisfy the response criterion at the last trial (such activations also remained at near-minimal levels during c alone as well, not shown in the graph). The respondent protocol could thus be replaced by one that consisted of 300 s activations for five moments, and the activation of s^* at the last moment *only* if the r activation was greater than 0.5. This protocol simulates a signaled operant reinforcement operation, characterized in Table 8.1 as a dependence of S^* on R and S. However, the simulation is atypical in that s^* was *simultaneous* with r responses at the last moment of s.

The upper right panel shows that this protocol promoted an increase in r activations to near-maximum maintenance levels that met the response criterion in all trials. This result simulates the effect of a signaled operant reinforcement operation, portrayed in Table 8.1 as a high R frequency in the presence of S. The protocol also promoted the maintenance of r^* activations by s activations at near-maximum levels, well above the response criterion. Therefore, the basic effect of respondent reinforcement is simulated in this phase as well. The implication of this last result is that operant reinforcement can maintain respondent conditioning. This implication is consistent with evidence that shows that operant reinforcement promotes respondent conditioning (see Henton & Iversen, 1978).

My main intention with this simulation was to show how the model can simulate signaled operant reinforcement as characterized in Table 8.1. However, extended exposure to the respondent protocol (s–s^* pairings) would have sufficed to increase the activation of r to levels comparable to those shown in the upper right panel of Figure 8.5. The implication is that respondent reinforcement also promotes operant conditioning. This implication is consistent with evidence that shows the acquisition and maintenance of emitted responses under respondent contingencies, autoshaping and positive automaintenance (e.g., Gonzalez, 1974; Stiers & Silberberg, 1974) being the most notable examples (see Burgos, 2007, for simulations of these effects).

Moreover, in these networks, respondent *reinforcement* (s–s^* pairings) is *necessary* for operant conditioning, which is not to say that respondent *conditioning* is. If respondent conditioning in these networks is defined as a change in r^* after respondent reinforcement, then respondent conditioning is not necessary for operant conditioning in this model. The reason is that r activations can increase under respondent reinforcement in the absence of r^* units. The model also predicts that, if the temporal scales of operant and respondent conditioning were comparable (as they are in the second simulation), respondent conditioning is faster than operant conditioning. Testing these predictions experimentally, however, is difficult at present, as current conditioning methods allow neither for comparable temporal scales nor minimal experimental controls.

Concluding remarks

The model thus allows for a reasonably unified treatment of the operant–respondent distinction at the neurocomputational level. Such treatment approximates the ideal of a single process underlying both types of conditioning, more so than any other model. It remains to be seen whether a complete computational unification is possible or even desirable. The model also preserves most of the basic behavioral categories of the distinction at the network level. Both tasks are accomplished in a purely neurobehavioral manner, without appealing to any of the usual cognitive categories found in other models.

My analysis, of course, suffers from limitations, although many are due to its simplified character. An obvious one is that the model cannot simulate unsignaled operant reinforcement or its basic effect. For operant conditioning, the model can only simulate signaled operant reinforcement and its basic effect, and only after respondent reinforcement (s–s^* pairings). This limitation is not a principled one, as the model can overcome it by using a maximal σ parameter (1.0) for r units (see logistic function of activation rule). This parameter allows occasional r activations of about 0.3, with zero s' activations (no explicit antecedent stimulus) and the same initial weights used in the simulations. Emission can thus be simulated by decreasing the activation criterion of the response rule to a value below that activation level. However, this strategy would require a justification of using such a σ parameter for r units, justification that is not apparent at this point.

A related problem is that operant reinforcement was simulated as a simultaneous occurrence of s^* with r responses. This admittedly atypical way to simulate an operant reinforcement operation was just a simplifying device, although it simulates the closest temporal contiguity possible in operant reinforcement. However, it is unclear exactly what it means vis-à-vis typical operant-conditioning situations in natural organisms. The simultaneity in question approximates operant contingencies that involve direct electrical stimulation of certain brain parts (e.g., Olds & Milner, 1954; Wurtz & Olds, 1963). This consideration, however, raises the difficult and yet unresolved issue of what makes reinforcers reinforcing, much discussed in the literature. Whatever the solution, it remains to be seen whether the model can simulate delayed operant reinforcement, where s^* is activated some moment after an r response. In any case, the way an operant reinforcement operation was simulated here shows that the model need not postulate any association of S^* with a decaying memory of R to simulate operant conditioning in a simple form.

Another issue has to do with differential operant reinforcement of desired responses and non-reinforcement of undesired responses. This issue is a complex one that remains to be investigated with the model. As a preliminary intuition, a network could simulate this in a simple way, by having at least two r units. Above-criterion activations of one unit could simulate a desired response, and activations of the other, an undesired response. To make the two responses mutually exclusive, the corresponding units could inhibit each other. Then, a training protocol could schedule s^* to be activated at a certain moment only when the first response occurs. The expected result, to be confirmed, is that the frequency of the undesired response will decrease. The problem is that both units would have to be assumed to have relatively high (above-criterion) activations, which raises the question of why they were high in the first place. The only possibility that is apparent from the present analysis is that r activations increase only after Pavlovian reinforcement (s–s^* pairings).

Also, I made no attempt to capture what some (e.g., Hearst & Jenkins, 1974) regard as another defining feature of skeletal responses acquired under respondent reinforcement, namely: "directedness." In the second simulation, r responses lacked directedness. However, as I have shown in a previous paper (Burgos, 2007), the model can simulate directedness as sensory feedback, in the form of r-dependent s activations. To simulate this in a way that allows the feedback to differ from the sensory stimulus used in the reinforcement operation, a network would be needed with at least another s input unit.

Finally, I have said nothing about two other distinctions that have been much discussed in relation to the operant–respondent distinction. One is between continuous and partial reinforcement. This distinction is believed to make important differences in acquisition, maintenance, and extinction from one type of conditioning to the other. The evidence in this regard, however, is too complex to attempt a full neural-network analysis in a single bound. A stepwise strategy would be wiser. As a preliminary intuition, continuous operant reinforcement can be simulated by a protocol where r responses in an experienced network activate s^* at every moment. This protocol would cause a high vta activation and, hence, a near-zero d_t at every moment, resulting in a significant weight loss. The result would be a decrement of r and r^* activations to near-zero values. The model thus predicts a deleterious effect of operant continuous reinforcement.

The other distinction is between appetitive and aversive conditioning. No previous research with the model has attempted to simulate aversive conditioning, but a preliminary intuition is possible here as well. Consider a particular phenomenon, like conditioned suppression of the bar-pressing response in rats. This phenomenon could be simulated with a network that has an additional s^* unit, s^{**}, and an additional r^* unit, r^{**}, unconditionally activated by s^{**}. In addition to this, the UR to the shock (a vigorous jump immediately followed by a brief post-shock period of freezing; e.g., Myer, 1971) could be hypothesized to be incompatible with bar pressing. The model could simulate this incompatibility with a network where r^{**} inhibits r (whose activation would correspond roughly to bar pressing), such that a high r^{**} activation would cause a low r activation. If s activations are paired with s^{**} activations, the former could acquire the ability to cause high r^{**} activations, and thus decrease the r activations. It remains to be seen whether the model can actually simulate this.

Author note

I thank Nestor Schmajuk for his kind invitation to participate in this symposium. I also thank John Donahoe, Peter Killeen, John Moore, and two anonymous reviewers for commentaries to previous drafts.

References

Asratyan, E. A. (1972). Conditioned reflex theory and motivational behavior. *Acta Neurobiologiae Experimentalis*, **34**, 15–31.

Bindra, D. (1972). A unified account of classical and operant conditioning. In A. H. Black and W. F. Prokasy, eds., *Classical Conditioning II: Current Research and Theory*. New York: Appleton–Century–Crofts, pp. 453–481.

Brown, P. L. & Jenkins, H. M. (1968). Auto-shaping of the pigeon's key-peck. *Journal of the Experimental Analysis of Behavior*, **11**, 1–8.

Burgos, J. E. (1997). Evolving artifical neural networks in Pavlovian environments. In J. W. Donahoe and V. P. Dorsel, eds., *Neural-Network Models of Cognition: Biobehavioral Foundations*. Amsterdam: Elsevier, pp. 58–79.

Burgos, J. E. (2003). Theoretical note: simulating latent inhibition with selection neural networks. *Behavioural Processes*, **62**, 183–192.

Burgos, J. E. (2005). Theoretical note: the C/T ratio in artificial neural networks. *Behavioural Processes*, **69**, 249–256.

Burgos, J. E. (2007). Autoshaping and automaintenance: a neural-network approach. *Journal of the Experimental Analysis of Behavior*, **88**, 115–130.

Burgos, J. E. & Donahoe, J. W. (2000). Structure and function in selectionism: implications for complex behavior. In J. Leslie and D. Blackman, eds., *Issues in Experimental and Applied Analyses of Human Behavior*. Reno, NV: Context Press, pp. 39–57.

Burgos, J. E. & Murillo-Rodríguez, E. (2007). Neural-network simulations of two context-dependence phenomena. *Behavioural Processes*, **75**, 242–249.

Burgos, J. E., Flores, C., García, Ó., Díaz, C. & Cruz, Y. (2007). A simultaneous procedure facilitates acquisition under an optimal interstimulus interval in artificial neural networks and rats. *Behavioural Processes*, **78**, 302–309.

Davis, H. & Hurwitz, H. M. B. (eds., 1977). *Operant-Pavlovian Interactions*. Hillsdale, NJ: Erlbaum.

Dickinson, A. (1979). Review of S. H. Hulse, H. Fowler & W. K. Honig (eds.). Cognitive processes in animal behavior. *Quarterly Journal of Experimental Psychology*, **31**, 551–554.

Donahoe, J. W. & Burgos, J. E. (1999). Commentary: timing without a timer. *Journal of the Experimental Analysis of Behavior*, **71**, 257–301.

Donahoe, J. W. & Burgos, J. E. (2000). Behavior analysis and revaluation. *Journal of the Experimental Analysis of Behavior*, **74**, 331–346.

Donahoe, J. W. & Palmer, D. C. (1994). *Learning and Complex Behavior*. Boston, MA: Allyn & Bacon.

Donahoe, J. W., Burgos, J. E. & Palmer, D. C. (1993). A selectionist approach to reinforcement. *Journal of the Experimental Analysis of Behavior*, **60**, 17–40.

Donahoe, J. W., Palmer, D. C. & Burgos, J. E. (1997a). The S-R issue: its status in behavior analysis and in Donahoe and Palmer's *Learning and Complex Behavior*. *Journal of the Experimental Analysis of Behavior*, **67**, 193–211.

Donahoe, J. W., Palmer, D. C. & Burgos, J. E. (1997b). The unit of selection: what do reinforcers reinforce? *Journal of the Experimental Analysis of Behavior*, **67**, 259–273.

Dragoi, V. & Staddon, J. E. R. (1999). The dynamics of operant conditioning. *Psychological Review*, **106**, 20–61.

Dykman, R. A. (1976). Conditioning and sensitization. *Pavlovian Journal of Biological Science*, **11**, 24–36.

Fukushima, K. (1975). Cognitron: a self-organizing multilayered neural network. *Biological Cybernetics*, **20**, 126–136.

Gibbon, J. & Balsam, P. (1981). Spreading association in time. In C. M. Locurto, H. S. Terrace and J. Gibbon, eds., *Autoshaping and Conditioning Theory*. New York: Academic Press, pp. 219–253.

Gonzalez, F. A. (1974). Effects of varying the percentage of key illuminations paired with food in a positive automaintenance procedure. *Journal of the Experimental Analysis of Behavior*, **22**, 483–489.

Gormezano, I. & Tait, R. W. (1976). The Pavlovian analysis of instrumental conditioning. *Pavlovian Journal of Biological Science*, **11**, 37–55.

Gray, J. A. (1975). *Elements of a Two-Process Theory of Learning*. London: Academic Press.

Grossberg, S. (1987). *The Adaptive Brain I*. Amsterdam: Elsevier.

Guthrie, E. R. (1935). *The Psychology of Learning*. New York: Harper & Row.

Hearst, E. (1975). The classical-instrumental distinction: reflexes, voluntary behavior, and categories of associative learning. In W. K. Estes, ed., *Handbook of*

Learning and Cognitive Processes: Vol. 2. Conditioning and Behavior Theory. Hillsdale, NJ: Erlbaum, pp. 181–223.

Hearst, E. & Jenkins, H. M. (1974). *Sign-Tracking: The Stimulus–Reinforcer Relation and Directed Action.* Monograph of the Psychonomic Society: Austin, TX.

Henton, W. W. & Iversen, I. H. (1978). *Classical and Operant Conditioning: A Response Pattern Analysis.* New York: Springer-Verlag.

Hineline, P. N. (1986). Re-tuning the operant/respondent distinction. In T. Thompson and M. D. Zeiler, eds., *Analysis and Integration of Behavioral Units.* Hillsdale, NJ: Erlbaum, pp. 55–79.

Hull, C. L. (1943). *Principles of Behavior.* New York: Appleton.

Killeen, P. R. (1994). Mathematical principles of reinforcement. *Behavioral and Brain Sciences,* **17,** 105–172.

Kimmel, H. D. (1976). Cherchez la difference! *The Pavlovian Journal of Biological Science,* **11,** 56–65.

Klopf, A. H. (1988). A neuronal model of classical conditioning. *Psychobiology,* **16,** 85–125.

Konorski, J. & Miller, S. (1937a). On two types of conditioned reflex. *Journal of General Psychology,* **16,** 264–272.

Konorski, J. & Miller, S. (1937b). Further remarks on two types of conditioned reflex. *Journal of General Psychology,* **17,** 405–407.

Logan, F. A. (1960). *Incentive.* New Haven, CT: Yale University Press.

Machado, A. (1997). Learning the temporal dynamics of behavior. *Psychological Review,* **104,** 241–265.

Mackintosh, N. J. (1975). A theory of attention: variations in the associability of stimuli with reinforcement. *Psychological Review,* **82,** 276–298.

Mackintosh, N. J. & Dickinson, A. (1979). Instrumental (Type II) conditioning. In A. Dickinson and R. A. Boakes, eds., *Mechanisms of Learning and Motivation: A Memorial Volume to Jerzy Konorski.* Hillsdale, NJ: Erlbaum, pp. 143–169.

Miller, S. & Konorski, J. (1928). Sur une forme particulière des reflexes conditionnels. *Les Compte Rendus des Seances et Mémoires de la Société Polonaise de Biologie,* **99,** 1155–1157. Translated by B. F. Skinner (1969) as "On a particular form of conditioned reflex." *Journal of the Experimental Analysis of Behavior,* **12,** 187–189.

Mowrer O. H. (1960). *Learning Theory and Behavior.* New York: Wiley.

Myer, J. S. (1971). Some effects of noncontingent aversive stimulation. In F. R. Brush, ed., *Aversive Conditioning and Learning.* New York: Academic Press, pp. 469–536.

Nutan, K. S. & Meti, B. L. (2000). Deficits in operant behavior and alteration of CA1, CA3 hippocampal dendritic arborization due to subicular lesions. *Journal of Neuroscience Research,* **59,** 806–812.

Olds, J. & Milner, P. (1954). Positive reinforcement produced by electrical stimulation of the septal area and other regions of rat brain. *Journal of Comparative and Physiological Psychology,* **47,** 419–427.

Pan, W.-X., Schmidt, R., Wickens, J. R. & Hyland, B. I. (2005). Dopamine cells respond to predicted events during classical conditioning: evidence for eligibility traces in the reward-learning network. *The Journal of Neuroscience*, **25**, 6235–6242.

Pear, J. J. & Eldridge, G. D. (1984). The operant/respondent distinction: future directions. *Journal of the Experimental Analysis of Behavior*, **42**, 453–467.

Pearce J. M. & Hall, G. (1980). A model for Pavlovian learning: variations in the effectiveness of conditioned but not of unconditioned stimuli. *Psychological Review*, **87**, 532–552.

Ray, R. D. & Brown, D. A. (1976). The behavioral specificity of behavior: a systems approach to procedural distinctions of classical and instrumental conditioning. *The Pavlovian Journal of Biological Science*, **11**, 3–23.

Rehfeldt, R. A. & Hayes, L. J. (1998). The operant/respondent distinction revisited: toward an understanding of stimulus equivalence. *The Psychological Record*, **48**, 187–210.

Rescorla, R. W. & Solomon, R. L. (1967). Two-process learning theory: relationships between Pavlovian conditioning and instrumental learning. *Psychological Review*, **74**, 151–182.

Rescorla, R. W. & Wagner, A. R. (1972). A theory of Pavlovian conditioning: variations in the effectiveness of reinforcement and noneinforcement. In A. H. Black and W. F. Prokasy, eds., *Classical Conditioning II: Current Research and Theory*. New York: Appleton, pp. 64–99.

Sánchez, J. M., Galeazzi, J. M. & Burgos, J. E. (2010). Some structural determinants of Pavlovian conditioning in artificial neural networks. *Behavioural Processes*, **84**, 526–535.

Schlosberg, H. (1937). The relationship between success and the laws of conditioning. *Psychological Review*, **44**, 379–394.

Schmajuk, N. A. (1994). Behavioral dynamics of escape and avoidance: a neural network approach. In D. Cliff, P. Husbands, J.-A. Meyerm and S. Wilson, eds., *From Animals to Animats 3*. Cambridge, MA: MIT Press, pp. 118–127.

Schmajuk, N. A. & Moore, J. W. (1986). A real-time attentional-associative model for classical conditioning of the rabbit's nictitating membrane response. In *Proceedings of the Eighth Annual Conference of the Cognitive Science Society*. Hillsdale, NJ: Erlbaum, pp. 794–807.

Schoenfeld, W. N. (1966). Editorial: some old work for modern conditioning theory. *Conditional Reflex: A Pavlovian Journal of Research and Therapy*, **1**, 219–223.

Schwartz, B. & Gamzu, E. (1977). Pavlovian control of operant behavior: an analysis of autoshaping and its implications for operant conditioning. In W. K. Honig and J. E. R. Staddon, eds., *Handbook of Operant Behavior*. Englewood Cliffs, NJ: Prentice-Hall, pp. 53–97.

Sharf, R., Lee, D. Y. & Ranaldi, R. (2005). Microinjections of SCH 23390 in the ventral tegmental area reduce operant responding under a progressive ratio schedule of food reinforcement in rats. *Brain Research*, **1033**, 179–185.

Sheffield, F. D. (1965). Relation between classical conditioning and instrumental learning. In W. F. Prokasy, ed., *Classical Conditioning: A Symposium*. New York: Appleton, pp. 302–322.

Skinner, B. F. (1935). Two types of conditioned reflex and a pseudo type. *Journal of General Psychology*, **12**, 66–77.

Skinner, B. F. (1937). Two types pf conditioned reflex: a reply to Konorski and Miller. *Journal of General Psychology*, **16**, 272–279.

Spence, K. W. (1956). *Behavior Theory and Conditioning*. New Haven, CT: Yale University Press.

Staddon, J. E. R. (2001). *The New Behaviorism: Mind, Mechanism, and Society*. Philadelphia, PA: Taylor & Francis.

Stiers, M. & Silberberg, A. (1974). Lever-contact responses in rats: automaintenance with and without a negative response-reinforcer dependency. *Journal of the Experimental Analysis of Behavior*, **22**, 497–506.

Stout, S. C. & Miller, R. R. (2007). Sometimes competing retrieval (SOCR): a formalization of the comparator hypothesis. *Psychological Review*, **114**, 759–783.

Sutton, R. S. & Barto, A. G. (1981). Toward a modern theory of adaptive networks. *Psychological Review*, **88**, 135–170.

Trapold, M. A. & Overmier, J. B. (1972). The second learning process in instrumental learning. In A. H. Black and W. F. Prokasy, eds., *Classical Conditioning II: Current Research and Theory*. New York: Appleton, pp. 427–452.

Tronson, N. C., Schrick, C., Guzman, Y. F., Huh, K. H., Srivastava, D. P., Penzes *et al.* (2009). Segregated populations of hippocampal principal CA1 neurons mediating conditioning and extinction of contextual fear. *The Journal of Neuroscience*, **29**, 3387–3394.

Wagner, A. R. & Brandon, S. E. (1989). Evolution of a structured connectionist model of Pavlovian conditioning (AESOP). In S. B. Klein and R. R. Mowrer, eds., *Contemporary Learning Theories: Pavlovian Conditioning and the Status of Traditional Learning Theory*. Hillsdale, NJ: Erlbaum, pp. 149–189.

Wurtz, R. H. & Olds, J. (1963). Amygdaloid stimulation and operant reinforcement in the rat. *Journal of Comparative and Physiological Psychology*, **56**, 941–949.

Yun, I. A., Wakabayashi, K. T., Fields, H. L. & Nicola, S. M. (2004). The ventral tegmental area is required for the behavioral and nucleus accumbens neuronal firing responses to incentive cues. *The Journal of Neuroscience*, **24**, 2923–2933.

Index

Printed in the United States
By Bookmasters

Printed in the United States
By Bookmasters